The Search for Certainty

Wilford W. Spradlin
Patricia B. Porterfield

The Search for Certainty

Springer-Verlag
New York Berlin Heidelberg Tokyo

Wilford W. Spradlin
Department of Behavioral Medicine
  and Psychiatry
University of Virginia School of
  Medicine
6 East Blue Ridge Hospital
Charlottesville, Virginia 22908, U.S.A.

Patricia B. Porterfield
Department of Behavioral Medicine
  and Psychiatry
University of Virginia School of
  Medicine
6 East Blue Ridge Hospital
Charlottesville, Virginia 22908, U.S.A.

Library of Congress Cataloging in Publication Data
Spradlin, Wilford W.
   The search for certainty.
   Includes index.
   1. Certainty. I. Porterfield, Patricia B.
II. Title.
BD171.S67   1983   121   83-14756

With 1 Figure.

Typeset by Bi-Comp, Inc., York, Pennsylvania.
Printed and bound by R. R. Donnelley & Sons, Harrisonburg, Virginia.
Printed in the United States of America.

9 8 7 6 5 4 3 2 1

ISBN 0-387-90889-7 Springer-Verlag New York Berlin Heidelberg Tokyo
ISBN 3-540-90889-7 Springer-Verlag Berlin Heidelberg New York Tokyo

Preface

Who are we? What are we? How do we fit into the world? Or into the universe? These and other questions pertaining to ourselves and our environment are as compelling to us today as they were to our primitive ancestors. Throughout our history we have developed paradigms of thought that have attempted to answer these questions, each conceptual framework being particularly relevant to its age. We are, in the twentieth century, witnessing a complete reorganization of our thinking. We are now, with the aid of technology, able to bring together both ancient and new patterns of thought and to observe the emergence of a kaleidoscopic world view that is uniting the once dissonant theories of philosophy, religion, and science.

This book sketches an historical picture of three world views that have shaped our ideas about ourselves. These conceptual formats that have so influenced us are not mutually exclusive and are present in all of us simultaneously, although to varying degrees depending upon our individual biases.

Perhaps the most ancient paradigm is that of The Anthropomorphic World of Words. With the instruments we call language and words we differentiated ourselves and our environment into entities. We utilized words to remove ourselves from our experiences and to see ourselves as objective observers in a world fashioned for our use. Our linguistic skills made it possible for us to extrapolate and predict certain events crucial to our existence, especially those of a temporal nature such as birth and death. Our awareness of our finiteness led to the evolution of religious philosophies and the espousal of an anthropocentric universe in which gods and other forces of nature were viewed as like ourselves. The belief system that incorporates the idea that a God or gods created the earth and then created us in His or their image has been an extremely efficient frame. It has served us well for thousands of years and is still of paramount importance to millions of individuals. The Anthropomorphic World of Words has a global quality that does not address detailed information specifically and holds tremendous appeal for the philosopher and the mystic.

Although the idea of a man-centered universe proved to be almost totally acceptable, there were a few dissenting opinions. Copernicus suggested that the Earth is not necessarily the center of the universe. Darwin and Wallace sought to prove that we are on a continuum with other animals. Freud validated Darwin by indicating that we are heirs to many of the primitive drives and instinctually influenced motivational patterns seen throughout the rest of the animal kingdom.

As instruments and ideas became available to quantitate and qualify events and entities, we became heavily involved in a system of measurement and observation that grew into the paradigm we term *science* and catapulted us into The Mechanical World of Form and Function. We began to postulate laws of nature that are immutably fixed and knowable and believed that we could learn these laws and unravel all the mysteries of living and nonliving systems. As scientific scholars used that language of relationships called mathematics to measure and observe, they found that some of their data fit poorly into The Anthropomorphic World of Words. They were not able to reconcile many of the old word-world beliefs with the linear sequencing of data that captivated the imagination with the promise of provable and testable answers to our questions about ourselves.

The gathering of information into predictable sequences became a threat to religion in that it implied the world was reasonable and a mechanical interaction that could be understood without the introjection of the magical or miraculous phenomena hitherto used to explain the soul and its world. Western religious thought and scientific thought were viewed as conflicting, and science was labeled by some as antithetical to religious faith because it suggested that man was not lord of the universe. Many of us were caught in the struggle between science and religion and felt forced to choose between them or to live in a dualistic world of conflicting and irreconcilable beliefs.

Around the turn of this century we entered another conceptual world—The Relative World of Process. This world view was catalyzed by the publication of Einstein's theories of relativity. Mathematicians, physicists, and other scholars involved in studying the microcosm and the macrocosm began to postulate about a four-dimensional universe in which mass and energy and time and space coordinates are interchangeable.

In one sense, the enormous emphasis on differentiation and measurement characterized in The Mechanical World of Form and Function has led to the paradoxical situation in which all measurement became relative with no absolutes. With this relativistic approach to ourselves and our world, form and function fused. Being and nonbeing, self and nonself became moot questions in that the answers might always be stated as relative to what. This new theoretical frame placed all living and nonliving systems on a continuum, thereby decreasing or even abolishing our justification of ourselves as special isolated and absolute entities.

Although its opponents criticize this new mode of thinking as being mechanistic, its emphasis on relativity, probability, and uncertainty makes this theoretical format much less mechanistic in nature than some of the previous ones that focused on entities involved in event sequences. Any absolutes or cause and effect sequences are seen as illusions that are testable only in a retrospect organization of events.

Some postulate that this new philosophic frame will eliminate that form of thinking called religion. Others see this new conceptual approach as a man–God merger in which the lack of differentiation allows a certain increased frame of reverence in the relativity of all being. Life and death are no longer seen as discrete entities or events but as a process phenomenon with a waxing and waning nature in which the individual self merges into a continuum with the rest of creation.

All the varied facets of nature take on the aspect of kaleidoscopic, harmonic, resonating fields of influence intermeshing in patterns with transient properties analogous to the harmonic interaction of a symphony. This is somewhat reminiscent of the music of the spheres concept whereby the Greek philosophers postulated the influence of the heavenly bodies on our existence. The new emphasis on relativity allows a flexible format for mathematical representation of harmonic influences and attempts to modulate these influences to increase the data base of information and the flow of this information, i.e., the effect of these influences on other patterns of influence to give a statistically probable, though never absolute, presentation of various harmonics.

By monitoring and modulating such fields of influence as electromagnetic activity, we have been able to expand our communication skills to a global extent and are attempting to move to establish information exchange throughout the universe by harnessing and modulating influences that can move away from the earth at the speed of light.

The new conceptual frames of the twentieth century have allowed us to address the microcosm of subatomic fields and the macrocosm of interstellar relationships using our instruments and perceptive organs as an integrated part of the information flow. We no longer stand on the outside and observe but now participate as part of the interacting events. The information processed by our protoplasm, whether this information comes from electron microscopes or huge radar telescopes and which in the word world would be called perception and cognition, must be viewed in The Relative World of Process as a transient harmonic of interacting force fields.

For many of us the death of the absolute comes as an inconceivable and heretical blow to our whole world of ideas. To others, it opens a new frame of reverence in which we rejoin the fluid harmony of all being and in the process become infinite. In this type of transcendence, we merge with the ultimate and may set aside the fears generated by contemplating the dissolution of the transient organization called the individual or the individual self. This philosophic relativism with its emphasis on uncertainty has the possibility of engendering tolerance in social interchanges by implying that there can be no right, wrong, good, or bad since these are all relative concepts predicated on the delusion that the individual or his social group are unique, absolute entities.

For our practical functioning in everyday social situations there can be little question that we will continue to rely on the "as if" proposition that we do exist as unique responsible individuals. However, the potential for realizing our participation in the unbounded infinite may provide a frame of reverence that avoids the split between science and religion. This relativistic approach to the concept of self in no way diminishes the beauty of artistic creation in which a transient pattern of organized influences that we call an individual catalyzes other influences into information sequences that we call art, science, and philosophy. The phenomenon we call an individual person is simultaneously a discrete system of organized influences and a harmonic of the entire universe.

In composing this book we relied very heavily on the work of many scholars and made extensive use of quotations. Since the anthropomorphic conceptual frame dominated our world view for thousands of years, we gave considerable time to its description. The mechanical world view has been dominant for only a few centuries and is evident in volumes of scholarly work. The relativistic world view has evolved in our present century and is only beginning to permeate our individual thinking. We have linked together the ideas of these different ages and different fields of endeavor to illustrate the theoretical paths we have traveled to reach our current views about ourselves and our place in nature. All these systems of thought or world views are important, and all have influenced our individual philosophies even though we may be unaware of their impact.

We would like to extend our appreciation to Jeanette Barnett who typed the manuscript and to Dr. Stuart Munro who spent many hours editing and encouraging.

Contents

The Search for Certainty

Chapter 1

The Birth of Certainty

> In every age there is a turning-point, a new way of seeing and asserting the coherence of the world. It is frozen in the statues of Easter Island that put a stop to time—and in the medieval clocks in Europe that once also seemed to say the last word about the heavens for ever. Each culture tries to fix its visionary moment, when it was transformed by a new conception either of nature or of man. [2:pp. 23–24]
>
> *Jacob Bronowski, 1973*

> The human sense of identity—the fact that we experience ourselves as agents, displaying volition, operating "our" body as if it were a machine distinct from the I which operates it, is the most familiar of all human experiences; and perhaps upon inspection, the oddest. [3:p. 23]
>
> *Alex Comfort, 1979*

Civilization and Its Concepts

The study of humanity and civilization is the study of evolving conceptual frames. During the centuries many conceptual frames have evolved that have revolutionized our view of ourselves and the universe as each age and each culture attempt to organize their own particular speculations concerning our place in nature.

Formats for arranging or organizing information have been rapidly evolving in our present industrial and technological society. The process we call civilization seems to hinge on our acquisition of new information and the subsequent alteration of conceptual formats. These two processes are concomitant. New information requires a new conceptual format, and new conceptual formats allow acquisition of new information. All these concepts that have shaped our world are products of the human mind. "The point," writes Jacob Bronowski, "is that knowledge in general and science in particular does not consist of abstract but of man-made ideas, all the way from its beginnings to its modern and idiosyncratic models" [2:p. 13].

In studying these man-made conceptual frames, we cannot follow a strictly chronological order. Some very old concepts persist side by side with very new concepts. As we examine a selection of twentieth century concepts we will notice that some of them have their roots far back in antiquity.

We will study the evolution of concepts with the purpose of determining how they affect our ideas about the human self and its world. Studying the evolution of concepts is a process somewhat analogous to studying biologic evolution. For example, some species that are phylogenetically very old continue to exist with newer species. Anthropomorphic concepts about the human self originating in the Stone Age are still very strong in a culture that is beginning to appreciate the concept of relativity.

The individual's world view and self view depend on the quality and quantity of information integrated, information that is sometimes frightening and not easily assimilated into preexisting patterns. New conceptual frames are often so different from previous formats that we consider them a new species of human thought. Most of us are unaware of the magnitude of some of the recent changes in world view, especially those occurring during our own time. We may accept the advent of new concepts as an historical event occurring in our time, but we remain unable to accept the actual conceptual frames as methods of organizing information in our everyday lives.

Those who do speculate about the nature and source of human knowledge, the philosophers who give birth to concepts, are often unappreciated in their own times or reach fame only to have their viewpoints attacked to the extent that sometimes they pass from fame to scorn in a few years. An example of the latter is Herbert Spencer, who for a while was considered the most famous philosopher of his time. The English-Hegelian reaction against positivism destroyed his reputation. According to Will Durant:

> Strange to say, his [Spencer's] fame vanished almost as suddenly as it had come. He outlived the height of his own repute, and was saddened, in his last years, by seeing what little power his tirades had had to stop the tide of "paternalistic" legislation. He had become unpopular with almost every class. [4:p. 399]

Spencer died in 1903 with the belief that his work had been a failure and that he would have had greater satisfaction in life had he never developed the ideas that had enjoyed such brief acclamation [4].

It has been speculated that the increasing egotism of Friedrich Nietzsche, with its accompanying delusions of grandeur and persecution, would not have occurred had he been more appreciated by his contemporaries. As Durant wrote:

> Perhaps a little more appreciation by others would have forestalled this compensatory egotism, and given Nietzsche a better hold upon perspective and sanity. . . . But when these bits of light came, Nietzsche was almost blind in sight and soul; and he had abandoned hope. "My time is not yet," he wrote, "only the day after tomorrow belongs to me." [4:p. 446]

And, so, he died with the label insane in 1900.

Baruch Spinoza, born in 1632, was excommunicated from his synagogue on July 27, 1656, with the following malediction:

> With the judgment of the angels and the sentence of the saints, we anathematize, execrate, curse and cast out Baruch de Espinoza, the whole of the sacred community assenting, in presence of the sacred books with the six-hundred-

and-thirteen precepts written therein, pronouncing against him the malediction wherewith Elisha cursed the children, and all the maledictions, written in the Book of the Law. . . .

Hereby then are all admonished that none hold converse with him by word of mouth, none hold communication with him by writing; that no one do him any service, no one abide under the same roof with him, no one approach within four cubits length of him, and no one read any document dictated by him, or written by his hand. [4:p. 153]

Spinoza died on February 20, 1677, at age 44, and his name was scorned for at least a generation following his death [4].

Perhaps changes in conceptual formats are so frightening that we actively work to deny their impact. Or perhaps we become so rigid in our thinking that we cannot conceive of the possibility of dramatic shifts. It may be that the passage of time is necessary for a gradual and most lasting appreciation resulting in the acceptance of thoughts once considered radical and heretical.

Examples abound of ideas that are now accepted but that caused their original expositors to be persecuted. One of the best known and most striking is evidenced by the story of Galileo Galilei (1564–1642), who insisted on trying to prove to the world that the Copernican theory of the earth revolving around the sun was accurate. He, being a scientist, believed that scientific data would be readily accepted and welcomed. He did not take into account the political power of the Roman Catholic Church and its ability to persuade the people of the value of religious dogma over scientific fact. History has shown that scientists often make the mistake of believing that their discoveries will be greeted with enthusiasm and do not understand the unwillingness of the establishment to accept data that do not validate its authority [2].

Galileo was tried in 1633. Bronowski wrote:

Galileo was confined for the rest of his life in his villa in Arcetri at some distance from Florence, under strict house arrest. The Pope was implacable. Nothing was to be published. The forbidden doctrine was not to be discussed. Galileo was not even to talk to Protestants. The result was silence among Catholic scientists everywhere from then on. Galileo's greatest contemporary, René Descartes, stopped publishing in France and finally went to Sweden. [2:p. 218]

To believe that the experience of Galileo could not be repeated today is to be as naive as he was at the time of his persecution. One of the reasons that scientists are not as readily attacked today may be that the public is not aware of the potential impact upon its value systems of the discoveries of modern physicists, astronomers, and mathematicians. It is predictable that there may be a movement to discredit new data from physics and halt the research when people realize that the new theories cast doubt upon established belief systems.

The current debate between the evolutionists and the creationists should give us some idea of the primitive and concrete quality of the thinking of many in our present culture and of the potential power of those who arm themselves with religious dogma. There is little difference between those who refused to accept the truth of the Copernican world system in 1633 and those who refuse to accept the fact of evolution in the 1980s.

The March 16, 1981, issue of *Time* carries the headline "Putting Darwin Back in the Dock" and part of the text reads:

> Indeed, it is happening. More than a century after Charles Darwin published his *Origin of Species* in 1859, more than half a century after the Scopes "monkey trial" in 1925 in Dayton, Tenn., the argument between evolution and divine creation has been revived. [10:p. 80]

And yet, the majority of us believe that we live in an enlightened age. Occasionally we read in newspapers and magazines that anthropologists and other social scientists have stumbled upon remnants of a Stone Age culture. These cultures are usually found within a relatively unexplored area in the tropics or on some remote and isolated island. We muse about how these living fossils conceptualize themselves and the world. We are fascinated by their naiveté and often animistic or anthropomorphic views of their environments. Their cultures are labeled Stone Age because of their lack of technology. It might be just as appropriate to label them Stone Age cultures because their conceptual frames are simplistic and concrete. The latter definition would be somewhat unfair, since most of our present cultures live with beliefs in Stone Age types of concepts.

It may be somewhat disconcerting to realize that we and the majority of persons with whom we associate daily continue to intersperse ancient and modern concepts in organizing our view of the world. We are word-world people, and many of our conceptual patterns still resemble those of the Stone Age. We invented stone implements and words many centuries ago and continued to refine both these instruments until our crude stone axes became laser beams and our words became complex printed symbols. Muscle power gave way to nuclear power, and the spoken word was implemented by writing and finally by telecommunication and data processing technology. Since all of us are engaged or involved by this technology, with the exception perhaps of a few eccentrics who have avoided involvement by retreat, we may state that there is an enormous difference between our life styles and those of persons in a Stone Age culture. We have automobiles, television sets, home computers, and other articles demonstrating our technological capability. Why then make the absurd statement that most of us still live in a Stone Age culture?

A key to this point of view lies in an exploration of our conceptual frames. A large number of us believe that our minds and bodies are two separate entities and that our minds control our bodies most of the time. We believe that there is some type of manlike God in the sky who is susceptible to our prayers and praises. We believe that, on death, the soul, which has always been separate, leaves the body and makes a journey to somewhere. We put great faith in knowledge of good and evil, right and wrong. We know that the time is kept by clocks and watches and that space and objects that occupy space can be measured in inches or miles or some unit of the metric system.

Although we are completely immersed in twentieth century technology and are able to speak about nuclear energy, few of us appreciate the theoretical concepts involved in this advancing technology. Relativity theory, systems theory, information theory, and cybernetics are left for the present-day priests, the scientists. Every school child knows about DNA, but few connect DNA with themselves. We still think in form and function and not in process. If we attempt to broaden our perspective by conceptualizing the world as being built of basic building blocks called atoms, we see in our mind's eye these atoms as being tiny marbles surrounded by other tiny marbles. If someone speaks of force fields, we are reminded of the forces of good and evil that permeate mythology, or perhaps we think of the force as an anthropomorphic abstraction utilized by science fiction writers. We consider artificial intelligence a rather scary possibility and ridicule it as a transient gimmick.

We are much more familiar with the names of politicians or television and movie actors than with such names as Copernicus, Darwin, Einstein, Bohr, Maxwell, Schrödinger, Eddington, Jeans, Weiner, Shannon, Bertalanffy, or von Neumann. If we are asked to think of history, we think of Alexander the Great rather than Plato or Aristotle, of Julius Caesar rather than Archimedes, of Napoleon rather than Immanuel Kant, of Hitler rather than Whitehead. We remember people who do things rather than people who think things. We are much more attuned to perceivable changes in the physical world than to changes in our conceptual world.

We like our world to be simple and predictable and describable by words that have definite meanings. We like our words to resemble the flint tools of our ancestors. Theories concerning relativity, nuclear physics, and computer science are as remote and frightening to us as is a low-flying jet aircraft to a Stone Age culture in New Guinea. Over time we have come to accept their existence, but they represent a different world we do not understand. We smile at the cargo cults of the aborigines who worship airplanes, but we reverently expect science to find the solution to our energy problems with little more appreciation of the concepts that permeate science than the aborigine has of the metal birds that occasionally lay valuable eggs.

Tracing the history of concepts is a fascinating occupation. First, we note that the conceptual frames we discard or attribute to primitive cultures are regarded with humor and sometimes dubbed myths. Those we use are called reality, and those that we are considering or beginning to use we call theories. Theories are the contemporary conceptual formats currently used by scholars and scientists. Some of these theories indirectly influence our lifestyles via technology, but they do not permeate the thinking of most of us concerning routine, day-to-day matters. We think of new theories as clever toys for physicists, mathematicians, chemists, biologists, physicians, and engineers, but they seem somewhat removed from our most important concept, that of ourselves.

As new conceptual frames or theories arise from the reorganization of existing information and the incorporation of new information, there are attempts to name these concepts, and we encounter terms such as Bunges' "emergent materialism" or Delgato's "triunism." We may become familiar with the names and have little understanding of their meaning. Most of us will be disappointed that all information cannot be well integrated into a new concept or that the concept generates more questions than answers. We are more comfortable, for example, with static relationships in three dimensions than with dynamic four-dimensional frames of reference in which all components are relationships within relative and uncertain systems.

We have a tendency to attempt validation of a particular concept to the exclusion of related concepts. Our need for rigid and concrete answers prevents the acceptance of what may initially appear to be mutually exclusive frames of thought. Persons involved in scientific endeavors seem to prefer concepts or theories that allow the measurement of probability. Those individuals involved in religion, art, and metaphysics sometimes work within frames of reference that defy measurement. It is difficult to state that any given format is right or wrong. All concepts may be judged, not as true or false, but on the type and amount of information they incorporate.

A hybrid term that might help us in our encounters with seemingly opposing concepts is *relative empiricism.* All information and concepts are relative, and all our conceptual frames of organized information must be judged empirically in terms of what effects they have upon other concepts and information. In one conceptual frame we might encounter demons and dragons. In another, we might find quanta and quarks. It does seem productive to consider whether a given conceptual frame allows measurement of its information, but this does not negate or perhaps even mitigate the influence of those conceptual frames that do not allow measurement.

Niels Bohr observed that in making any statement about the struggles of the ego we leave the scientific realm. This is another way of saying that by using anthropomorphic information arrangements we preclude our ability to measure. This does not mean that terms like ego should not be used as designating an abstract process, but we must note that empirically an abstraction such as ego may preclude integrating information from physiologic and psychologic measurements.

Persons who prefer conceptual frames that are not given to measurement may be comforted by appreciating that the building blocks of theoretical frames are not discrete objects or entities. Alfred North Whitehead, in *Adventures of Ideas*, discusses the abandonment by modern physics of the doctrine of simple location. We like to speak of and must at times consider a focal region or entity as a thing itself, but in actuality, the separation of the phenomenon we are describing from the external stream is not possible. We cannot accurately conceive a physical thing as an instantaneous fact. Whitehead states quite clearly:

> The physical thing is a certain coordination of spaces and times and of conditions in those spaces at those times, this coordination illustrating one exemplification of a certain general rule, expressible in terms of mathematical relations. [13:p. 162]

Although many theories are being developed that affect us technologically, we tend to pay little attention to them as long as they make our lives easier or more pleasurable. We do not concern ourselves with whether the conceptual frame lends itself to measurement, but rather with how it affects our day-to-day living, especially our ideas about ourselves. Sometimes we lack the language to express our thoughts or we lack the data base to understand what we are seeing or hearing.

Everyone has heard about the theory of relativity. We have some understanding of its importance in the realm of physics and of one of its more frightening results, the atomic bomb. Since this theoretical concept is unfamiliar except in very general terms and since its implementation only attracts our attention on occasion, we stand in awe of such events as an atomic explosion. We endow this phenomenon with magical or supernatural properties outside the comprehension of ordinary folk. In this case, we lack the specific knowledge to apply the theory to ourselves.

We know that atomic things are dangerous if not handled correctly, but we rarely realize that we ourselves are atomic reactors. If we were in close proximity to a sufficient number (critical mass) of restless and unstable (radioactive) atoms as occur in a nuclear blast, our own atoms would stampede along with the rest and we would participate in the explosion. But this is rather melodramatic. Our own atoms of carbon, hydrogen, and oxygen are not like those wild uranium atoms. Our atoms are gentle—they are more civilized. They like organizing themselves into systems rather than stampeding off into chaos. These orderly systems of atoms are organized by information or blueprints so that they appear rather predictable.

Because we cannot always apply developing theories to ourselves, we fail to understand when a conceptual revolution is taking place or the impact it may have on our lives. Many of us do not see any reason to explore new conceptual frames if they do not noticeably influence our lives or our often rigidly defended value systems.

We usually follow habit patterns and theoretical frames that we have inherited from past individual and social systems without much concern about their origin. We defend our rather pragmatic stance by saying, "If it works, why bother?"

Most of us learned in elementary school about Copernicus and Galileo and their theories. We understand that the universe does not necessarily revolve around our planet, but we still envision that the sun comes up in the east, shines on our world, and goes down in the west. The stars come out at night. If questioned, we admit that they are probably up there all the time. Up there? What do we mean by up there? Everyone knows up from down and night from day, so why all these questions? If we persist in our interrogation, we may ask something even more absurd, "Who is it who knows about time and space?" We answer, "I do" or "I don't," which leads us to the most ridiculous question of all, "What is the 'I' that does or does not know about these things?" At this point, you may object, "Look here, we went through all this years ago and what did it get us? Philosophers have argued these types of questions for centuries and have gone around in circles. Why reopen a closed issue or attempt to clarify a hopelessly clouded one?"

Perhaps our unending desire to solve the riddle of who we are, our self-concept, may be as human as our aptitude for speech. We do not tire of comparing ourselves to the rest of the animal kingdom, wondering how we became aware of our differentiation. Alex Comfort writes:

> If a pig had a "sense of identity" comparable to that of man, it would presumably experience it from birth. Being precocial, this is to say, born able to walk and forage, birth for such a discursive piglet would have to be an experience closely similar to that which we normally experience in waking. The human experience is clearly different; we are altricial mammals born with much less, or a much more selective, immediate grasp on our environment—chiefly touch, sound and possibly odor, plus taste. Accordingly, we "wake" gradually:

if there is an incident in which I-ness first becomes concrete, as there may be an incident in which we first discover we can walk, or read, it precedes memory and we do not explicitly recall it. [3:pp. 23–24]

What we do know is that from our beginnings we have lived in a self-centered world. We are told that we are created in God's image and the universe revolves around us. Who are we? We are ourselves. The human self is seen as the apex of creation. With little thought we talk about our minds and bodies, implying that they are our possessions, and again, when we question the possessive pronoun, the "our" or "mine" refers to ourselves. We speak glibly of self-confidence or self-doubt, self-consciousness, selfishness, self-assuredness, selflessness, self-destruction, self-indulgence, and self-pity. We admonish others to be themselves, to take care of themselves, to put others before themselves. We hear frequently, "Know thyself." All these self references seem to be reasonable, and yet if the question is asked, "What is a self?", we begin to experience difficulty. We seem to have less trouble in discerning what is not a human self than in delineating the boundaries or properties of a self. To say that the human self consists of a body and mind still leaves a number of questions. Even though we say, "I am not myself today," we usually do not mean to imply that we are some other self. There seems to be an unspoken assumption that one could "lose one's mind" or markedly alter one's body and still have an intact self.

Most of us are at somewhat of a loss if we attempt to answer the childish question, "What happens to my 'self' when I go to sleep?" One might expect that the field of medicine, which studies almost every aspect of man, both in health and in disease, might have developed a philosophic if not a scientific approach to the question of self. However, it seems that medicine has in the past largely bypassed this question by relying on the division of man into two categories—mind and body, or psyche and soma. Those in medicine who have a biologic orientation address physiologic and body systems, and others in medicine, who are concerned about the psychologic and behavioral aspects of man, address the mind or psyche, the so-called mental phenomena, leaving the self to go with whichever discipline happens to be in focus. In emotional disturbances the self is equated with ego function. In physiologic disturbances the self is equated with the perception of pain and other uncomfortable stimuli.

It is somewhat puzzling that study of the evolution of the self concept has not been a focus for the hard sciences. Only recently has a scientific approach been applied to the phenomenon of self. In spite of enormous advances in information concerning man's internal and external environment, the self has been largely the domain of philosophy, religion, and healing practices. Theories stemming from these sources have not lent themselves well to scientific investigation.

Language and the Concept of Self

How did the concept of self originate? Perhaps the "I" is related to language. There is some indication that young children differentiate, i.e., develop a sense of self as different from others, at the same time they are developing language. If we assume that ontogeny recapitulates phylogeny, and therefore that the developing child reflects some of the stages humans went through during evolution, we could state that man differentiated himself from his environment with the help of language, or at least that language and self-differentiation occurred simultaneously.

It is interesting to speculate whether we had a sense of self before we developed language. We can suppose that we did and that we had some way of communicating our ideas to other people. But we get no real feeling for the self until we are able to hear it expressed in verbal terms. We can even speculate as to whether animals have a sense of self. We discuss such questions in beginning philosophy classes: "Does a cat have a self?" We read expressions on the faces of our pets and feel we can communicate with them. But we have no way of knowing whether our dog thinks, "Here comes my master," when he sees us coming because he can't verbalize it. He may show us signs of recognition by running toward us, wagging his tail, licking our hands, barking in appreciation of our recognition, but we have no reason to think that he forms concepts or thoughts such as those that we entertain.

With the advent of language we began to say "my tree, my hands, my mother, my cave, my shadow, my self." We then left the world of other animals. Abstraction and differentiation are abilities that seem more evolved in us than in other animals. The size of our brain, our longevity, flexible hands, and upright posture are all given credit for our ability to process information, learn, and solve problems. The evolution of a syntactical operation for data organization associated with vocal capabilities to develop language also contributed to our unique position among animals. Thus we witness the emergence of those properties that we call human.

In 1801, Jean Baptist de Lamarck, a French biologist, proposed the theory of the gradual evolution of man from prehistoric primate ancestors. Charles Darwin, in 1858 in the *The Origin of Species* and in 1871 in *The Descent of Man*, developed the theory of the mechanism of evolution that is now widely accepted [14].

According to the theory of evolution, our prehuman ancestors included the primates, a group of animals that includes the monkeys and apes. Our development is supposed to have taken millions of years. Two types of prehistoric species include *Proconsul*, the ancestor of the higher apes, and the hominids, the first manlike creatures. The hominids were not apes. They existed at least 12 million years ago and are believed to have originated in Africa [14].

The Age of Man is called the Quarternary period and includes the Pleistocene epoch (1,000,000 to 8000 B.C.) and the Holocene epoch, which is also known as the "Wholly Recent" epoch (8000 B.C. to the present) [1]. The hominids, who date back far before these periods, and who are believed to be our direct ancestors, gradually evolved so that they possessed many qualities or characteristics similar to our own: the ability to make and use tools, binary vision, the ability to walk upright, an easily manipulated opposing thumb and forefinger, a more highly developed central nervous system, and the ability to speak [14].

The earliest hominid identified to date is *Australopithecus*. However, recent discoveries and the results of ongoing investigations may test all our old theories. For example, Donald C. Johanson and Maitland A. Edey published *Lucy: The Beginnings of Humankind* in 1981, which identifies a new species, *Australopithecus afarensis*, named after the Afar triangle in Ethiopia where the fossils were found. This would set the date of our human ancestors at some 3,500,000 years ago [6].

Currently accepted theory places the appearance of the first human species about 1,000,000 years ago during the geological time period known as the Pleistocene. Some species associated with that time period include Java Man (500,000 B.C.), Peking Man (also 500,000 B.C.), Rhodesian Man (dated somewhere between the middle and late Pleistocene), Heidelberg Man (350,000–300,000 B.C.), Neanderthal Man (most prominent from 40,000 B.C. to 25,000 B.C.), and *Homo Sapiens*, or modern man (believed to have existed as early as 20,000 B.C.) [1].

The development of language, the ability to communicate through speech, is dated during the lower Paleolithic stage, which ended about 30,000 B.C. C. F. Hockett speculates that human language evolved between 150,000 and 50,000 years ago. Neanderthal Man, who flourished during this period, also hunted, fished, made tools and weapons, used fire, painted, lived in caves, produced spearheads, and may have developed some rudimentary religious sense as evidenced by the burial of their dead with food, indicating a belief in the hereafter [1].

What was life like for the Neanderthal? When we use present conceptual formats to organize information about the past, we are putting ourselves in a situation similar to that of the hero in Mark Twain's *A Connecticut Yankee in King Arthur's Court*. We may speculate about a Neanderthal social group living in a cave. We may even call it a family. But we cannot use the Neanderthal's data processing format and see the world as he sensed it. Since the Neanderthal brain was as large as or larger than the present human brain, we might assume they organized the information coming to them from the world similar to the way we do, but this assumption does not take into account social factors.

Most of us have thought about the world of primitive people such as the Neanderthal. How many of us as children imagined a prehistoric world populated by strange and scary predators, a world of swirling mists and swamps and steamy jungles inhabited by little cave families huddled together for protection? We thought of a father, mother, children, and perhaps various other relatives who felt the same kinds of emotions we experience—love, hate, fear, jealousy.

We have no way of knowing what the individuals in a Neanderthal social group talked about or thought about or even what their environment was really like. We know little of prehistoric social systems or the ability of ancient people to organize information into abstract concepts because they did not have the ability to record their symbolic systems for future reference.

If we had the opportunity of meeting our ancestors before the emergence of language, we would probably depend largely on nonverbal communication, such as facial expressions and gestures. If we could meet them today, that is, we with our language and they without, the confrontation might be similar to that which occurs when we observe apes in a zoo. They would seem human, but there would be an awesome chasm between us. Why would they be so different from us? They would have the same anatomic and physiologic equipment. They would have all the potential for knowing everything that we know. Their brains would be receiving the same stimuli or perceptive information as ours, as far as we know.

The difference would be the conceptual format for organizing information. Without language they would be unable to share information of an elaborate nature with us. They would be locked in a world of their own experiences, a here-and-now world that could be shared only through the gestures and cries still prevalent throughout the remainder of the animal world. Children could apprentice with adults to learn various experiential skills of hunting and seeking shelter, but it would be difficult to anticipate events that one had not experienced.

When the animals we call human developed the capability to process information into symbolic units we term words, they could use these word tools to share their information with other humans. They could also store experiences in a logical sequence and use this arrangement to better predict future sequences of events. This was quite different from those animals whose information was locked into a type of format that did not allow sequential storage of data. Those animals with information processing systems that were locked into a form that did not allow efficient data transfer from one individual to another were limited to a here-and-now format that makes learning slow and dependent upon perceived environmental stimuli.

If you visit a zoo and have the time to stand silently in front of one of the great apes, our nearest relatives, look silently into his eyes. It appears to be a frustrating experience for both parties. We can almost feel a kinship, a time before the parting of the ways. We quickly slip into our differentiating format, anthropomorphizing the ape's condition and then feeling a bit guilty about what we are doing to him. Because we are locked into our differentiating format, just as the ape is locked into his undifferentiated paradigm, we cannot communicate with him to our satisfaction.

The development of language was of enormous magnitude. If we were to write a story called "Primordia" we might begin: "A hairy, dirty, blood-stained hand lifted a stone and hurled it at a shadowy form. They say we began here, but perhaps our beginning came with discovery of another tool, a far more potent weapon against the unknown. The tool was invented by long trial and error and is still in the beginning phases of development. The tool first came into being without our actual awareness. No ancestor had used it before. The tool was a word."

Since language evolved as an information exchange system before we learned ways of recording our word symbols, we can only speculate as to how it came about. Undoubtedly the biologic equipment was a prerequisite for this complex data processing activity. But we have only recently begun to study this aspect of ourselves.

Hockett, in *Man's Place in Nature*, discusses the development of language, listing several points common to all languages. Every language has developed word forms that differentiate between *I* and *you*, the perceiver and the perceived. Every language includes the use of kinship terms, such as aunt, uncle, cousin, and daughter. These facts validate the importance of the idea of self throughout the world and throughout the ages of man, considering that our species has developed some 4000 to 5000 different languages [5].

Although we may have discovered characteristics common to all languages, we cannot trace the actual invention of language. According to Charlton Laird, Hebrew was considered by Christians for centuries to be the language used by Adam and therefore the language that would naturally be common to all individuals if they were not taught another language. Other early thinkers theorized that language was not invented at all but was a gift given by God directly to man [7].

Two prominent and current theories of the basis of language are those of B. F. Skinner and Noam Chomsky. Skinner's view is that language is learned just as other performances are learned, and that nothing additional is needed to learn language than is needed to learn anything else. Chomsky's view is that language is an innate neurological phenomenon [8].

What do we know about languages? We know that they are born and die and that each individual helps invent his or her particular language each day. We also know that women are the chief transmitters of language, for they traditionally have been the ones who stay at home with the children and teach them to speak [7].

One interesting feature of language development, as indicated by Joseph Lyons and James J. Barrell, is that once we have learned as children the name for an object, we no longer consider it a name. We consider the name to be the object. For example, if we are taught to say sky, we will, when hearing the Spanish word *cielo*, think, "That's the Spanish word for sky." Once we have learned to name objects in our native tongue, we will forever be able to think or know in that language. We will not be able to recall how we learned to name various things. As Lyons and Barrell describe it:

> There is absolutely no way that I can go back behind my own knowing in English and apprehend this object as nameless. My learning of the English word is now buried beyond recall. [8:p. 292]

Laird points out that when we speak of language and its uses throughout the world, we must be aware that it is spoken language that is most prevalent. Even extremely sophisticated and literate individuals, such as teachers and writers, speak many thousands more words than they write. Language was invented as spoken language and remained spoken language for millenia [7].

It was not until sometime between 4000 and 3000 B.C. that writing was invented by the civilizations that emerged in the Nile Valley of Egypt and the Tigris-Euphrates Valleys of Mesopotamia. The Akkadians of Mesopotamia, as well as other Near Eastern peoples, acquired cuneiform writing, which the Sumerians had developed prior to 3000 B.C. The Egyptians developed several systems of writing, including hieroglyphics and hieratic and demotic script. Hieroglyphics included 600 signs and was sacred. Hieratic was a cursive script used for public and commercial affairs. Demotic was an abbreviated script used by the commoners [1].

In 1922, Sir John Marshall discovered the existence in northwestern India of a great pre-Ayran civilization that utilized a pictographic script on parchment, cotton cloth, birch bark, and palm leaves. This script has been only partly deciphered. These early civilizations of the Indus Valley existed between 4000 and 2500 B.C. [1].

We take both spoken and written language as a given, a part of ourselves. We feel horror when a friend suffers brain damage sufficient to obliterate his or her ability to speak or understand language. The lack of ability to communicate through the medium of language erects an almost insurmountable barrier between our self systems and the self system of the afflicted individual. To emphasize the importance of language to our present self concept, let us perform a little experiment. Close your eyes and try to think without words. Be careful that your tongue isn't moving. If you think about what you are doing, you are cheating. *I* is particularly difficult to get rid of. We take ourselves, or our *I*, for granted. If we are asked what the *I* is, we usually come up with another word for the same phenomenon. For example, it is me, myself. We realize we are being tautological, but we see no other way to express it. If we are not careful, we make statements like "my body, my mind, my self," without realizing that we are implying by the possessive pronoun *my* that the *I* possesses a self, a mind, and a body without being any of these things.

Let's try a second experiment. See how long you can go in normal conversation without using the word *I*. It is not only the egocentric or egotistic person who uses constant self-referencing words. We are all engaged in references to self in order to differentiate perceiver and perceived or speaker and listener. It seems somewhat paradoxical that language, being the great unifier of men into cultural groups, is also the tool by which we differentiate ourselves, not only from other people but from all other things.

> Language is fundamental to the development of culture.
> If culture is a river, then language is the bed in which the river flows.
> [9:p. 14]

Culture is a learned phenomenon, a social heritage. It is promulgated by the sharing of ideas, beliefs, knowledge, customs, skills, and ways of behaving.

A peculiar facet of language consists in its being an instrument for individual use that requires a social system to be of continued value. Words must represent the same relative phenomena to the people using them, or there is no exchange of information. Take the word *it*. We have agreed that *it* is a rather general word that can be used in many ways. The cosmos can be labeled it when we say that, "It (the cosmos) is all there is." A tiny electron can be referred to as "it" by saying, "It is a small electric charge." We may even refer to the word *it* by saying: "*It* can refer to almost anything." The social system serves as the language bank. New words have to be validated by the social system if they are to be more than personal idiosyncrasies.

An individual may originate a sound or combination of sounds and give it an abstract or symbolic meaning, but this uniquely personal symbol dies with the individual unless other individuals adopt the same sounds as representing the same concept. Thus, we have individuation dependent on communication and abstraction and the communication system dependent on the group.

And yet, we all develop patterns of language peculiar to ourselves. Although the words may have shared meaning and be linked together in acceptable grammatical frames, we all develop individualized vocabularies and manners of speaking that are born with us and die with us. Laird describes this phenomenon:

> First we noticed that language relies upon a body of human agreement bewildering in its complexity. Human beings can speak, and can be understood, only because they have at their call millions of meanings and countless ways of putting these meanings together to produce larger and more exact meanings. These meanings and means of meaning, although they may later become codified, rest upon an agreement unconsciously entered into, signed, and sealed by all of us. Language is language only because it has currency; the giving of currency is an act of social faith, the utilizing of the common by-product of many minds busy with their own affairs. Thus looked at from one point of view, language is a common product made by all of us, in process of being remade by all of us, and understandable only if studied as the commonality of many minds over many generations.
>
> On the other hand we have seen that language as it exists is always the possession of individuals. Vocabularies are individual vocabularies, and ways of individuals. A man's speech is as peculiar to him, as inseparable from him, as is his own shadow. It has grown with him, and most of it will die with him; like his shadow, it is to a degree made anew every day. He inevitably speaks a dialect, his own dialect, which is in turn a compact of many regionalisms, a linguistic goulash which every man brews after his own recipe. Looked at from this point of view, language becomes a pattern of infinitely blending dialects. [7:p. 22]

That which makes us unique in the animal kingdom, the ability to communicate by speech, also places us in a state of differentiated dependency. We must depend upon the social group for validation of the symbols we use at the same time that the use of these symbols differentiates us from the group.

Although the use of words differentiates individuals within cultural groupings, it also serves to emphasize the enormous variations among cultures. The word symbols within a culture are indicative of the importance of certain behaviors to that particular social group. Most of us are conscious of time, and we place great value upon knowing what time it is. We have socially validated such symbols as late, early, prompt, and tardy, and their use is habitual and frequent. The Sioux were said to have had no word for time and would not have readily understood the concept of being "on time." Having a language does not in itself mean that an individual will be understood even by other individuals speaking the same language. The problems are many times multiplied for those speaking different languages and trying to communicate with one another.

Agreeing upon a broad meaning for a certain word does not ensure complete understanding within any given social system. Symbolism is a condensation of data into a complex unit. The more the condensation, the greater the distortion. The word *father* may merely denote a male parent or it may, at times, be used to incorporate all the aspects of a particular male human being and the complex relationship with another human who is his progeny. In the latter case, the amount of data contained in the word is enormous and varies with each individual, making definitive social validation difficult if not impossible.

Words are sounds used to represent a unit of human experience. Since each experience is different for each individual, each word is only a rough generalization of a delineated experiential phenomenon. A word contains a varying amount of information different for the speaker and the listener but has been socially validated as expressing the same general experience. Speech communication is much more complex than it might appear. Within each individual there is a continuous, dynamic, fluid process of interacting influences. These influences include genetically and experientially coded information in continuous interaction. Some of these patterns of influence have the emergent properties we call thought. If these patterns are experienced in sufficient magnitude or in repeated fashion, we may label or pair the experience with a social symbol or word that we can use as a cue in recalling events or in the commerce of social interchange.

However, what we think and what we say may be so different that the results of our speech are not at all what we may wish. A thought may be a kind of picture with layers of abstractions, a gestalt or symbolic configuration that cannot be segmented into the units of speech required to convey that thought to another person. L. S. Vygotsky addresses this problem by stating:

> Thought, unlike speech, does not consist of separate units. When I wish to communicate the thought that today I saw a barefoot boy in a blue shirt running down the street, I do not see every item separately: the boy, the shirt, its blue color, his running, the absence of shoes. I conceive of all this in one thought, but I put it into separate words. A speaker often takes several minutes to disclose one thought. In his mind the whole thought is present at once, but in speech it has to be developed successively. A thought may be compared to a cloud shedding a shower of words. Precisely because thought does not have its automatic counterpart in words, the transition from thought to word leads through meaning. In our speech, there is always the hidden thought, the subtext. Because a direct transition from thought to word is impossible, there have always been laments about the inexpressibility of thought:
> "How shall the heart express itself?
> How shall another understand?"
> Direct communication between minds is impossible, not only physically but psychologically. Communication can be achieved only in a roundabout way. Thought must pass first through meanings and then through words. [11:pp. 209–210]

Whenever we unitize a continuum, such as a thought, we distort. Whenever we unitize the continuum of human experience, we distort the experience by chopping it into blocks or units and labeling the block with the socially agreed upon symbol or word. This chopping of experience into blocks necessitates drawing boundaries around the individual block or unit, which we may define as the process of *differentiating*. In a forest, we may focus on a unit of the forest and call it a tree. We have differentiated the tree from the forest. To say that the forest is composed of trees is a distortion, since each tree is not exactly like the one we have singled out to call a tree. This seems quite simple. It becomes more complex when we use a word to represent an experience that is not readily perceived. The word *beauty* is much more difficult to delineate or bound. Yet, we readily say something is beautiful or not beautiful.

We take such abstractions as beauty for granted. In some primitive languages there were no words for even broad categories, such as trees and animals, no general classifications. Each tree had a name and each animal had a name but they were not grouped together. Words denoting such qualities as soft, hard, cold, and warm were also unknown. To describe hardness, the individual would have to use an analogic descriptive form, such as "like a rock" [12].

Once a language has assumed abstract forms, it is necessary to suppose that there is a general agreement as to the meaning of words, or speech would be impossibly cumbersome. If we stopped to explain in detail the meaning of each word we utter, we could never complete a sentence. In describing a trip into the desert, the returned vacationer may say, "I saw the most beautiful flowers," and it is unlikely that she will find it necessary to describe them in detail or that any of her listeners will question her at length as to her definitions of beautiful and flowers. Her listeners may nod and act as if they had total understanding of the beautiful flowers. It would probably be most disconcerting to examine the picture in each person's imagination and find that no two people were imagining the same flowers. Some may imagine a cactus, others a buttercup.

Construction of the Word World

As we continued to chop our experiential world into word blocks, we began to utilize these blocks more and more as though they were actual units of reality. We began to construct a word world. This world consisted of a series, or sequential arrangement, of blocks of experience, with each block as differentiated as possible from other blocks in order to avoid confusion in communicating with others.

Our world, unlike the continuous experiential flow of other animals, now took on the characteristics of a world built of discrete units. In some respects, our concept of words resembles our concept of atoms. Originally we conceived of the world as built of immutable atoms, each like tiny marbles, discrete and self-contained. Recently we have begun to conceive atoms as probability centers of influence whose boundaries cannot be definitely delineated without distortion—so with words.

In the early construction of our word world, we became convinced that experience could be delineated into discrete blocks that were true or false. Our concepts, which were composed of these words, were true if the correct words were put into the proper sequence. Ultimate truth could be obtained if we stacked our word-world blocks in the correct alignment. We then set about to make sure that each block had clear and well-defined boundaries. The first problem was the realization that the blocks were of different sizes. This is another way of saying what we have alluded to previously—that words contained varying amounts of information since they represented different experiential phenomena.

The first major cleavage in this world of words was the differentiation of the self, or subject, from the nonself, or object. The world was cut into two blocks, the me and the not-me. Each of these blocks was then further subdivided into smaller blocks. The not-me block continued to be divided and subdivided as our experiences grew, and these experiences were recorded and validated so that they could be utilized by subsequent generations.

An individual could observe the recorded words, the blocks of experience of another individual who existed even centuries before. An individual might also share an experience of another individual separated by long distances if the recorded experience were transported from one site to another. We may presently read about the Lewis and Clark Expedition to the Northwest and participate in that experience many decades later, even though we have not visited the Northwest ourselves.

Dividing the not-me part of the world was an extremely productive and successful enterprise, allowing for rapid advance in culture and freedom from the time-space lock of experiential learning. The division of the not-me world into smaller and smaller units was the beginning of science and technology. Individuals did not have to have the experiences of other individuals to share the information as long as they participated in the cultural system's word-block world.

The division of the me block of the world was equally important since it represented the other half of the experience. This process proved more complicated. The difficulty arose in the use of perceptive organs to differentiate experience into blocks. We could see, hear, feel, touch, and taste the not-me world. When these perceptions were applied to the me part of the world, we were limited to our external body surface and crude pain and pleasure sensations from within. We divided our external anatomy into block experiences and said, "my arms, my legs, my body, my eyes."

When we addressed the fluid internal world of the me in which all experiences were recorded or taking place, we had no perceptive boundaries. We represented this territory as "myself," which we crudely divided into mind and body, or soul and body. Since the experiencer was called a self and the experience was termed the nonself, we occasionally confused properties that occurred in the experiential interaction of the self and nonself. We attributed selflike properties to the blocks in the nonself world, and vice versa. We assumed that the self was a concrete entity, like a tree. At other times, we attributed selflike qualities to the external world and spoke of the soul of a tree.

The inclination to confuse the self and nonself experiences has been quite prominent in our conceptual patterns. If one were to define *mind* as organized patterns of information, or perhaps patterns of information processing, we may extrapolate that all living systems process information in fairly standardized patterns, so we may say that all living systems have mind. This would then allow us to talk about the mind of a cell, the mind of an insect, a fish, or a mammal. Without stretching the definition, we could even speak of the mind of an oak tree. The problem with equating mind, psyche, and soul and in discussing the minds of various living systems is that we might be accused of panpsychism.

Panpsychism is an ancient theoretical concept in which human thought processes were attributed to plants, animals, and inanimate objects. We might smile at the aborigine praying to the soul of a rock or a tree or placating the soul of an animal that he has killed. We state that this is a primitive anthropomorphic way of thought. If we examine modern conceptual frames, we find vestiges of this so-called naive thinking to be quite prevalent in our self concepts. Although we would be reluctant to talk about the psyche of an ant when referring to its information processing activities, we quite readily speak of the human psyche, and a large portion of the population still refers to the human soul as though it were a well-defined entity.

We have the paradoxical situation of anthropomorphizing processes within ourselves, just as the ancients anthropomorphized processes outside themselves. We have further concretized an abstraction called the *psyche* into an entity with its own anatomy, including its ego, its superego, and its id. We use these terms as nouns and assign these named entities various activities. We may say that a weak ego struggles against the overwhelming drives of a relentless id. During its struggle the ego is continually goaded by the merciless and punitive superego. We can see from this type of terminology that we continue to separate the human psyche into anatomic parts and further concretize these anatomic parts into entities that in themselves have human traits.

We have moved the panpsychism from the external world into the internal world. We refer to information stored in our memory banks as having personal characteristics, for example, the internalized or introjected nurturing mother in conflict with the rigid and regimenting introjected father. The psyche becomes an internalized cast of characters that in themselves have psyches. The scenario for these interacting anthropomorphic characters is said to be driven by libidinal energy. This libidinal energy, to some degree, resembles the driving forces of fate and magic seen in the rituals of primitive persons. We can discuss the similarity of primitive drama, in which animals and inanimate objects are endowed with magical powers to react in an anthropomorphic manner, and our internalized anthropomorphic entities driven by a mystical libidinal energy.

Older cultures spent a great deal of effort trying to decipher the hidden meanings of runes and magical terms. Our culture spends an equal amount of time delving into the symbolic meaning of our psychic operation. An educated person of today might scoff at the machinations of a shaman or a witch doctor who is attempting to placate or remove anthropomorphized evil forces in the external world. The same educated person may spend hours in psychoanalytic sessions attempting to reconcile the internalized anthropomorphic forces that disrupt his psyche. We will address the issues of our propensity to anthropomorphize and its results and the impact of analytic thinking in later chapters. For now, we wish to stress that these characteristics are emergent properties of language.

Another important facet of the word world concerns the binary system of opposites. Once we had developed a human symbolic operation based on a unitized data processing paradigm and dependent upon differentiation, we had to rely on a binary system. Differentiation depends on polar extremes. Once we differentiated, we had to say that a thing either "is" or "is not." We were forced to say "yes" and "no." These opposite extremes are mediated by gradations of differentiation. Light and dark are mediated by twilight. Yes and no are mediated by maybe. Good and bad are mediated by neutral.

Binary differentiation distorted experiences by making them preconceived patterns. We took as opposites male and female and then forced other phenomena into this particular binary pattern. Varying amounts of previously experienced information made the male-female differentiation fall into stereotyped patterns. These patterns remain firmly ingrained in our thinking even though there are social pressures that attempt to alter them from time to time (for example, the women's liberation movement).

For example, if we are asked, of a lion and a cat, which is male and which is female, most of us would say that the lion is male and the cat is female. The list can be extended to include verbs, adjectives, or objects. A buffalo is male, a deer female. Pink is female, black is male. Playing football is male, and playing music is female. We think of the moon as female and the sun as male. To test your own tendency to divide into male and female even those words that are normally not thought of in sexual terms, see how easily you differentiate between the following pairs of words.

poetry–prose	more–less	digital–analog
in–out	hot–cold	up–down
soft–hard	zero–one	north–south
word–number	passive–aggressive	sweet–sour
rock–pebble	bland–bitter	aroma–odor
one–two	red–green	black–brown
flesh–blood	drum–piano	blood–water
pink–purple	purple–orange	yellow–orange
green–yellow	hammer–nail	nail–board
ice–fire	ice–water	mystery–fact
precise–inexact	faithful–unfaithful	bedroom–den
feeling–unfeeling	indulger–abstainer	

When we utilize a binary system of dividing concepts, entities, and experiences into such categories as male and female, we have been tricked by the system into using stereotyped information to make our differentiation. Obviously, a buffalo could be male or female and a color is sexless. Perhaps size, strength, or some other quality has led us to lump unrelated entities into categories that have nothing to do with the entities themselves or even with their characteristics.

The building of a word world by the use of a binary system of differentiation was accompanied by another phenomenon. At some time after we began to build our word world, we invented another set of language tools. To some degree, the new tools resembled the old word blocks of experience, but there was a subtle difference. The new language consisted of neat blocks that could be applied to the word blocks to make them fit more precisely. These new blocks could unitize relationships among experienced events and could be used to divide space and time into blocks. We invented numbers.

Although these neat little number blocks did not represent anything in themselves, they were enormously helpful in correctly sequencing events, in quantitating experiences, and in describing relationships. We began to say two nights ago, four elephants, a three days' walk, or one spear throw away.

We could describe the distance from our boat to the shore as two moose lengths.

By standardizing this number language, we were able to measure our words. We could make our word blocks more accurate, validating our belief that ultimate truth could be attained if our word blocks were correctly aligned and measured. How could we have foreseen that this language tool that helped to solidify our word-block world would eventually destroy it?

With the evolution of language and the reification of a world of words, we became certain that we existed as a unique entity, apart from the rest of the universe. With the birth of the certainty of our own importance and our own uniqueness came the search for certainty in all aspects of our endeavors. If you know that you are, then you can know that you know. We began to look for answers, for proof of our speculations about ourselves and our place in the universe.

Our search for certainty can be arbitrarily divided into three broad areas, which we have characterized as The Anthropomorphic World of Words, The Mechanical World of Form and Function, and The Relative World of Process. Most of us have a belief system that places us predominantly in one of the three paradigms, although we may experience considerable overlap. As we review the history of our concepts, we may ask, "What have we learned? Who are we? Of what can we be certain?"

References

1. Bernstein, P, and Green, R: *History of Civilization, Volume I; To 1648.* Totowa, New Jersey: Littlefield, Adams, 1963
2. Bronowski, J: *The Ascent of Man.* Boston: Little, Brown, 1973
3. Comfort, A: *I and That: Notes on the Biology of Religion.* New York: Crown, 1979
4. Durant, W: *The Story of Philosophy: The Lives and Opinions of the Greater Philosophers.* New York: Washington Square Press, 1953
5. Hockett, C: *Man's Place in Nature.* New York: McGraw-Hill, 1973
6. Johanson, D C, and Edey, M A: *Lucy: The Beginnings of Humankind.* New York: Simon and Schuster, 1981
7. Laird, C: *The Miracle of Language.* Greenwich, Connecticut: Fawcett, 1953
8. Lyons, J, and Barrell, J J: *People: An Introduction to Psychology.* New York: Harper & Row, 1979
9. Oliva, A (Editorial Consultant): *Monarch Review Notes in Sociology.* New York: Monarch, 1963
10. Pierce, K M: Putting Darwin back in the dock. *Time,* March 16, 1981, pp. 80–82
11. Vygotsky, L S: Thought and word. In Adams, P (Ed): *Language in Thinking.* London: Penguin Education, 1972
12. Wells, H G: *The Outline of History: The Whole Story of Man.* Garden City, New York: Doubleday, 1971
13. Whitehead, A N: *Adventures of Ideas.* New York: Mentor, 1955
14. Wines, R, Pickett, R, Toborg, A, and DiScala, S (Editorial Consultants): *Monarch Review Notes in World History, Part 1.* New York: Monarch, 1963

The
Anthropomorphic
World of Words

Chapter 2

Spirits and Gods

Bit by bit the mythical universe comes to rule all aspects of life. There are in fact societies which regard myth as reality itself, more real than the objective universe. [7:p. 10]

Pierre Grimal, 1965

We were provided with folklore in our early years—stories of fairies and imps, ghosts and devils and mystic meanings in simple things. We accepted them on the authority of our parents, or the even more compelling authority of our older playmates. Throughout life they remain as part of our common culture pattern. Because they were learned early and during our most impressionable years, they have a firm hold and, no matter how unreasonable, are often difficult to shake off. [15:p. vii]

Gerald Wendt, 1979

The Creation of Spirits as Causal Agents

The crown jewel of the human symbolic operation was the self. Once the self was established and differentiated from the rest of the world, the word blocks were set up in a cause-and-effect sequence. Perhaps the biologic processes involved in segmentalizing our experience into blocks resulted in a sequential arrangement of events into a space and time pattern, leading to a type of linear logic. With language, whether an innate biologic structure or a learned phenomenon, we developed the concept of cause and effect. "If I (the self) act in a certain manner, then I will cause certain things to happen." It was only a short step from that idea to believing that if I or my self can cause events to occur, other events are probably caused by other selves.

The ability to organize information in a logical cause-and-effect sequence had enormous advantages. "If I start a fire, then other animals will stay out of my cave. If I set a trap, I will snare animals for food." This linear sequencing of information also allowed curiosity about events not so readily perceived to be voiced logically in a cause-and-effect pattern. "If I have a self and other persons have a self, maybe everything has a self. Just because the self is hidden from me does not mean it is not there. If I can cause things to happen, maybe these hidden selves are causing things to happen."

We began to extrapolate from our experiences and speculate about the interworking of the objects and individuals in our environment. We began to organize information about animals, trees, rocks, mountains, streams, storms, and all other natural phenomena. We began to project our self concepts onto all the events and objects around us. This anthropomorphic conceptual frame made everything like us.

We can speculate that our early ancestors lived in an even more hostile world than we do. They did not have access to the opinions of numbers of others as readily as we do. The population was extremely sparse, and trying to survive was a monumental task. Life expectancy was very short. They attempted to find reasons for the things that were happening to them and to others. They tried to make the world comprehensible.

In their attempt to gain control of a forbidding environment, our forebears began to name the innumerable selves or spirits that they imagined populated their world. In naming a spirit or self, such as that of a volcano, and endowing the mountain spirit with human qualities, there was a chance that they could exert some influence over it, if not completely control it.

It would be easy to call this spirit-naming process a religion or a form of worship, but it was also very pragmatic. Early cultures did not have a heritage of testable theories and sought an explanation for natural phenomena that would allow them to understand their experiences. Anthropomorphism was a way of organizing information about the world and might be called the birth of reason.

Sigmund Freud described our early reasoning very succinctly:

> With the first step, which is the humanization of nature, much is already won. Nothing can be made of impersonal forces and fates; they remain eternally remote. But if the elements have passions that rage like those in our own souls, if death itself is not something spontaneous, but the violent act of an evil Will, if everywhere in nature we have about us beings who resemble those of our own environment, then indeed we can breathe freely, we can feel at home in the face of the supernatural, and we can deal psychically with our frantic anxiety. We are perhaps still defenseless, but no longer helplessly paralyzed; we can at least react; perhaps indeed we are not even defenseless, we can have recourse to the same methods against these violent supermen of the beyond that we make use of in our own community; we can try to exorcise them, to appease them, to bribe them, and so rob them of part of their power by thus influencing them. [6:pp. 25–26]

Our ancestors, in their search for the reasons things happened and for the means by which they happened—the how—took the experience of their senses as the source of their knowledge. They added to this the human penchant for imagination and love of the magical to create a universe inhabited by quixotic spirit selves who possessed all the human qualities as well as superhuman characteristics.

They created legends that explained events on the earth before it was populated by man, legends which have impacted upon our thinking to this day. Allan Scott and Michael Scott Rohan point out that:

> Somewhere in the depths of the oldest memories of our race, a swirling source of dreams and madness, lingers a presence that still touches the borders of the

everyday world: a memory of the secret peoples. In myth and legend, fairytale, and folklore, they live on, sometimes shrunken, sometimes grotesque, yet always with an aura of unique power. And the memory is tinged with ancient wonder—and fear. [10:p. 23]

The secret peoples were gnomes, imps, dwarves, elves, trolls, and other magical beings who could do many wonderful things and who seemed to be closely allied with nature and therefore able to exert control over events not usually influenced by humans. How did these secret peoples originate? They were descendents of the "elementals," creatures who evolved from the basic elements of nature. Air, fire, water, and earth were given names and spirits and then human qualities and even human forms and are probably the oldest of the spirits created by man.

The story goes that the elementals were developing at the same time man was evolving and that when they began to realize that there were other life forms upon earth which could think, they began to try to assume human shape because they were both jealous and afraid of the power of primitive man. As well as being the forefathers of the secret peoples, the elementals are directly related to the beings who would later be thought of and described as gods by the Greeks and Romans as well as by other peoples [10].

Primitive people attributed natural phenomena, such as storms, thunder, winds, and lightning, to the work of the elementals. In order to better understand and shape our world, we created beings or selves out of the elements and attributed to them the qualities we found in ourselves. And, to make them not so fearful and more accessible, we gave them a human form. Legends relate that sometimes the elementals had enormous problems taking on and keeping this human form.

One of the more interesting accounts of our attempts to give human spirit and life to the elements is written as if to tell the story from the point of view of the elementals. It appears as if the elementals shaped themselves, a reflection of our need for a creator. They were reluctantly changing to suit themselves to our world.

> Their first attempts were clumsy in the extreme. The problem was that the elementals regarded flesh—protoplasm—as something too weak and too needlessly complex to suit their requirements. Instead they tried to sculpt themselves bodies out of the elements they were most at home in, or out of things native to those elements. It was not a simple process. The earth elementals had the easiest task, but the rest found that even with the aid of magic a physical body was a devilishly tricky thing to hold together. The giant Ymir, father of the Norse gods and giants, was supposed to have been born out of a mixture made from the mists and ice of Nifheim and the fires of Muspellheim. Legend speaks of his body being torn to pieces by his grandsons, the gods, but it is more likely that he simply fell apart. Later his bones were used to build mountains, so Ymir must have put some earth in the mix, as well as water and fire. [10:p. 40]

We can see from this passage that the elementals were also credited with the creation of the world or that they were used in some way to create the mountains, the oceans, the plains, and the sands. Egyptian, Assyrian, and Greek legends describe elementals as the joint creators of the world [10].

Another aspect of the story of the elementals is that in their attempt to enter our world, they created chaotic conditions because of their battles with each other. The geological changes that occurred upon the earth were attributed to the fierce fighting of armies of elementals [10]. Again, we see beginning attempts to put some order into an otherwise hostile and alien world. If there was an earthquake or a flood, there had to be a reason for it.

Since imagination was vivid and modern scientific checks were not placed upon reason, our ancestors often fancied that they actually saw spirit beings. In the early days of our existence, we were supposed to have had very close communion with the various manifestations of nature. We could talk to the forest animals and we could converse with nymphs and naiads, or so the stories indicate. Although we had differentiated ourselves with the use of linguistic symbols, we yet remained in touch with the world around us. We did not readily distinguish between what was real and what was unreal, letting these categories blur into each other. Our stories about the spirits reflect this inability to differentiate between our imagination and our perceptions. We must have had, however, a feeling of closeness with all of nature, which we have lost in the ensuing years. "The real interest of the myths," says the great mythologist, Edith Hamilton, "is that they lead us back to a time when the world was young and people had a connection with the earth, with trees and seas and flowers and hills, unlike anything we ourselves can feel" [8:p. 13].

At the time that the elementals and the secret peoples were communicating with us, they were very real. And they were also terrifying. We created spirits who exemplified the worst of the anthropomorphic creatures and not the beautiful, often whimsical, beings whom the Greek and Roman poets would immortalize. The spirit creations of primitive people were vengeful and destructive and required considerable skill in appeasement in order to avoid the consequences of their anger. As Hamilton emphasizes, primeval forests were places of horror and not the homes of the lovely nymphs and naiads of Greek and Roman vision. The only defense against the awesome power of the more terrifying spirits was magic. And the magic was often accompanied by human sacrifice. "Mankind's chief hope of escaping the wrath of whatever divinities were then abroad," writes Hamilton, "lay in some magical rite, senseless but powerful, or in some offering made at the cost of pain and grief" [8:p. 14].

In ancient times, we were faced with the difficult task of trying to stay alive without the benefit of modern medical knowledge. We were almost certain to die early and often violently. The selves or spirits we created to help us explain death and put our experiences into a cause-and-effect sequence had to be considered, or their wrath was quick and terrible. We developed rituals and other patterns of behavior that enabled us to make peace with these other selves who were simultaneously human and other than human. Although the spirits exhibited all our more fearful characteristics, such as rage and jealousy, they were also capable of doing wonderful and magical favors for those individuals who pleased them.

Differentiation of Spirits into Polar Opposites

The binary quality of language forced the anthropomorphic spirit creatures to be endowed with qualities that were polar opposites—good and bad, light and dark, loving and hating, friendly and hostile. Since each spirit was human with regard to its characteristics, it was rare to find one that was wholly good or wholly bad. The spirit selves were as unpredictable and quixotic as their human creators. They were also ambivalent, a characteristic that Jeffrey Burton Russell, Professor of Medieval Studies at the University of Notre Dame, attributes to "the unconscious."

> Seldom in myth is anything seen as wholly evil, for myth is very close to the unconscious, and the unconscious is ambivalent. What comes from the unconscious is basically perception of self, and the self is perceived as both good and evil. Only the rational, intellectual conscious separates the natural ambivalence of good and evil into polarities, opposite absolutes. Myth is complex and ambiguous. . . . The struggle between the polar opposites can be expressed in the ambivalence of traditional deities. The great gods of India, such as Kali, Shiva, and Durga, manifest both benevolence and malice, creativity and destructiveness. [9:pp. 56–59]

But, even before the appearance of gods upon our horizon, the elementals also showed evidence of unpredictability. They were capricious and as likely to be harmful as helpful. It was a time of enormous insecurity for primitive people, as is apparent in the numerous rituals and acts of magic they invented to help them deal with these spirit selves.

Some of the elementals were believed to have taken trees or mountains as their forms and as their homes instead of adopting human shape. The tree folk were known as dryads. They were thought of as generally calm and lovely, but were known to become monstrous if threatened. Different varieties of trees were given different qualities. According to the Greeks, the cypress tree could rob you of your intelligence if you slept beneath it. You might even lose all your memories. The holly and the oak trees had the same reputation in England. Some of the Slavic tree spirits, called *Leshy*, are described as having "a face the colour of fungoid wood, a green, mossy beard, and staring green eyes" [10:p. 155]. They were said to play practical jokes on travelers, such as leading them out of their way and then scaring them by appearing suddenly before them [10].

The tree spirits did not really like humans and tried to stay away from them. They liked staying in one place but would move to another glade if too many humans moved in too close. Their two greatest enemies were people and fire. Legend has it that, as the centuries passed, the tree spirits, at least some of them, became more tolerant of people and some were even friendly. Tapio, the Finnish forest divinity, is believed to have been the model for J. R. R. Tolkien's ents in *The Lord of the Rings* [10].

Tolkien, the most gifted modern writer to use an anthropomorphic format, has Merry, one of the Hobbits in his magnificent tale, describing the forest to his friends:

> And the trees do not like strangers. They watch you. They are usually content merely to watch you, as long as daylight lasts, and don't do much. Occasionally

the most unfriendly ones may drop a branch, or stick a root out, or grasp at you with a long trailer. But at night things can be most alarming, or so I am told. I have only once or twice been in here after dark, and then only near the hedge. I thought all the trees were whispering to each other, passing news and plots along in an unintelligible language; and the branches swayed and groped without any wind. They do say the trees do actually move, and can surround strangers and hem them in. [13:pp. 156–157]

Later in the same story, Merry is overpowered and almost swallowed by Old Man Willow, a rather malevolent tree who overpowered those whom he wished and then dragged them into his cracks.

Before artificial lighting, night was extremely frightening. As darkness fell upon the earth, its human inhabitants could not see and were at the mercy of the spirit selves, who were fortunate enough to be able to see in the dark. Knowing that we could not see, the spirits waited until night to snare us. The anonymity the night offered was coupled with the terrors it concealed. Only the boldest, or those who had something to hide, ventured forth after dark.

The shape shifters, who appeared in their most menacing form at night, also exhibited opposite characteristics, generally changing from a benign to a malignant form. These were descendents of the elemental creature, Proteus, a titan who could change swiftly from one form to another. The shape shifters included the vampires and werewolves. The ability to fly and tremendous physical powers were often attributed to the shape shifters. Several theories have been offered as to why they assumed such horrible characteristics. One of these is that the shape shifter was viewed as a primitive example of the results of mental disturbance. The disturbed person chose the monstrous shape that he assumed as a result of a troubled mind. One of the most famous examples is the fictional *Dr. Jekyll and Mr. Hyde*, written by Robert Louis Stevenson, who was supposed to have modeled his story on a recurrent nightmare. "His description of Mr. Hyde," claims Scott and Rohan, "reads like that of a shape-shifter frozen in the moment of his transformation, as if by the last weak remains of an inherited ability boosted, perhaps, by the infamous potion" [10:p. 105]. They go on to point out that a few shape shifters were somewhat attractive and that not all were harmful.

The shape shifters are indicative of the tendency of primitive people to give human form to animals or to allow humans to take on animal form and so acquire the advantages of animals while maintaining the intellectual ability of humans. It is understandable that early people wished to learn the secrets of the animals so that they could hunt them more easily or so that they could gain an advantage over their human peers, who were not so cunning as the animals they hunted or as adaptable to the ways of the mountains and the forests.

The division of male and female was also evident in the spirit selves we created. We can speculate that this differentiation was probably one of the earliest and most basic. When the elementals took on human forms, they made themselves into male and female, just as their human counterparts. This was not always for purposes of reproduction but sometimes just for division of roles.

In the race of dwarves, who were hard workers and who loved to mine and make things which they then hoarded, the women worked at forges. Legend claims that the dwarf wives soon tired of all this drudgery and rebelled against their husbands. After spending time depressed and unable to produce their beloved metals, the males resorted to violence and chained the women back to their forges. It is speculated that the reason no one ever saw a dwarf woman was that they were kept prisoners at their bellows. Eventually, the females decided to put an end to their slavery, and they allowed their bodies to fall apart, resuming their elemental state. Some decided to explode. Whatever their method of obtaining their freedom, the female decision to give up human form caused a lack of interest among the males in the continuation of their work, and the race gradually decreased in number and was generally unheard of after the nineteenth century [10].

It would appear that the females of other secret people were also very elusive. The female troll, for example, was reported to rarely appear above ground. The reason given for this is that she was so ugly she didn't want to come out into the light but wished to remain where she was appreciated. Troll males much preferred the hideous troll female and shied away from human females because they were never ugly enough. "Mortal women are usually far too attractive to interest male trolls—besides, their skin is not leathery enough to give a good grip—but occasionally a human woman almost ugly enough to be desirable may turn up" [10:p. 64]

There are several records of marriages among the races of elementals. The sea god, Njord, married a titan giantess named Skadi. Poseidon married Amphitrite, the daughter of the titan, Oceanus. The marriages also assumed very human characteristics. Skadi supposedly complained constantly about not being able to sleep because of the noise of the sea gulls, and she convinced Njord that he should spend half of his time in the mountains with her. Njord evidently tried to comply but was unable to adapt to the mountains, and the marriage ended. Poseidon is reported to have had many affairs with other titan females. The offspring resulting from one of these affairs is said to have been the race of the cyclopes [10].

Many stories have been handed down through the generations concerning mermaids, but the mermaids were only half of the race of merfolk. Their male counterparts were called tritons. These were very large elementals. A mermaid would average six and one-half feet in length, and a triton would be nine feet tall. Since encounters between sailors and mermaids almost always resulted in disaster for the sailor, sea-faring men tried to avoid even the sight of any of the merfolk. An old ballad relates:

> T'was on Friday morn when we set sail
> And our ship not far from land
> When the captain he espied a lovely mermaid
> With a comb and glass in her hand. . . .
> And up spake the captain of our gallant ship
> And a fearful man was he
> "I have wedded a wife in fair Bristol town
> And tonight she a widow will be." [10:p. 144]

Although many of the female elemental forms were said to be beautiful and alluring, the mythological female was often portrayed as harmful to men. Russell theorizes that when opposites are expressed sexually and split, they are seen as conflicting. The yang, or female, principle, when in contention with the yin, or male, principle has been made to appear evil and inferior.

> Whether this is because men rather than women have made the myths as well as written the theology is unclear. Some efforts have been made to trace male domination over the female to a successful revenge of the male patriarchy after the female gods of agriculture had replaced the male gods of the hunt. The sky god or High God deposes the Great Mother and rules in her place. [9:pp. 61–62]

Russell goes on to explain that male domination of the female is almost worldwide in mythology and theology.

Even in the domain of evil, the female is not allowed the dominant role. The Devil is always thought of as a male figure. However, when it comes to the question of who is going to be punished for the evil, the female is at once granted a more prominent position.

The original division of the spirit selves into male and female forms was a natural one for primitive people to make. If the selves that occupied the streams, hills, trees, rocks, and mountains were going to assume human forms and human characteristics, they must of necessity be both male and female. The issue of reproduction was probably a crucial factor. The elementals and the races that followed them had to have some means of assuring their survival.

Splitting the spirit selves into anthropomorphic sexual opposites also allowed for greater control over such essential activities as hunting and the growing and reaping of plants. If mating of male and female resulted in the birth of other males and females, the creation of and subsequent attention to male and female spirits might ensure their cooperation in promoting the abundant reproduction of the plant and animal life needed for survival.

The marriage of woodland sprites was supposed to guarantee the growth of vegetation. Mock ceremonies between humans representing sprites were celebrated in Europe to quicken the growth of plants and trees [5]. Sir James Frazer, author of *The Golden Bough*, discusses the possibility of such rites occurring today:

> At the present day it might perhaps be vain to look in civilised Europe for customs of this sort observed for the explicit purpose of promoting the growth of vegetation. But ruder races in other parts of the world have consciously employed the intercourse of the sexes as a means to ensure the fruitfulness of the earth; and some rites which are still, or were till lately, kept up in Europe can be reasonably explained only as stunted relics of a similar practice. [5:p. 157]

In such widespread areas of the world as Central America, Australia, New Guinea, Java, and Europe, the human sexual act is believed to have a direct influence upon the growth of crops. Some customs require regular intercourse between husband and wife during the growing season, and others deny any contact between them during the same period of time, indicating a belief in the efficacy of self-denial. Because women are the bearers of the children, a barren female was considered by many to be unlucky and could even be banished from her home lest she prove a malevolent influence upon the vegetation [5].

Magic and Religion

To primitive people, all the elements were mysterious and seemed to be alive, willful, and capricious. The naming of the spirits of the elements, spirits that were also a human invention, allowed us to communicate with them, to address them, and to appeal to them. Some have chosen to regard our early endeavors to commune with nature as a religious activity. However, as was indicated earlier, this also might be considered a very practical means of sequencing events into a cause-and-effect pattern in order to exert control or influence and better explain the experiential world. It is difficult to establish when religious aspirations emerged in our thinking.

Among the fundamental psychological preconditions of religion are (1) some idea of survival after death and (2) some notion of the divine. The Neanderthal, who flourished in the Middle Paleolithic period, did bury some of their dead with artifacts, perhaps pointing to a belief in the hereafter. Primitive people were obsessed with hunting and might have thought that the spirits of the dead would aid them in the hunt or perhaps even reemerge as the spirits of animals that might then cooperate with their hunters. It is impossible to be certain what they believed. We believe that the conditions surrounding our ancestors and their anthropomorphizing of the elements, objects, and animals around them eventually led to conceptual forms we term *religions*. This idea is validated by Pierre Grimal, a professor at the Sorbonne and an expert in world mythology.

> The constant and primitive demands on these prehistoric men resulted in a dependence on perceptions that modern man does not need: thanks to these perceptions the savage lives in a world in which spiritual forces appear to be essential reality, and in this way the spirit becomes more important, almost more real than the physical body. This spirit world, which is peopled and ruled by invisible forces, prepares the mind for religious beliefs. [7:p. 20]

In the early panpsychic world, relationships were diffuse. The spirits were seen as immanent in all things and could be identified with all the forces and workings of nature. People appealed to any and all the spirit selves for help in hunting or protection from the elements or, perhaps, deliverance from disease and death. The dryad, a tree spirit, might be as helpful as the naiad, a water spirit, depending on the occasion or on which particular spirit self was available.

We can also speculate that when we first differentiated and named the early spirit selves, the elementals and the secret peoples, all individuals who desired to do so could speculate about their nature. Anyone was free to attempt communication with the nymphs, water sprites, and dryads.

Because of the elusive quality of the spirit selves, our early life was dominated by magic and the supernatural. This was especially true as the spirit selves came to be thought of as gods or divine personifications who responded to ritual and sacred rites. As we began to formalize our relationship with the spirit world, certain spirits were given divine status. Panpsychism evolved into pantheism and polytheism, and we have the emergence of religion.

We thought of the god selves in the dualistic terms of good and evil, light and dark, the same binary paradigm with which we first created the early elemental spirits. Evil and good spirits were manifestations of good and evil gods. Most of our thinking in ancient times was centered on the evil aspects of the spirit world rather than the good. However, the split between the two was not so definitive at first, as ancient religions were inclined to perceive evil as being part of the divine. They accepted the intermingling of the good and evil principles.

> How can one measure the good without knowing the bad? How can one long for light without knowing the anguish of darkness? In what an unpleasant land of plenty would one live were there no bad. Evil causes suffering and from pain springs the desire for something better; deficiencies cause us to want improvement, evolution and to set up ideals. It can safely be said, as it has often been, that God would cease to exist if there were no devil, or as a French theologian expressed it: "God and the devil are the whole religion." [11:p. 150]

Evil, for the ancient Hebrews, represented by Satan or the Devil, carried with it knowledge but also death. Satan was seen as the great rule breaker, the rules supposedly having been made by God as the principle of good. Social regulations were attributed to God's will. We had only to view our own behaviors to validate our ideas about the existence of good and evil forces both within and without. Earlier religions allowed us to worship both the light and the dark powers, recognizing that they were equal in strength.

Kurt Seligmann, author of *Magic, Supernaturalism, and Religion*, writes:

> In the primitive dualistic world the powers of light and darkness are worshipped alike. The equal strength of both good and evil may have arisen in the mind of man when he observed nature and meditated upon his own life. Man is inhabited by contradictory forces; in his thought and action, good and evil are so intimately mingled that he cannot always distinguish between them. [11:p. 12]

Attempts were later made to reconcile these opposing forces. Zoroaster clearly defined the problem of living in a world populated by good and evil spirits who were the "rulers of a split universe" and foresaw a time when the opposing hosts would be reconciled. The Gnostics were also clear in their belief in the necessity of both good and evil and the synthesis of these two forces.

> Can we mould him (Satan) and his opponent into a synthesis? The Zoroastrians did not achieve this, but they made us believe it possible. Ormazd and Ahriman will be reconciled at the end of time. Side by side, they shall enter the new kingdom as brothers. The Gnostics made it clear that the universe exists only through this everlasting antagonism and, the universe being one, good and evil are united in the divine. [11:p. 151]

The later concern with a reconciliation between the opposing forces of the split universe presupposes a dualistic attitude toward human behavior. Each individual was subject to the influences of demons and angels, and each individual had to attempt a reconciliation within himself, the "me block," of both dark and light forces, which were a product of the "not-me block."

In addition to emphasizing the idea of a split universe of good and evil, the ancients espoused a belief in the existence of demons and angels and in the reality of magic. Although the Hebrews forbade the practice of magic as contrary to the will of Jehovah, they did not deny its power.

The Scriptures speak of magic as something whose existence no one doubts. Here, magic is a reality. The widespread condemnation of the occult does not arise from the suspicion that its magical operations are exploited for deception, but because magic is morally and socially harmful, indulging in what is forbidden and doing violence to divine teaching. . . . The Mosaic religion, like the Christian, opposed magic as an illicit tampering with God's power. But being itself an outgrowth of magic, its rituals contain many elements whose magical origin can hardly be denied. [11:p. 26]

Most of our activities in very early times centered around the sorcery or magic necessary to exist under the conditions imposed by the exceedingly frightening, evil spirit selves. Frazer argues that it was quite natural for primitive people to grasp magic as the means for changing their environment, as they were not attuned to conceptual frameworks that looked beyond the obvious to a mode of thinking that required a more sophisticated approach.

It became probable that magic arose before religion in the evolution of our race, and that man essayed to bend nature to his wishes by the sheer force of spells and enchantments before he strove to coax and mollify a coy, capricious, or irascible deity by the soft insinuation of prayer and sacrifice. . . . The shrewder intelligences must in time have come to perceive that magical ceremonies and incantations did not really effect the results which they were designed to produce, and which the majority of their simpler fellows still believed they did actually produce. [5:pp. 63–65]

Magic was one of the tools we used to ensure order in our communication with these gods. Although we may today interpret magic as a mixture of charms and spells designed to produce supernatural effects, it was used in early religious practice to lend predictability to natural events. The practice of divination, for example, among the Chaldeans, Egyptians, Romans, and Greeks, was a science. Seligmann says:

We find similar "superstitions" among all these peoples, where divination is the logical application of their theory of magic. To the magus, there exists no accidental happening; everything obeys the one law, which is not resented as a coercion but rather welcomed as a liberation from the tyranny of chance. The world and its gods submit to this law, which binds together all things and all events. *Certa stant omnia lege:* everything is established solidly by that law which the wise man discerns in happenings that appear accidental to the profane. The curve observed in the flight of birds, the barking of a dog, the shape of a cloud, are occult manifestations of that omnipotent coordinator, the source of unity and harmony. [11:p. 5]

As more of the spirit selves became personified as gods, it appears that they were no longer as accessible to everyone. Specialists were required, priests who possessed the knowledge necessary for communion with these divine powers. It would seem, then, that with the rise of religious practices, the common people lost their ability to commune with the forces of nature. In Chaldea, for example,

A caste of priests was founded in whom all occult knowledge was concentrated. They were masters in the arts of prescience, predicting the future from the livers and intestines of slaughtered animals, from fire and smoke, and from the brilliancy of precious stones; they foretold events from the murmuring of springs and from the shape of plants. Trees spoke to them, as did serpents, "wisest of all animals". Monstrous births of animals and of men were believed to be portents, and dreams found skilful interpreters. [11:p. 4]

In tracing the history of the emergence of religious practices and beliefs from the more primitive and ancient magical paradigms, we are impressed by the numerous and irrefutable examples that illustrate the magic-to-religion continuum and the implacable hostility priests have shown toward magicians.

The controversy between magic and religion is explained by Frazer to be one of the attitudes and motives of the respective practitioners more than of the subsequent results of their teachings. The magician believes that the world obeys certain natural laws that reveal an order and uniformity, a belief somewhat analogous to that of the scientist. The magician is convinced that as long as he adheres to certain rules and rituals, he will always obtain the results he wishes unless some other sorcerer intervenes. He does not evince any belief in a higher power to which he must submit. The priest is convinced that there is a higher power than man and that he can find ways to please or propitiate his gods or god [5].

This radical conflict of principle between magic and religion sufficiently explains the relentless hostility with which in history the priest has often pursued the magician. The haughty self-sufficiency of the magician, his arrogant demeanour towards the higher powers, and his unabashed claim to exercise a sway like theirs could not but revolt the priest, to whom, with his awful sense of the divine majesty, and his humble prostration in presence of it, such claims and such a demeanor must have appeared an impious and blasphemous usurpation of perogatives that belong to God alone. [5:p. 60]

There might also have been an element of jealousy and competition between the opposing parties. The priest claimed to be a mediator between God and man and the only acceptable means to achieve some degree of peace of mind, and the magician made promises of similar results without having to resort to pleasing the gods. Whether labeling themselves magicians or priests, these individuals maintained that they were able to translate the sacred languages and to influence events accordingly.

When the shaman first emerges in the historic period he appears as the guardian of the sacred temple and the mediator between men and gods. It was his duty in the early morning to break the clay seal which protected the sacred room wherein the god was housed and to attend the deity with the necessary ritual— washing, anointing and filling the chamber with the perfume of incense. He greeted the worshipers, led them in chanting hymns, in bowing in adoration and in making sacrifices and libations; he alone interpreted the sacred books and spoke for the divinity. . . . He alone could mediate between men and gods because he alone knew the histories and the wishes of the supernal beings. [12:pp. 22–23]

Much of the power of the shaman lay in his ability to deal with the demons that plagued mankind. These demons were thought to actually invade the body of an individual, taking up residence inside the person. This belief, as we shall see in Chapter 3, carried over to the Christian world, where for centuries one of the functions of the priest has been to exorcise demons.

Scott and Rohan suggest that the secret peoples who had been so much a part of early mankind were turned into demons by the medieval church, which tended to label everything not human a demon. "The classic image of a demon . . . was created out of dim memories of trolls and semi-humans of an earlier age" [10:p. 191].

Zoroaster is credited with being the first magician, and many of the doctrines of Zoroastrianism are contained in the Christian doctrine, especially in their beliefs concerning demons and angels and the magic required to exorcise these entities. Although the theological tenets of Zoroastrianism can be labeled religious, the rites concerning exorcism are definitely magical. The followers of Zoroaster had elaborate beliefs and instructions concerning human hair and nails, which are contained in the collection of books called the *Venidad*, along with numerous other examples of antidemoniac folk wisdom [11].

Wizards used nails and hair for conjuring up the dead. Claudia de Lys explains that the belief that hair and nails have a separate existence and individual lives of their own stems from the fact that, after death, the body tissues shrink away, giving the illusion that the hair and nails have continued to grow. The magic surrounding hair and nails made them very powerful instruments, for it was believed that a person could be bewitched through the possession by one or the other of these specific parts of the body [4]. This is a direct result of the view that any objects that have once been conjoined continue to have an influence upon one another even after they are separated.

We have utilized the example of hair and nails because it seems to be a universal consideration, even among very primitive tribes. Seligmann reports that hair and nail superstitions are still prevalent, as demonstrated by the Turks and the Chilean gauchos, who hide their hair in walls, the Armenians, who conceal it in hollow trees, churches, and columns, and French peasants from the Vosges Mountains, who mark the spots where they bury their hair so that they may recover it on the day of resurrection [11].

> Christianity, like Zoroastrianism, correlated hair and hell. Pious Jews think similarly about nails, a belief which causes them to pare them as short as possible. They profess that nails are abodes of evil, and that they are the only part of the body incapable of serving God. [11:p. 18]

Seligmann explains further that the terrible superstitions surrounding hair are evidenced in the treatment of witches, for it was thought that witches could cast spells through the use of hair.

> Before going to the torture chamber, suspected witches had all their hair shorn, a practice which made many a witch confess before the torture was applied. The French legal authority Jean Bodin (1530–96) records such an instance. In 1485 forty witches in northern Italy simultaneously confessed their crimes, after having undergone this procedure. [11:p. 18]

The Zoroastrian cleansing rituals that were used to cast out the fly demon are analogous to the Catholic rites of exorcism performed upon persons possessed by demons.

In A.D. 1582 Jerome Mengo published his *Whip for the Demons*, which deals with this difficult matter (exorcism). . . . At the end of the exorcism the patient is bathed in a mixture of holy water and other liquids so as to cleanse him of some malignancy against which no remedy has been foreseen, some spell which may lie hidden in the hair of the enchanted. [11:p. 20]

It is probable that most of the magicians, sorcerers, and priests were aware of their charisma and their ability to control their trusting followers while remaining cognizant of the flimsy foundations upon which their methods rested. These were the politicians who saw a way to control the masses through playing on their superstitious natures. The evidence of superstition, which began very early and has remained in vogue, can be found in the history of astrology, which we will discuss further in the next chapter.

The Sumerian and subsequently the Babylonian and Assyrian priests were the forefathers of the pattern of thought we today call *astrology*. They observed the stars and the movements of the planets and claimed that their knowledge of the planet gods aided them in predicting what would happen on earth. The interpreter gods, of which there were seven, were lead by Jupiter-Marduk, the creator. The others included the moon, or Sin, who governed growth; the sun, or Šamaš who was responsible for life and light but could also bring drought; Mercury, or Nabû, who was the god of wisdom; Saturn, or Adad, who officiated over hunting; Mars, or Nergal, who was an evil god responsible for war, pestilence, and death; and, finally, Venus, or Inanna (Ishtar), who was the beneficent goddess of love and motherhood [11].

Even in the planet gods one could see both evil and good, except for Nergal, who seemed to be wholly evil. Beneficent Ishtar could prove harmful to sucklings and widows. Nebo, the god of wisdom, could exert harmful influences, because all knowledge has both its good and evil components [11].

The signs of the zodiac had their beginnings in Sumeria, also, and the relationships of the star configurations to the planet gods were used to predict earthly happenings and to determine various courses of action [11].

The priests were evidently quite jealous of the secret knowledge they possessed and were determined that the symbols, allegories, and language they used remained mysteries to the uninitiated.

These enigmatic images were expressed in the old tongue of Akkad or Sumer, the "language of the gods", in which only the initiate conversed. The cosmic secrets were hidden from the people, because of the fear that knowledge of the future might either discourage them or cause them to abandon their daily work from joy. Those who had knowledge of the stars were more influential than king's ministers, and foreign rulers consulted them frequently. [11:p. 6]

With the evolution of these formal religious rituals and the appearance of a special class of interpreters, the priests, our lives became even more complicated. We entered a world of morals and rules where our behavior was the ultimate criterion for determining our relationship to the universe. We were judged to be in or out of harmony with the gods, depending upon our conduct as judged by the religious ruling class.

Good, evil, life, death, pain, pleasure, and other dualistic, self-orienting conceptual frames allowed increased self-reflection and anticipation of future events, the ultimate of which was the death of the individual. Death itself was preceded by pain, fear, and loneliness. All that composed the not-me block of the world took on the aspect of a god or gods. The unknown was personified as a god or gods. The gods created and destroyed; therefore, the gods had power. If we pleased the gods, that is, did what they expected or wanted, perhaps the deities in return would protect us from fear, loneliness, and death, which seemed inevitable.

We became responsible for the happiness of our gods. Elaborate rituals evolved to placate and please. We were now at the mercy of rules, regulations, laws, sacrifices, rituals, dogma, and liturgy to ensure a good life here and/or, perhaps, a good life after death. Our budding awareness of our own finiteness, coupled with our tendency to anthropomorphize, resulted in the emergence of religious beliefs and practices as attempts to put naturally occurring phenomena in a cause-and-effect sequence.

These ancient religious paradigms were the working formats for the individuals who created them. They constituted our interpretation of reality and gave us the rules by which we lived.

In trying to build our world of rules in a cause-and-effect sequence using word blocks, we used our powers of observation to determine those facts that governed our behavior. Through intermittent reinforcement we were conditioned to validate certain phenomena. If, only occasionally, the recitation of a magical formula resulted in the desired happening, that was enough to convince us of its accuracy. If appealing to the wind god to cleanse the air of disease was followed by fewer people becoming ill, this cause-and-effect sequence validated our belief that the wind god was responsible and that careful recitation of an appeal to that divinity was effective.

All cultures throughout the world began to develop myths and religious practices that governed the lives of the people and directed their thoughts toward a self-orienting world of words.

> Sumerian myth conforms to the patterns set by mythological archetypes throughout the world, both in civilisations contemporary with that of Sumer (or, at least, of ancient date), and equally in so-called primitive cultures of modern times. Thus Sumer had cosmological myths and myths of origin, which, like myths everywhere, are in this case both a reflection on the cosmos they are meant to explain, and at the same time a justification of the particular type of society from which they proceed. . . . The primitive or traditional societies of our own time in which myth is still current as a statement of sacred realities merely produce myths that, when all is said and done, are the end-product of an evolution of several thousands of years. [7:p. 56]

The written records of Sumerian beliefs and practices are not complete, and some of the writing seems obscure because we do not have all the pieces for full interpretation, but we have enough data to make several observations. For the Sumerians,

> Spirits lurked everywhere. Larvae and lemures lived beneath the earth; vampires escaped from the dead to attack the living; Namtar (pestilence) and Idpa (fever) plagued the cities. Night was ruled by the demons of evil, of the desert, of the abyss, of the sea, of the mountains, of the swamp, of the south wind. There were the succubi and the incubi, carriers of obscene nightmares; the snare-setting Maskim; the evil Utuq, dweller of the desert; the bull demon Telal; and Alal the destroyer. [11:p. 1]

The Sumerians, concomitant with their belief in the various demons sent by evil gods, believed that *within* us could also exist the evil powers of the demons. The sorcerers did not have to obey religious commandments and laws but could cast spells or, with the possession of an evil eye, could slay their victims by looking at them. An individual could fall under the spell of a sorcerer and be overcome by a demon spirit.

> The imprecation acts upon man like an evil demon. The screaming voice is upon him. The maleficent voice is upon him. The malicious imprecation is the cause of his disease. The maleficent imprecation strangles this man as if he were a lamb. The god in his body made the wound, the goddess gives him anxiety. The screaming voice, like that of the hyena, has overcome him and masters him. [11:p. 2]

It is important to note that the sorcerer's incantations had to be spoken exactly or they were ineffective. The demons would not obey unless the verbal formulas were followed explicitly. By the time the Sumerian legends were recorded, we were so dependent on words as a way of formulating the world that those anthropomorphic creatures we called gods were impotent to interact in natural events without their having the proper words.

A Reverence for Words

The Sumerians implied that nothing existed before its name was formulated. They created special gods, called *functional gods*, who were responsible for the naming of objects so they could exist. This implies that the words must exist before the entities can exist. A thing was without form or function until it was named. To pronounce the name of a thing was equivalent to creating it.
Ancient Sumerian records relate:

> Because the name of Ashnan (the grain-goddess) had not been born, had not been fashioned, because Uttu (the goddess of clothing) had not been fashioned, there was no ewe, no lamb.
> Because the names of Ashnan and Lahar (the cattle-god) . . . were not known, grain did not exist. [7:p. 62]

Seligmann states that naming was also of maximum importance in Egypt.

> Nothing could come into being before its name had been uttered. Not before the mind had projected its idea upon the outside world would a thing have true existence. "The word," the hieroglyphics tell us, "creates all things: everything that we love and hate, the totality of being. Nothing *is* before it has been uttered in a clear voice." [11:p. 39] [italics added]

The Egyptians went even further in their dependence upon naming and the emphasis of its importance by giving two names to every individual. Only the so-called lesser name was known to others. The individual's greater name was kept secret, as it carried with it all the magical qualities of that person [9].
The Egyptian influence upon the ancient Hebrews is seen in the Hebrew obsession with the name of their god, which was endowed with supreme magical powers superior to those of any other existing entity.

The Egyptian belief in the magic power of a god's secret name, so well exemplified in the legend of Ra and Isis, had probably inspired the Israelites with that people's excessive reverence of the name of Yahweh, an epithet which was never to be pronounced except by a holy priest. The force of this tradition on the Judaic side, combined with the reverence still accorded sacred names in Alexandria and in all the Roman temples of Isis and Serapis, enabled the Pauline doctrine to propound that when Jesus was risen from the dead and made to sit on the right hand of God, God exalted him highly, and gave unto him a name which is above every name: that at the name of Jesus every knee shall bow, of things in heaven and things in earth, and things under the earth.' This meant angels and devils and demons of every sort, and the "name" in question was Christ, which exalted its owner to the summit and sovereignty of all the angelic and demonic creations. [12:pp. 199–200]

The value placed upon language is obvious. Nothing could be given life unless it was differentiated and named. To know its name might even allow control of that entity or individual. The magic incantations or formulas that accompanied the rituals utilized in worshipping the gods were imbued with tremendous powers. The word world was supreme. We were growing increasingly more dependent on our word blocks. People began to equate words with events and at times placed more value on the word for the event than on the actual experience of the event. This was particularly true when a revered person, such as a shaman or sorcerer, expressed an experience in words. His devotees attempted to synchronize their experiences into the same words. We began to trust our words as much as our experiences and to revere the word system.

Curses and blessings originated from the practice of priests and shamen of articulating names when conversing with the spirits, names that were automatically coupled with magical messages. The name or uttered word was much more than a sound. It represented a system of beliefs concerning the relationship of name, supernatural power, and subsequent event.

People developed a fear of calling out a dead person's name because the utterance itself might disturb the ghost or spirit. This applied to all deceased, but if the deceased were known to have been evil there was the additional liability that the awakened evil spirit would actually hurt someone. The current expressions "Bless his soul" and "May he rest in peace" are directly related to these early beliefs [4].

Onomancy, the practice of divination by the letters of one's name, was a respected tool utilized by magicians.

Names were very important to the Pythagoreans who taught that the minds, actions and successes of men were dependent upon their fate, genius and names. Plato himself inclined to the same opinion. It was Pythagoras who popularized the superstitious idea that blindness, lameness and similar misfortunes would fall upon a man's right or left side according to the odd or even numbers in his name. An ancient rule in divination by names was that the one in whose name the letters added up to the highest sum would be the happiest and most fortunate. [4:p. 429]

Many religious rites centered around the use of names. Some early magicians specialized in psychomancy, or sciomancy, which is described as the art of calling up or raising the souls of the dead to predict events in the future.

This form of magic is analogous to the seances regularly performed by many persons in the world today.

The sound of a word often carried magic properties, especially potent when spoken by the right person at the right time and in the correct manner. Some individuals refused to expose themselves to knowledge of magic formulas in the fear that they might use them incorrectly and have to suffer very dire consequences. In societies that allowed the inheritance of the priesthood, once in a while the favored son would declare himself uninterested in accepting the mantle, so tremendous a responsibility accompanied this legacy.

Just as words were powerful for us, they were even more important to the gods. Words were, in fact, considered synonomous with the ultimate. For the Cabalists, as described by Seligmann,

> The material form of intelligence, represented by the twenty-two letters of the alphabet, is also the form of all that exists; for, outside man, time and the universe, only the infinite is conceivable. . . . As in Genesis, the beginning of the world is His Word; and similarly to the Gospel of St. John, the Word became flesh. But to the Cabalist the Word is not *with* God, but *is* God, or a part of the threefold Jehovah. . . . The Cabalists attribute still greater power to the Word. To them, words are the principles and laws which we distinguish in the universe. In the Word they discover the invariable signs of thought which repeat themselves in every sphere of existence, and by which all that exists can be reduced to one plan. [11:p. 243]

Sir Francis Bacon was impressed with the power of words and is reported to have said:

> We must consider that it has great force; all miracles at the beginning of the world were made by the word. And the peculiar work of the rational soul is the word, in which the soul rejoices. Words have a great virtue when they are pronounced with concentration and deep desire, with the right intention and confidence. For when these four things are joined together, the substance of the rational soul is moved more quickly to act according to its virtue and essence, upon itself and upon exterior things. [11:pp. 148–149]

Here, in the words of Bacon, we see clearly expressed the belief that the speaker must be a prepared and qualified individual who is cognizant of the conditions necessary for the proper use of the language. The implication is that the words themselves carry the force, that they are intrinsically powerful.

The ancient Egyptians equated the power of Thoth with his knowledge of language, letters, and numbers.

> He was the god who knew all the right "words of power," the prayers, the ceremonies, the formulas for all occasions, using them in the "correct voice" and with the proper gestures. He even knew the secret names of the deities and hence could command the supreme beings to his will. In power as a sorcerer he was exceeded by none, and rivaled only by the clever Isis, who had come into her command of magic by stealing the "secret name" of Ra. [12:p. 20]

The written word was also sacred and its form was significant. Different civilizations revered selected linguistic forms as "the language of the gods."

Mohammed composed the Koran in verse, the rhythmic prose called *sadj*. This he had done for a weighty reason, for the Arabic seers had always offered their oracles in the *sadj*, and the people would not have accepted Mohammed's laws had they not been written in the language of the gods. [11:p. 132]

Smith, in discussing the development of Egyptian hieroglyphics, says:

The scribes by whose genius the art was transmitted and perfected were no doubt deemed to possess a superhuman talent, and to the end of their history the inhabitants of the Nile Valley never abandoned the conviction that written symbols possessed unlimited magic power, that an amulet or a slab of stone could move all things in earth or heaven to a chosen end. [12:p. 17]

A rune is a magical form of writing, which is often seen in conjunction with magical signs, such as the cross and the swastika. The runic stones of Sweden were supposed to be endowed with magical powers and were sacred to Odin. Odin was the patron of poets and seers. Many runic stones have been found in the Scandinavian countries and in Germany. Many Germans believed, even before Hitler adopted a reversed swastika as a political emblem, that the swastika had magical properties and associated it with runic inscriptions [7].
Of Odin, the god who knew about all the runic signs, it is written:

Odin knew where all treasures were hidden. He knew the songs that opened up the earth, mountains, rocks, funerary mounds, and he could banish all that dwelt therein by the mere use of formulas; then he would enter and take what he wished. [7:p. 370]

As we became more differentiated from nature and more aware of self, we also became increasingly obsessed about death, the ultimate threat to self. Many of the rules of conduct we invented, especially those concerning the spirit selves or gods, were directed toward self-preservation. All animals have built-in programs to avoid injury, but we were able to go beyond this immediate response to threat and to anticipate our own deaths. Cause-and-effect reasoning was never more poignant than is evidenced by our ancestors' attention to death and all the rituals surrounding burial. We assume that they must have believed in an afterlife because they went to elaborate measures to ensure that the deceased persons had the items necessary for life buried with them. Or perhaps they reasoned: "If I bury enough articles with the body, then it will be able to survive somewhere else. If it survives after death, then my 'self' will also survive after death."
All cultures have been concerned with the question of death. Perhaps it did not start out as concern about death, for previous concepts of death might have been completely different from present ones. Prehistoric people may have assumed that the state of death was simply a state of sleep. Perhaps the food buried with the body was put there so that the spirit of the one asleep could benefit by continued communication with the plant and animal spirits [16]. It is likely that deceased individuals sometimes appeared in dreams of others and were, therefore, assumed to be still alive in some shadowy spirit realm not immediately visible but nonetheless very real.

Perhaps as early as 100,000 to 50,000 years ago, and certainly as early as 40,000 to 25,000 B.C., Neanderthal people associated with the Mousterian tool industry buried their dead with food. Later, during the same age, artifacts were also buried with the body. The early Sumerians did not believe in resurrection and did not erect elaborate tombs or mummify their dead. In Egyptian civilization during the period of the Old Kingdom (2750–2270 B.C.), it was believed that only the Pharaoh was ensured of immortality. This was changed during the time of the Middle Kingdom (2160–1788 B.C.), when other people were also granted an opportunity for immortality. The priest sold magical formulas and prayers from the *Book of the Dead*, which, if recited accurately, might please the gods enough to allow the reciter life after death. That accuracy was of prime concern is evident from the following quotation:

> The priests filled papyrus scrolls with magical formulas enabling the deceased to withstand his judges in the world beyond. The *Book of the Dead* told precisely what the soul would encounter during its journey into the shadowy kingdom, and how the deceased might plead his cause. . . . The answers to the examiners' questions were transcribed word for word, and knowing them was sufficient to obtain a favourable verdict. . . . These answers, uttered with the correct intonation and in the prescribed phraseology, would pass for truth. [11:p. 35]

The early Egyptian description of the self is an excellent example of our growing obsession with our differentiated state not only in this life but in the life to come. The individual consisted of seven separate parts that were quite distinct in their functions. They included the body, *khat;* a name, *ren;* a shadow, *khaibut;* a heart, *ab;* a primordial life spirit, *aakhu;* a ghost, image, spirit, or personality, *ka;* and a spectral, reassembled, resurrected person, *ba.* The spirit was born with the individual, stayed with that individual for a lifetime, and preceded the body into the tomb. The resurrected person began to exist only at or after death, when all the other parts rejoined the body. The various functions and activities of the spirit help explain the practice of supplying the deceased with provisions [12].

> The *ka*, or double, continued after death to perform all the functions of human life, sharing the same joys and sorrows as the living, delighting in the same amusements, requiring the same nourishment, suffering the same risks, even that of death. It continued to exist rather from an instinctive horror of annihilation than from any joy of life. At night hunger, thirst, loneliness and misery might drive it from the tomb to prowl about fields and villages, greedily devouring whatever food might have been discarded. It did not permit its family to forget it, but entered their houses and their bodies, struck them with disease or madness and, if ravenous, even sucked their blood. The only effectual means of preventing these visitations was for the living to keep the *ka* well supplied with provisions in the tomb. [12:pp. 24–25]

It is apparent from this description that the spirit was considered capable of causing such catastrophes as sickness and insanity if not properly appeased. These ghosts, which went abroad at night, must have been a tremendous source of fear for the living. However, they also allowed an explanation for natural phenomena that was otherwise lacking. A seizure was the work of a ghost who was powerful enough to invade the living. The dead exerted enormous power, and their ghosts were terrifying. Numerous were the incantations that had to be recited to ward off their evil influence, for the prevailing belief was that the magic of the word could be combatted only with more powerful or more magical words.

The *Book of the Dead* was the source of all knowledge concerning treatment of the deceased. It contained all the necessary magic spells and formulas to assist the deceased on this trip to the underworld and to revitalize his or her mummy. Among the many spells to help a person on the journey were those designed to protect the resurrected individual against decapitation, keep him from dying again, and help him to walk upright rather than upside down, all reflective anthropomorphic ideas about death and its consequences.

> If the *ba* followed the prescriptions of the *Book of the Dead* to the letter, he reached his goal without fail. On leaving the tomb he turned his back on the valley and, magic staff in hand, climbed over the hills which bounded it on the west and plunged boldly into the desert, then across the land of the sacred sycamores and a terrible country infested with many dangers, until step by step he ascended the mountains which surround the world and came to a great river across which he was carried by a ferryman. On the further shore he was met by the gods and goddesses of the court of Osiris, who acted as a guard of honor to convey him into the Judgment Hall. [12:pp. 41–42]

Greek Gods Made in Man's Image

The utilization of an anthropomorphic paradigm in the creation of myths and stories about the world reached a zenith in Greek thought. Unlike the Egyptian gods, who often resembled animals, the Greek gods were made in man's image. The Greek gods were glorified human beings who were not expected to control the lives of their creators or to perform miracles. They were approachable and they could be reasoned with, laughed at, and perceived much the same as peers. Greek poets fashioned a literary world around their gods. They had legends of origin, biographies, and family histories. They were born and sometimes died, fell in and out of love, married, fought wars, argued with each other, took revenge, held grudges, and in general, behaved very humanly. Because they were so human, they did not command the fear and terror surrounding many of the Mesopotamian gods [7,8]. Hamilton emphasizes the familiar atmosphere of the Greek heaven:

> Human gods naturally made heaven a pleasantly familiar place. The Greeks felt at home in it. They knew just what the divine inhabitants did there, what they ate and drank and where they banqueted and how they amused themselves. Of course, they were to be feared; they were very powerful and very dangerous when angry. Still, with proper care a man could be quite fairly at ease with them. He was even perfectly free to laugh at them. Zeus, trying to hide his love affairs from his wife and invariably shown up, was a capital figure of fun. The Greeks enjoyed him all the better for it. Hera was that stock character of comedy, the typical jealous wife, and her ingenious tricks to discomfit her husband, punish her rival, far from displeasing the Greeks,

entertained them as much as Hera's modern counterpart does us today. Such stories made for a friendly feeling. Laughter in the presence of an Egyptian sphinx or an Assyrian bird-beast was inconceivable; but it was perfectly natural in Olympus; and it made the gods companionable. [8:pp. 16–17]

The Greek world was also populated by river gods and by numerous nymphs who lived in trees and streams. The river gods could change shape, and nymphs were perceived as loving and having children and behaving very much as mortals. Everything in nature had its spirit, but these spirits were viewed quite differently from the way the early civilizations of the Near East viewed the spirit selves they created.

No desert was too terrible to have spirits, and their whims were loved and feared. All were active in their own field, conceived passions like those of men, loved and suffered although they were immortal. There were deities of this kind not only in the world of nature, but also in cities, where they presided over public and family life. They were often referred to vaguely as *daemones*—a word made infamous by the Christian religion, but it originally conveyed overtones of respect and often of affection. [7:p. 111]

According to Hamilton, Greek myth was relatively free of the terrors of magic and sorcery. The great Greek myths were integrated with their religious beliefs to explain natural phenomena. Writes Hamilton:

It [myth] is an explanation of something in nature; how, for instance, any and everything in the universe came into existence: men, animals, this or that tree or flower, the sun, the moon, the stars, storms, eruptions, earthquakes, all that is and all that happens. Thunder and lightning are caused when Zeus hurls his thunderbolt. A volcano erupts because a terrible creature is imprisoned in the mountain and every now and then struggles to get free. [8:p. 19]

The entire Greek universe was divided among their twelve major gods, who were each given dominion over his or her particular sphere. Zeus was the supreme god who held more power than all the others combined. He was lord of the sky, the rain, and the clouds and possessed the thunderbolt as his weapon. Hera was Zeus's wife and sister and was the protector of marriage and married women. They were the divine couple whose marriage proved to be as human as any marriage of mortals [8].

Poseidon was the god of the sea and was second only to Zeus, his brother. Hades, the third brother, ruled over the underworld and the dead. Pallas Athena, who was the daughter of Zeus only, having sprung in full armor and full grown from his head, was the goddess who first tamed horses and invented the bridle. She was the protector of agriculture, handicrafts, and civilized life, the goddess of the city [8].

Phoebus Apollo and Artemis were brother and sister, the twin son and daughter of Zeus and Leto. Apollo was a master musician, a very beautiful god who was lord of the silver bow and of archery. He was also known as the healer. In addition, he was named the god of light and the god of truth. It was stated that there was no darkness in him and that he had never uttered a false word. Artemis was the hunter-in-chief to the gods, the lady of wild things, and the protector of youth. She is also identified with Hecate, the goddess of the dark of the moon. She personified most clearly the evil and the good seen in all the divinities [8].

Aphrodite was an alluring and irresistible goddess of love and beauty who was known for her laughter and winning ways. She was said to have sprung from the foam of the sea. Hermes was Zeus's messenger and was thought to be the most cunning of the gods. He was also a master thief, the protector of traders, and god of commerce and the market. In addition, he was the divinity who guided the dead to their last home. Ares was the god of war and the most hated and ruthless of the gods. Hephaestus, also known as Vulcan and Mulciber, was the god of fire and the only one of the gods who was ugly and lame. Yet, he was an extremely popular god and was considered to be kind and peace loving. Hestia was Zeus's sister, the goddess of the hearth, the symbol of the home [8].

Although most scholars agree that the ancient Greeks were not as superstitious as perhaps were other early cultures, such as the Egyptians and Assyrians, they do note the Greek interest in prophesy. The common people believed that the philosophers, such as Socrates, were magicians who knew the future. The psychic power of Socrates is noted by Xenophon, Plutarch, and Apuleius. Philosophy, magical practices, clairvoyance, and religion were all intertwined.

In their quest for answers concerning the future, individuals and statesmen consulted oracles, the most noted of which was the one at Delphi, where the female oracle would go into states of religious ecstasy believed by the observers to be divinely inspired. All government business was conducted with the help of oracles and omens. No event was too insignificant to be considered an omen.

The art of necromancy was also practiced. Those who conjured up the deceased were called psychogogues. Belief in apparitions, ghosts, and specters was also widespread. Among those who professed a belief in these phenomena were Thales, Plato, and Democritus. Demons, as well as ghosts, occupied the thinking of the ancient Greeks. The later Greek philosophers were practitioners of demonology and devised elaborate ceremonies to repel the innumerable demons they believed populated their world.

Dreams were viewed as a source of premonitions and divine revelations. Medical science was also heavily invested in dream analysis, and records of dreams, their interpretations, and the resultant cures were recorded either by writing them down or carving them on temple walls. It would appear that the physicians of that time practiced what would later be the province of psychiatry.

> The importance of dreams is reflected in the stress placed upon their correct interpretation. . . . Many dreams, say Artemidorus, represent a simple and direct image of the event which they foretell. Others show symbols whose meaning must be ascertained. The interpreter should know every detail of the dream which he wishes to explore; if the beginning is confused, he should start his interpretation at the end and reascend to the source. Moreover, he should know the dreamer's state of mind, his social standing and his state of health. It is important to know whether the dreamer is a master or a slave, a rich man or a pauper, an old man or a youth. They may have similar dreams which should, however, be interpreted in various ways. [11:p. 50]

The Gods of Rome

The ancient Romans also worshipped many spirit selves and thought that spirits were everywhere and in everything. The lares were the spirits of the fields and the land and the penates were the spirits of the household stores and food. They also adopted many of the Greek gods, making the Roman pantheon as anthropomorphic as the Greek pantheon. There were gods of the sea, gods of the earth, and gods of the underworld. The flower and fruit goddesses were known as Florae. There were also nymphs, satyrs, and sirens. Nine famous goddesses were the muses, who were patrons of the fine arts and protectors of all artists and performers. Some of the names of the Roman gods are more familiar to us than their Greek counterparts. They include Jupiter, Juno, Neptune, Pluto, Minerva, Diana, Venus, Mercury, and Mars.

Rome also had a state religion, and religious ceremonies were an important part of the political arena. Astute politicians were aware of the importance of religion to the management of the state. Polybius in his *Histories VI*, written around 125 B.C., stated:

> The quality in which the Roman commonwealth is most distinctly superior is in my opinion the nature of their religious convictions. I believe that what maintains the cohesion of the Roman state is the very thing which among other peoples is an object of reproach: I mean superstition. . . . Since every multitude is fickle, full of lawless desires, unreasoned passion, and violent anger, the multitude must be held in by invisible terrors and suchlike pageantry. For this reason I think not that the ancients acted rashly and at haphazard in introducing among the people notions concerning the gods and beliefs in the terrors of hell, but that the moderns are most rash and foolish in banishing such beliefs. [3:p. 111]

The early Roman religious practices were based on numerous superstitions, and the rulers of Rome realized that religious festivals consolidated the state so the superstitions were encouraged. The religious rites and official events allowed the common people to be aware of their past and take pride in their government as blessed by the gods. The Romans were very practical people, and the Roman emperors used the beliefs of the people in magic and in various gods as ways to ensure their jurisdiction.

The avowed concern of the emperors that magic was antithetical to the best interests of the people was, in fact, an attempt to keep the magicians and their secrets for state use only. The Roman emperors officially opposed the practice of magic and issued decrees against it, although they practiced it regularly. The citizens were forbidden to have access to information that might affect the state, or particularly its rulers.

Nero, who was publicly contemptuous of magic, consulted magicians regularly and, upon the advice of an astrologer, had many of his subjects slain. Tiberius had his own astrologer, Thrasyllus, and yet banished from the empire during his reign all other magicians and astrologers.

The magic that the rulers opposed was private magic, not the public magic or religious rites regularly practiced by priests. Haruspicy, the interrogation of the entrails before making state decisions, was abolished by Tiberius but had been required until that time. The priests were thought to be able to predict the future through other practices, including the interpretation of many natural events, such as lightning, storms, and the flights of birds. Since the priests were an integral part of the official state religion, the magic they practiced helped to unify the populace in their endorsement of the power of the Caesars [11].

The Roman rulers were acutely aware of the power of religion, and strict laws governed the practice of any faith. The paranoia of the emperors concerning religion was somewhat justified, as any cult could become dangerous if its adherents preached rebellion against the government. Rome served as a kind of religious melting pot, since the Roman tentacles pulled worshippers from many faiths into the city. The newcomers brought with them more intellectually stimulating and interesting gods than the ones Rome had included in its pantheon.

The Roman rulers were especially concerned about the introduction of more appealing gods because Romans, beginning with Julius Caesar, had begun the practice of making gods out of their emperors. This was not a foreign idea to the Greeks, but the Romans adopted it rather reluctantly. Perhaps Cleopatra, the hereditary goddess, inspired Julius Caesar to attempt the attainment of divine status. He did adopt the throne and ivory scepter, he allowed his image to be carried with the images of the traditional gods, and he had a statue of himself set up in a temple with the inscription "To the Unconquerable God." There were also priests appointed for his godhead. Subsequent Caesars also proclaimed themselves divine and joined the ranks of the gods. Therefore, bowing the knee to Caesar was tantamount to kneeling before a god [14].

The three great religious movements that swept into Rome—the cult of Isis, Mithraism, and Christianity—were of considerable threat to the Caesar gods. The new mystery cults, as all three were termed, entered the Roman Empire at a time when the common people were miserable and cared little for the empire. The population was decreasing because the people refused to have children. They showed tremendous apathy toward the oppressive government and lived under its strict laws in appalling conditions of poverty. Gradually, the Roman masses became disenchanted with their gods.

One of the first Asian goddesses to make an official appearance was Cybele, the Great Mother. Rome was ordered by the Sibylline oracle to welcome Cybele if the people wished deliverance from Hannibal. Even then, her worship was under the direction of a commission. The people were not allowed to take part in the more exotic rituals.

The three mystery cults, so called because they involved elaborate rituals, including the burning of candles before altars, were especially appealing to the masses because they promised immortality. The people were eager to believe in an afterlife that would be far better than what they were enduring in the present life. The earlier Roman gods had not offered immortality to the common people.

Of the three mystery cults, Christianity was to prove the most influential and the most feared by the Roman rulers. Although the Christian religion was similar to the cult of Isis and to Mithraism in its belief in life after death, it was different in that it demanded loyalty and claimed that it was the *only* true religion. It was dedicated to the worship of one god, a divinity who did not permit worship of the Caesars. Exclusive devotion to Christ was a requirement that took precedence over obedience to the state. This religion, with its requirements of loyalty and devotion to Christ, was to become a power in the Western world that would permeate every aspect of Western thought.

References

1. Barraclough, G (Ed): *The Times Atlas of World History*. Maplewood, New Jersey: Hammond, 1978
2. Bernstein, P, and Green, R: *History of Civilization, Volume I: To 1648*. Totowa, New Jersey: Littlefield, Adams, 1963
3. Cunliffe, B: *Rome and Her Empire*. New York: McGraw-Hill, 1978
4. de Lys, C: *The Giant Book of Superstitions*. Secaucus, New Jersey: Citadel, 1979
5. Frazer, J: *The Golden Bough*. New York: Macmillan, 1922
6. Freud, S: *The Future of an Illusion* (Scott, W, Translator). Garden City, New York: Doubleday, 1927
7. Grimal, P (Ed): *Larousse World Mythology*. New York: Hamlyn, 1973, p. 10
8. Hamilton, E: *Mythology*. New York: Mentor, 1940
9. Russell, J B: *The Devil: Perceptions of Evil from Antiquity to Primitive Christianity*. Ithaca, New York: Cornell University Press, 1977
10. Scott, A, and Rohan, M S: *Fantastic People*. New York: Galahad Books, 1980
11. Seligmann, K: *Magic, Supernaturalism, and Religion*. London, Pantheon, 1971
12. Smith, H: *Man and His Gods*. New York: Grosset and Dunlap, 1952
13. Tolkien, J R R: *The Fellowship of the Ring*. New York: Ballantine, 1965
14. Wells, H G: *The Outline of History: The Whole Story of Man*. Garden City, New York: Doubleday, 1971
15. Wendt, G: Preface. In de Lys, C: *The Giant Book of Superstitions*. Secaucus, New Jersey: Citadel, 1979, p vii
16. Wines, R, Pickett, R, Toborg, A, and Di Scala, S (Editorial Consultants): *Monarch Review Notes in World History, Part 1*. New York: Monarch, 1963

Chapter 3

Christian Concepts

> When we look about us with the physical senses, Nature seems to be in continual warfare with herself. In fact, it seems utterly impossible to find anything not in deadly conflict with something else. Observing this mankind has unconsciously, from time immemorial formulated the idea of two great powers—the "good" and the "evil." From this idea the grand dogma of all theology—"God" and the "Devil"—sprang into existence. It soon became the chief cornerstone of every sacerdotalism which the world has witnessed. [31:p. 113]
>
> *Zolar, 1970*

> From all evil and mischief; from sin, from the crafts and assaults of the devil; from thy wrath, and from everlasting damnation.
>> Good Lord, deliver us.
> From fornication, and all other deadly sin; and from all the deceits of the world, the flesh, and the devil,
>> Good Lord, deliver us. [3:p. 40]
>
> *The Book of Common Prayer*

The Rise of Christianity

Christ was a different kind of god, a god perhaps more anthropomorphic than any of the other gods in that this divinity actually became human in order to share fully the human experience. This was quite unlike the Roman Caesars, who started out as men and elected to become gods. In addition, Christ (or Jesus) promised a new kingdom upon earth that was to occur almost immediately, replacing the oppressive Roman government for the masses. Although this doctrine understandably proved to be most pleasing to the multitude, it was frightening to those in power. Most of the converts to Christianity came from the urban lower and middle classes, and the high urban and rural classes remained polytheistic in their beliefs [6,28].

Although most of the Roman world was at least tolerant to Christianity even from the beginning, the Christians were not particularly popular because of their fanaticism, their rites concerning the eating of the flesh and blood of a son of God, and, most of all, their so-called atheism (because they did not worship the Roman gods). The old gods were still considered very powerful and deserving of respect and worship. The Roman rulers took advantage of the impiety of the Christians to blame them for all natural disasters, such as fires, floods, and earthquakes, and persecuted them accordingly, saying that they had angered the gods and brought their wrath down upon the Empire [6].

Christianity, in spite of its atheistic taint, continued to win converts as the traditional Roman cults lost favor with the populace, so that by the end of the third century, they had become a force within the Empire. The Emperor Constantine, early in the fourth century, declared Christianity the official religion of the Empire, making a political move to increase his power. Constantine and his family had been followers of the sun god, Apollo, and Constantine himself was essentially a tolerant individual. In the Edict of Milan in 313, he declared all religions equal. In 326, he decided to form a new capital, Constantinople, where there would be no worship of pagan religions. He also began to pass laws favorable to the Christians [1].

It is estimated that Christians comprised only about a twentieth of the population of the Roman Empire, but they had excellent organization, in that the structure of the Christian church was modeled after that of the empire. Constantine evidently recognized the potential political impact of this religious group and decided to take advantage of its growing power. His own conversion is questionable, as he continued to allow himself to be labeled on coins as a worshipper of Apollo, Mars, Hercules, Mithras, and Zeus. Whatever his personal convictions, the recognition of Christianity bestowed upon it the full power of the empire and assured its propagation throughout the civilized Western world [25].

It is speculated by some that if Constantine had not endorsed the Christian church, it would have been torn apart by internal strife concerning the nature of Jesus. It was impossible for some to believe that Yahweh would actually take human form, and so they denied the divinity of Jesus. Although the concept of Yahweh remained anthropomorphic in its insistence upon strict rules of conduct necessary in the split universe of good and evil, it was inconceivable that he would become human in any actual sense. Others felt equally strong in their conviction that Jesus was god. The doctrine of the virgin birth was adopted to allow Christ a way of becoming divine. It also allowed Mary special qualities.

> The doctrine of the virgin birth, which served primarily to endow Jesus with divinity, served also if secondarily to purify Mary of carnality, and the doctrine soon came to specify not an accidental, but a perpetual virginity. Thus elevated by the divine afflatus, Mary soon began to compete in popular affection with Isis, Cybele and Demeter. It required but slight and easy changes to transfer to her the stately ritual of the goddess Isis, with its shaven and tonsured priests, its matins and vespers, its tinkling music, its jeweled images of the Mother of God; and the ancient portrait of Isis and the child Horus was ultimately accepted not only in popular opinion, but by formal episcopal sanction, as the portrait of the Virgin and her child. [25:p. 216]

By the time Constantine came into power, Mary had been made a goddess in Thrace, Scythia, and Arabia. Homer Smith labels Yahweh, Jesus, Mary, and the assorted numbers of saints fast coming into being as the Christian pantheon.

The Council of Nicaea was called by Constantine in 325 to settle the dispute called the Arian heresy as to the divinity of Christ. The Arians, followers of Arius, a priest in Alexandria, held that Jesus was not divine like God. The Council decided otherwise, and the Nicene Creed they designed became the official Church doctrine [30]. But this was not the end of the official dispute. After nearly 400 years of conflict, it was decided that three Gods, the Father, the Son, and the Holy Ghost, would constitute the Holy Trinity [25].

The followers of Christianity also validated the existence of many anthropomorphic spirit selves called devils, demons, and angels, who owed their existence and their functions to the powers of light and darkness. Every individual was subject to the influence of the evil powers of darkness, which could take up their abode within the person, turning her or him into a witch or wizard. Conversely, there were humans who could become saints through real or legendary martyrdom. There were as many or more anthropomorphic spirit selves in the world of Christianity as had peopled the pre-Christian world.

> The transfer from pagan to Christian worship represented but little change. The statues of Jupiter and Apollo were readily christened St. Peter and St. Paul, and by the middle of the fifth century Christianity had acquired numerous pagan deities as saints. . . . A host of lesser pagan deities were as easily turned into devils and demons. [25:p. 227]

The recognition of saints and their subsequent veneration was an established fact by the sixth century. These godlike persons were thought to have entered the kingdom of heaven, truly validation of the resurrection of the body, an anthropomorphic ideal realized by the Christian faith.

> By the sixth century all Christian temples had statues which spoke, wept, perspired, or bled, these prodigies being officially approved. The saints listened to the people's prayers and rewarded them with miracles, and holy relics were taken onto the battlefield, or carried in long processions to avert drought, epidemics and other disasters. . . . The fortune was assured of any church that had the whole body of a saint: even a single bone or bit of apparel endowed an alter with additional supernatural power, and where relics could not be obtained an image was erected as a substitute. [25:p. 217]

The new state religion was permeated with magical thinking, as is strongly illustrated by the reverence shown by the Roman Catholic Church toward relics. Countless numbers of objects received religious veneration because they were thought to carry tremendous influence with higher powers.

> In the Middle Ages, when every tourist was a pilgrim, what mattered was relics—fragments of saints, which could range from a tiny splinter of bone to a whole skeleton. . . . Saints were cut up, they were sold, they were even stolen. . . . When St. Elizabeth of Hungary was lying in state in 1231, the mourners cut off her hair, her nails, and even her nipples. Each tiny portion would later inspire the faithful in some local church. [10:pp. 94, 96]

It is apparent that the buying, selling, and collecting of relics was a thriving business and that the church gained a prodigious amount of credibility among the believers by encouraging an emotional cathexis toward objects that were blessed by the priesthood and therefore must be valid. The church at Canterbury was able to persuade pilgrims that the clay on display there was the amount remaining after Adam's creation. The churches and many individuals who became collectors also became enormously wealthy [10].

> One small reliquary at Chartres suggests very well how naive, or how literal, the whole business of relics had become. It was designed to hold a relic of Jesus himself. As he had ascended into heaven, you could not have his skull or his bones as with an ordinary saint; you had to make do with parts of his body which he had shed before his death. This meant his milk teeth, various tears that he had wept, drops of blood. Most awe-inspiring of all, it meant the relic of his circumcision, and that was what the Chartres reliquary was designed to hold—what the French call *Le Saint Prepuce*, or in English the Holy Foreskin. At the height of the Middle Ages there were no less than fifteen foreskins of Jesus being worshipped in various churches around Europe. [10:p. 96]

Some of the more famous relics included the Holy Tunic, or undergarment, that the Virgin Mary wore at the time she gave birth to Jesus; the Crown of Thorns in its entirety, or only one thorn from the crown; fragments of the cross; the swaddling clothes of Jesus; bits of the skull of John the Baptist; and the rod of Moses. All these and many more were knelt before, prayed to, kissed, fondled, and carried in processions [10].

The worship of relics was accompanied by the practice of pagan customs. Numbers of the converts to Christianity brought with them and kept their earlier allegiances to other gods and the practices that accompanied their worship. These were adapted by the church in order to solidify its position. This is well illustrated by the actions of Gregory the Great, who allowed the Germanic barbarians to continue worshipping war gods and nature spirits at pagan shrines [24].

> This informal arrangement became the key to official Church policy during the pontificate of Gregory the Great (590–604). That practical and far-sighted Pope likened Christianity to a steep mountain that had to be climbed step by step, not in a single leap, and he instructed his missionaries to desist from their efforts to obliterate ancient pagan customs "of a sudden." Instead, he said, they were to infuse heathen practices with Christian meaning and to adapt pagan temples to the worship of the True God. This policy slowly transferred local religious loyalties to the Church, and assured the continuing growth and vigor of Christianity. [24:pp. 88–89]

Because of this attitude a type of religion evolved that was a blend of Christian and pagan, called *popular* or *folk religion*. Folk religion was responsible for the growing worship of saints and relics and the subsequent increased power of the Church, which played upon the superstitions of the masses. The feast of St. John's Day had its beginnings in the pagan celebration of Midsummer's Night, and December 25, Christmas, was the celebration of the pagan festival of the winter solstice [24].

The struggles of the saints (who eventually numbered more than 25,000) against the powers of darkness were appealing to the warlike barbarians, and stories of the saints replaced their stories of warriors. At first the Church opposed the worship of saints and relics but gradually gave in to popular demand. In 787, a general Church council declared that no temple could be consecrated unless it contained holy relics and any bishop who did so would be removed from office. There was no longer any clear demarcation between church and state, and many warriors were appointed bishops, a title that did not make them any less warlike in their thinking or practice.

The church hierarchy, many of whom were becoming quite wealthy and enormously influential, used more than their wealth to maintain power. They made liberal use of fear. Throughout history, as we have seen, there have been those who have capitalized on our anxiety and our belief in the use of magic, ritual, and religion to quell our fears. The priests of the now well established Christian religion were no exception. As society's leaders, they learned to take advantage of the format presented by belief in a split universe of good and evil to maintain established rules and cultural norms.

Reward and Punishment

Just as in pre-Christian times, the prevailing belief was in a special language, which was divinely inspired and which could be translated only by an expert. The expert was the priest who functioned in the same manner as the previous magicians, seers, and sorcerers. He alone could translate the words of the Scriptures or sacred writings and he alone could interpret them. The common person was discouraged from reading the Scriptures and was prevented from any attempt at interpretation. "When, in effect, Gregory the Great prohibited the laity from reading the scriptures," says Homer Smith, "he was moved by a deep concern lest Christians misinterpret the sacred allegories and thereby fall into dogmatic error" [25:p. 253].

The advantages to the priesthood of this type of prohibition are obvious. The priest was guaranteed a credulous and fearful following, for who would dare to contradict the words of the literate and all-knowing mediators between God and man? The Christian priesthood was similar to the priesthoods of all religions in the power that its initiates assumed over the minds of their followers. The priest had the power to condemn or reward his followers, for he set the rules by which their lives were governed.

The principles of good and evil were elaborated into a heaven and hell hereafter. Persons who followed the rules were to be rewarded in an afterlife. Those who broke the rules were promised punishment by torture. Rare was the credulous individual who did not feel terror when confronted with the realities of hell as described by those even more credulous persons who, utilizing vivid imaginations, painted horrible pictures of the fate awaiting rule breakers. It was not only the religious fanatics who seemed to thrive on the gruesome descriptions of hell. Artists and writers of the Middle Ages were obsessed with the possibilities. One portrayal in a thirteenth century encyclopedia reported:

> There is in the middle of the earth a place which is called Hell. Thus much say I to you of this place, that it is full of fire and of burning sulphur. And it is overhideous, stinking, full of ordure and of all evil adventure. And there is the fire so overmuch ardent, hot and anguishous that our fire and the heat thereof is no more unto the regard of that fire of Hell than a fire painted on a wall is in comparison to our fire. [10:p. 90]

Although that presentation shows conviction, it lacks the detail written in the second century by the author of the Apocalypse of Peter:

> In a place of chastisement directly opposite paradise . . . blasphemers are hung by their tongues above a flaming fire; women who adorn themselves for the purpose of adultery are hung by the hair over a bubbling, stinking mire; murderers are cast into a pit of reptiles; mothers who forsake their children are immersed in a pit of gore and filth; persecutors of the righteous are burned in fire up to the waist while their entrails are devoured by worms; other evildoers are punished by having their eyes burned out, by being rolled on swords and spits, by boiling in pitch and blood, by being hurled from high cliffs, or by careful, protracted roasting. [25:p. 265]

One may wonder what peculiar joys rewarded those individuals who took such great pains to invent these ludicrous tortures. We may speculate that they were so enraged at being forced into leading joyless lives that their revenge was to ensure that as many others as possible would be frightened into doing the same. Those who dared to disobey could do so only at the great risk of eternal damnation. We may also marvel at the type of mentality that would achieve happiness upon beholding the sufferings of others. And yet, this was precisely the case.

> It was believed that one of the pleasures of the blessed in heaven would be to behold the torment of the damned. A writer in about 1200 enumerated the joys of life hereafter, and listed this as the sixth: "The sixth and last cause of joy will be to behold the damned on the left hand, to whom the Judge will say Depart, ye accursed, into everlasting fire!" [10:p. 91]

Lest some more rebellious and independent thinkers question the accuracy of these speculations about hell, many persons reported more direct contact with the damned that validated the prevailing beliefs. Saint Bridget claimed to have a vision in which a soul in torment lamented:

> My feet are as toads, for I stood in sin: a serpent creepeth forth by the lower parts of my stomach unto the higher parts, for my lust was inordinate; therefore now the serpent searcheth about mine entrails without comfort, gnawing and biting without mercy. My breast is open and gnawed with worms, for I loved foul and rotten things more than God. My lips are cut off. Mine eyes hang down upon my cheeks. [10:pp. 90–91]

Although such descriptions of an imagined place of punishment might seem rather preposterous to us today, they were evidently taken as truth by the early Christians. It seems ironic that a god, especially one reported to be synonomous with love, could be so vengeful. Yet, these accounts have left an imprint, and even today, there are those who prescribe to the concept of a literal hell and who rejoice at being among the saved at the expense of the damned. Once the self was differentiated from all the rest of nature and placed in a binary paradigm of good and evil, reward and punishment were easily envisioned as being necessary to the split universe. The only arguments put forth were those concerning the exact location of heaven and hell, not their respective qualities.

The intertwining of ethics, morals, and social rules of conduct was often subtle and often explicit, as in the Hebrew tradition. God gave laws. The priesthood enforced and elaborated on God's laws. Crafty politicians and rulers capitalized on this phenomenon and formed liaisons with the priests, as exemplified when the Emperor Constantine embraced Christianity as the state religion. Both factions gained power.

Occasionally rule making became such a preoccupation that every aspect of life was regulated. Christian tradition has it that the Jewish social system at the time of the Roman conquest was stringently regulated by volumes of codified laws that were debated by the priestly caste.

One of the interesting paradoxes of human history was precipitated by a social movement now attributed to Jesus, which in essence rebelled against strict regulation of man's conduct focusing more on love of fellow man and love of the Hebrew god [29]. Early leaders in this movement were exterminated by the rule makers. The death of a major figure, Jesus, was conceived as martyrdom by his followers, who, in the course of a few centuries, built one of the great religious conceptual frames of the world and the dominant religious frame in the Western world.

The paradox becomes evident when we study the way in which a conceptual frame originally designed to decrease regulation grew into a paradigm with even more rules. Heaven and hell and the fate of the human soul in the hereafter became the cornerstone. Belief in the sacrifice of Jesus as God's son in a man-God-conspiracy was necessary for saving one's self or soul from burning in hell for all eternity. If the chief problem for the individual had been the quality of the life he led, perhaps Christian history would not have been so bloody. But, in addition to feeling responsible for their earthly deeds, Christians became convinced that their souls or spirits were in abiding danger of being possessed by demons through no fault of their own. Evil demons were disciples of the Devil, who, during the Middle Ages, assumed tremendous power over the minds of Christians, leading them to be suspicious of every action that might be defined as a sign of possession or witchcraft. Jeffrey Burton Russell, in his excellent book, *The Devil*, writes:

> The relationship of demons to the Devil has always been somewhat blurred, and the demons of the New Testament are a composite of different elements. One element is the fallen angels. To the extent that the demons are fallen angels, their origin is the *bene ha-elohim*, the sons of the God. In this context the demons share a common divine origin with the Devil, and there is reason to refer in one breath to "The Devil and the other Demons," for the Devil is the first and greatest of the fallen angels. But the demons have roots in other ancient traditions as well. They are menacing spirits of the thunderstorm or the lonely grove, avenging ghosts of the dead, bringers of disease, and violent spirits who possess the soul. [20:p. 252]

No matter how blameless a life the individual might lead, he or she might not be spared the loss of the soul through the actions of the Devil and his hordes.

The argument for possession was strong, and evidence for it was believed to be found in the New Testament. Russell holds the opinion that demonology is a central teaching of the New Testament. The demons, and sometimes Satan himself, possess individuals as one of their chief means of blocking the Kingdom of God, and through the business of casting out demons or devils, Jesus was able to show his power over the forces of evil [20].

Jesus made it clear that it was his mission to oppose Satan and to cast devils out of men. "He healed many that were sick of divers diseases . . . and suffered not the devils to speak, because they knew him"; the "unclean spirits, when they saw him, fell down before him and cried, saying, Thou art the Son of God." Jesus expels an unclean spirit from a man in Capernaum; he casts seven devils out of Mary Magdalene; in Peter's house he casts out the spirits of "many" who were possessed with devils; and he casts the devils out of two Gadarenes and into a great herd of swine nearby, which thereupon throw themselves down a steep cliff into the sea and perish. [25:pp. 233–234]

Satan is also reported to have tempted Jesus and was rebuked and to have actually entered into Judas. Satan was conceived as a general whose army was composed of supernatural beings against whom humans were powerless without the help of the Holy Spirit. Although healers and magicians could exorcise demons, they did not do it by using the power of the Holy Spirit as did Jesus [25].

One of the more frightening aspects of the Devil as tempter was his ability to change shape. Quite unlike God, who was always seen as representative of goodness and light, the Devil, although the Prince of Darkness, could appear as a beautiful girl, a handsome youth, any human or animal form. He had been dubbed the ape of God because he could copy all the different forms created by the deity. However, he could not copy or imitate anything exactly. He always erred by leaving something out. For example, it was thought by some that devils in human form did not have buttocks because they could not create that part of the anatomy accurately, so that, in place of the backside, there was another face [22].

In addition to being able to imitate all animal and human forms, the Devil could change personality. He could be very charming as a young girl or very commanding as a soldier or very conniving as a merchant. No one was immune to his wiles because he was inordinately clever, able to determine the weaknesses of his intended victims and then to tempt them accordingly [22].

The most awesome characteristic of the Devil was his ability to seduce his victims sexually and even to reproduce. The devils were able to assume the shapes of incubi or succubi and visit persons in their beds. The incubi were male and the succubi female, and they were associated with fertility and sexuality as well as with death and evil. The Devil's horns, which became a Western tradition, were symbols of fertility and signs of wild, unmanageable, and destructive sexuality [20].

Witchcraft and the Persecution of Witches

Christian tradition aligned the body with the material and sin-filled world, which was the kingdom of the Devil. This necessitated a clear-cut dichotomy between body and soul, with the body being seen as sinful because of its very nature. The attitude engendered by the church toward sex was one of distrust and even repulsion. Saint Paul believed that sexual desire is in conflict with God, so that to indulge in the pleasures of the flesh or even to admit to an interest in sex is tantamount to enmity toward the Creator. Because of this teaching the Church became extremely paranoid in its crusade against sex, this paranoia reaching a zenith during the Dark Ages with the persecution of witches, who were almost always linked with sexual practices.

A interesting account of the fall of the *bene ha-elohim* from angel status is found in the Apocalyptic Book of Enoch. The Watchers were the fallen angels who had indulged their lust for human females. Two other Apocalyptic books, the Testament of Dan and the Testament of Reuben, are important in any survey of a history of witches [20].

> As Eve tempted Adam, Reuben says, so did women allure the Watchers by using seductive makeup and hair styles: the burden of sin is placed upon man, or rather upon woman. The Watchers, being spiritual creatures, cannot themselves beget children, so they appear to women while the women are having intercourse with their husbands. Lusting after the Watchers, the women conceive alien forms from the seed of men. A variant of this incubus myth appears frequently in the history of medieval witchcraft: the witch conducts her revels while appearing to be safely in bed with her husband. [20: p. 194]

Witches were clearly in league with the Devil. They were part of the hordes of Satan through their association with the Prince of Darkness. If the prevailing attitude of the Middle Ages was, as Tertullian phrased it, that woman is the gate to hell, then it is not surprising that most witchcraft was believed to have been practiced by women, and women were persecuted in alarming numbers.

Women were held in such low esteem that any kind of a crime was seen as preferable to giving in to the lust that resulted in sexual liaison. In the year 386, the Roman synod decreed that bishops, deacons, and priests who were already married must practice sexual abstinence. In the years 1030 to 1051, all clerics were commanded to cast out their wives and sell their children into slavery. In Spain in the year 600, men were encouraged to sell their wives into slavery and donate the proceeds from these sales to the poor [25].

The Church took as its task the business of ferreting out witches, thus protecting men against these followers of the Devil. No less a personage than Saint Augustine validated that witchcraft depended upon a pact with the Devil. The Church utilized its weapons of sacred magic to war against the enemies of God. Smith lists among those protective devices the sight or manual sign of the cross, the reading of the Scriptures, and the use of charms, incantations, amulets, prayers, and exorcisms. Agobard, Archbishop of Lyon, is reported to have said in the ninth century that "the wretched world lies now under the tyranny of foolishness; things are believed by Christians of such absurdity as not one ever could aforetime induce the heathen to believe" [25:p. 260].

Several scholars have given opinions as to the primal roots of witchcraft. Some evidenced the belief that all the heresies stemming from Gnosticism were responsible and that the Gnostic sects were the source of witchcraft and satanism. Others saw witchcraft as being a natural result of the pagan practices of the folk religions [25]. Seligmann strongly suggests that witchcraft is associated with the once permitted and even encouraged worship of the old deities, a type of worship that was much more appealing to the impoverished masses than the humorless and guilt-evoking worship of the Christian god. What had once been widely accepted was now looked upon as evil [22].

With the devil's establishment of his power, the ancient survivals, the amusements of serfs, the most innocent stories, were henceforth Satanic, and the women who knew about the old legends and magic traditions were transformed into witches, or evil fairies, as the old stories call them. The traditional gatherings, the Druids' festival on the eve of May Day, the Bacchanals, the Diana feasts, became the witches' sabbath; and the broom, symbol of the sacred hearth, though retaining its sexual significance, became an evil tool. The sexual rites of old, destined to stimulate the fertility of nature, were now the manifestations of a forbidden carnal lust. Mating at random, a survival of communal customs more ancient than the Old Testament, the judges now decided to be an infringement of the most sacred laws. [22:p. 177]

Throughout Europe before and during the Middle Ages, the practice of witchcraft was a religious custom. Sometimes the worshippers mimicked wild animals and involved phallic symbols in their ceremonies. The covens were religious units consisting of twelve elders headed by a priest, sometimes a Christian priest who continued to worship as his forefathers had done. The wearing of animal masks and hides were a carry-over from the bacchanalia [9,12]. The meetings of the witches were public and were called *sabbats*, from *s'esbattre*, which means to frolic. The ceremonies involved dancing around fires and pleasurable sexual orgies. The members of the group would sometimes pretend to ride brooms in imitation of horses [25].

Drugs such as aconite, poplar, cinquefoil and deadly nightshade, as well as bat's blood, animal fats and soot were rubbed into the skin and may have aided the illusion of real flight. Witches took to themselves particular animals, dogs, cats, weasels, toads and mice as familiars or incarnations of magic power, to aid them in their sorcery. The esbat was a secret meeting of the elders when waxen images, candles, and "flying ointments" were prepared by expert hands, and a cat, dog, cock or an unbaptized child supplied by its witch-mother or stolen, was sacrificed. [25:p. 271]

Scott and Rohan suggest that a history of mankind's belief in witchcraft might reveal the idea that the owls, rats, dogs, cats, bats, and other birds and animals utilized by witches were creatures possessed by the last of the air elementals who wished to enter the physical world. They were not gifted enough to take human form or to fabricate bodies of their own. Once they took the form of some animal or bird, they could serve witches as scouts, advisors, or guards. The elementals were thus able to influence the witch cults of the Dark Ages [21].

As the Church grew more menacing, those witches who were engaged in performing ancient religious practices reacted by turning their coven meetings into parodies of the rites of the church. They would have black masses in which they used profane wafers and holy water. Sometimes they made human sacrifices, either using a willing victim or consipiring with the public executioner to obtain a victim legally. Smith believes that some of the witches may have enjoyed making fun of the saints [25].

The most prominent feature of the sabbat was the worship of the Devil, and records of the Inquisition are full of the sexual practices involved in Devil worship. One must remember that the confessions extracted from the accused witches were obtained by the most horrible forms of torture and words where put into their mouths, words they gladly accepted since only confession would stop the torture.

Those religious rituals, which had long been customary, especially among the peasants, were now regarded as evidence of satanic possession, and the worshippers were tortured and condemned once they fell into the clutches of the dreaded witch finders. Witches did exist, but certainly not in the form recorded by the Inquisition. By the sixteenth century, however, so thorough had been the Church, that all the classes of Europe, from peasants to judges, were united in the conviction that witches must be hunted down and destroyed [22].

The sexual paranoia of the Church was never more evident than when it conducted its crusade against the witches. All the Church Fathers, from Saint Augustine to Saint Thomas Aquinas, were in agreement that incubi and succubi existed and that it was indeed possible to have intercourse with Satan. Under torture, the witches described their union with Satan [25]:

> The devil's caress was variously described as brutal, painful, lacerating, torturing, although there are abundant testimonies, some from girls but twelve to sixteen years of age, as to its delights. On one point there seemed to be well-nigh universal agreement: the devil was cold all over, like a creature of stone, yet his touch imparted an atrocious, delicious joy. [25:p. 273]

The activities of the *concubitus daemonum* (the incubi and succubi) were the most dreaded of all the activities of the armies of evil, and the demons did indeed compose an army. In 1568, Johann Wier claimed to have counted the demons and found that there were 1111 legions of 6666 each, making a grand total of 7,405,926 [25].

The church saw its chief order of business as the stamping out of evil. The Christians took this very seriously. The Calvinists declared that all happiness was sin. Since the church and state were one, witchcraft was made a penal offense by both Catholics and Protestants. If anyone voiced an opinion contrary to the government, he was likely to be seen as under the influence of Satan and prosecuted accordingly. The growing persecution also produced resistance, and Satan became a political figure because he represented the forces of freedom, nature, and antagonism toward the established order. As the Church encountered more resistance, it increased its persecutory practices and the witch burnings turned into horrible orgies. The witch hunts that produced the victims were unimaginably gruesome [25].

> Among the objective evidences of league with Satan were the "devil's mark," which might be a supernumerary breast, a suspicious looking mole (devil's teat) or an area of the skin which was insensitive to pain when pricked with a needle. In his search for devil's teats the howls of the accused did not stay the hand of the witch-finder: quite the contrary, since the object was to find a place where the needle could go in without causing pain; and when he failed he sometimes remained convinced that the devil's mark was there, but hidden in such parts and places that it would be necessary to tear the body to pieces to discover it. [25:p. 274]

Witch finders became respected professionals and witch persecution an industry. This industry employed so many people that its dissolution would have precipitated an economic crisis. Not only the witch finders made their living in this manner, but torturers, jailers, judges, exorcists, woodchoppers, and scribes. The torturers, who were the professional hangmen, became enormously wealthy because they received an honorarium for every witch they tortured and burned. They soon caught on to making the victims name their accomplices so that they were assured of a steady supply. These experts in torture were also protected by the law, and any person dying while tortured was considered a victim of Satan and not of the hangman [22]. They operated under the authority of God. They were commanded to go about their work joyfully and not in any way to show that they were disturbed by the cries and screams of the tortured [25].

The paranoia increased, and according to the followers of Luther, it was essential because the hordes of Satan were growing daily. These disciples of Luther estimated in Feyerabend's *Theatrum Diabolorum* that there were 2,665,866,746,664 existing devils [25].

Others said that there were at least 10,000,000,000,000.

> Calvin had said, "Whoever shall now contend that it is unjust to put heretics and blasphemers to death will, knowingly and willingly, incur their very guilt." To Luther, the devil was a living personality who interfered with his work and rest, and once, so it is related, this preacher threw his inkstand at His Satanic Majesty. Luther subscribed to the belief in incubi and succubi and demonic changelings, and asserted that to deny the reality of witchcraft was to deny the authority of the Bible. [25:p. 293]

Smith gives a thorough description of the ordeals of the accused. The accusers were encouraged to make their accusations secretly, and the accused were taken by surprise and allowed no defense. They were assumed guilty. They were allowed to say nothing except to name their accomplices, and they were not told who accused them. The judges were commanded to make their examinations last and not to conduct them too quickly. The victims were stripped, and usually all the hair was shaved from every part of the body. They were then put to torture [25].

Although Smith's description of the methods of torture is lengthy, it is so thorough that we will quote it in its entirety:

> There were heavy pincers to tear out the fingernails, or to be used red-hot for pinching; there was the rack, a long table on which the accused was tied by her hands and feet, back down, and stretched by rope and windlass until the joints were dislocated; to this were added rollers covered with knobs or sharp spikes, which were placed under the hips and shoulders, and over which the victim was rolled back and forth; there were the thumbscrew, an instrument designed for disarticulating the fingers, Spanish boots to crush the legs and feet, metal shirts lined with knives, the Iron Virgin, a hollow instrument the size and figure of a woman, with knives so arranged inside that when the two halves of the figure were closed under pressure the accused would be lacerated in its deadly embrace. This and other devices were inscribed with the motto *Soli Deo Gloria*, "Glory be only to God." In addition there were a variety of branding irons, horsewhips, pins to be thrust beneath the nails, and various devices for suspending the accused in space, head up or head down, with weights attached. . . . When the torturer and his assistant grew tired, the hands and feet of the accused were tied, the hair was cut off (if it had not already been shaven)

and brandy was poured over the head and ignited, or sulphur was burned in the arm pits or on the breast. [25:pp. 286–287]

The documentary evidence concerning the witch persecution centers almost entirely upon women, since the authorities, who happened to be male, estimated that there were at least twenty female sorcerers to every male [22]. It is impossible to know exactly how many individuals were persecuted for witchcraft by the Christians, but the number is estimated to be several million [25].

We must not delude ourselves into thinking that this mass sadism was promoted and executed by the ignorant. It was promulgated by the most learned individuals of the period. As Seligmann phrased it, they represented "the flower of learning." He names some of the more noted participants, who include Pierre de Lancre, a scholar and patron of the fine arts; Henri Boquet, an eminent legal expert, judge of the province of Burgundy, and president of the tribunal of St. Claude; and Nicholas Remy, legal expert and secretary to Duke Charles III of Lorraine [22]. Every list must include Henry Kraemer and James Sprenger, Professors of Theology in the University of Cologne, Order of Friars Preachers, who authored the *Malleus Maleficarum* (*Witches' Hammer*) as ordered by Innocent VIII. The *Malleus* was, according to Smith, "a manual treating the subject of witchcraft under thirty-five topics, instructing the faithful as to the position they should take in regard to this evil and detailing how accused persons should be examined, prosecuted and condemned" [25:p. 283].

However, rather than placing the blame upon these men, Smith chooses to place it upon the Church and its tradition, which included many persons both Christian and pagan. The Christian premises rested upon a long heritage. The Egyptians had given mankind the idea of "the talismanic power of righteousness, of doing that which the gods loved" [25, p. 291]. The Hebrews gave us their God. The absolutes of good and evil came from the Persians. Socrates added the immortal soul, and Plato "a doctrine of physical imperfection striving to achieve spiritual perfection" [25, p. 291]. The Babylonians donated the person of Satan. Saint Augustine is credited with integrating all these elements, or as Smith goes on to say:

> Augustine had woven all these threads together into a fabric of sin stretching from generation to generation without end. It was these men, and not a fifteenth century pope and his two zealous Dominican priests, frightened half out of their wits by boils, hailstorms and epidemics of sick pigs, who are to be blamed for man's descent into the lowest depths which the human intellect has ever reached. [25:p. 291]

We may ask why this violent phenomenon was allowed to proceed, but we are reminded that the *Malleus* warned against skepticism as heresy. Those who dared to raise a voice against the slaughter were themselves tortured and burned. As the Church threw its awesome power into witch persecution to the point that the economy rested upon it, it is surprising that Western civilization ever recovered from it. Recovery was rather slow in some areas. In 1768, John Wesley said, "The giving up of witchcraft is in effect the giving up of the Bible." In 1775, an earthquake was attributed by the Reverend Thomas Prince to Benjamin Franklin's kite flying. Two witches were burned in Poland in 1793, a wizard was drowned in England in 1865, and in 1900 an attempt was made in Ireland to roast a witch [25]. In America, the Salem witches were hanged rather than burned, and this occurred in the 1690s. Their number was few, and some of those responsible later repented and recanted in writing [22].

An accounting of some recent events are noteworthy in their validation of the aura of superstition and religion that yet surrounds our Western culture and of the legacy we have inherited from our Christian forefathers, as well as from the Egyptians, Persians, Babylonians, and Hebrews.

Modern Religion and Magic

Christian fundamentalists have become increasingly more active in the past few years. The battle of the creationists versus the evolutionists is once more in the courtroom, as we mentioned briefly in Chapter 1, a reminder of the famous "monkey trial" of 1925. In March 1981, a group of "scientific creationists" complained in a California courtroom that the state was teaching evolution as fact in public science classes and that this infringed on the free exercise of religion. They argued that the state should take the position of "neutrality" concerning the question of the origin of life. They did not demand that the scientific creationist view also be taught, but this is essentially the only way that the state could be neutral [17].

Although many argue that there is absolutely nothing scientific about the creationist viewpoint, the term "creation science" is now being used, many scientists feel, as a device for getting the Genesis account of creation into school curricula under the guise of science [17].

In the California case, Judge Perluss stated that the particular textbook statement concerning evolution did not infringe the free exercise of religion and could stand unamended. However, he also reminded editors and textbook publishers of a 1973 state board of education policy directive asking that evolution be presented as theory, not as dogma [17].

Legislators in at least fourteen states have introduced bills that would require that creationism be taught in the classroom along with evolution. Arkansas passed a bill declaring that both must be taught if either is taught and that they must be given equal weight. On July 21, 1981, the governor of Louisiana signed into law the Balanced Treatment Bill. Louisiana thus became the second state to require that whenever evolution is taught, creation science must also be presented [4].

The battle between the evolutionists and creationists is being viewed with alarm by many who see it as indicative of a combined religious-political movement, which may be a violation of the First Amendment separation of church and state. It is also seen by many scientists as an attack upon the nature of scientific inquiry itself [4].

Harvard professor Stephen J. Gould, a distinguished paleontologist, reminds us that, because of the nature of the creationists' belief system, no amount of scientific data will ever make any impression upon them. He quotes Dr. Duane Gish, one of creationism's leading intellectuals, as saying:

By creation we mean the bringing into being by a supernatural Creator of the basic kind of plants and animals by the process of sudden, or fiat, creation. We do not know how the Creator created, what processes He used, *for He used processes which are not now operating anywhere in the natural universe.* This is why we refer to creation as special creation. We cannot discover by scientific investigations anything about the creative processes used by the Creator. [11:pp. 35–36]

Gould then writes:

"Scientific creationism" is a self-contradictory, nonsense phrase precisely because it cannot be falsified. I can envision observations and experiments that would disprove any evolutionary theory I know, but I cannot imagine what potential data could lead creationists to abandon their beliefs. Unbeatable systems are dogma, not science. [11:p. 35]

Many of us cannot accept the idea that we occupy only a tiny place in the universe and that it is entirely possible the cosmos does not revolve around us. Some scholars worry that we are moving toward a merger of state and religion through legislation that is forcing teachers and publishers to present religious dogma as scientific theory. Kenneth M. Pierce points out in an article in *Time* that this is an age when medical quackery and astrology are also on the upswing [17]. He says about the creationism versus evolution controversy:

The relation of science and mortality is an important matter. Creationism may belong in social studies or the history of religion, but it should not be pushed into biology classes or textbooks, especially not by legislative fiat. [17:p. 82]

The Bible, as the Word of God, is still the leading seller among books in the United States, and sales are increasing. Some people think this indicates a return to "old-time religion." Many of the more modern translations are being fought by those of us who insist that the King James version is the only true translation. We are incensed at attempts to introduce new information based on more accurate translation, such as that which would delete the term *virgin* in connection with the virgin birth [16].

The 13.6 million Southern Baptists in the United States elected, in June 1981, the Reverend Bailey Smith as their leader. Smith is a professed believer in the theory that the Bible is free of any historical or spiritual error and is, therefore, inerrant [2]. This is in direct contrast to the beliefs of numerous biblical scholars who claim otherwise if, for no other reason, than the growing evidence that newer translations based on later information may change much of the text. Concerning the King James version, for example, Richard N. Ostling reports in *Time:*

More important, biblical scholars insist the King James is no longer accurate enough. It was translated from relatively late medieval manuscripts in Hebrew and Greek, the best available then, but 20th century research has turned up texts that are as many as 1,000 years closer to the originals. The ending to the Lord's Prayer in *Matthew 6:13*, for instance, beginning with "for thine is the kingdom," is not in the earliest manuscripts. [16:p. 62]

The inerrantists hold unwaveringly the viewpoint that the Bible is indeed the language and word of God and that no human embellishments must be allowed to alter its message [2]. As with the creationism versus evolution argument, scientific data have no place in the controversy, for the matter has been settled by faith by those individuals who claim they have the knowledge necessary to make the decisions.

The interaction of religion and politics can also be illustrated in the anti-abortionist argument that legislation should reflect the right to life as based on moral and theological tenets. The right to life movement implies that a woman's body becomes the property of the state once she has conceived and that the state should be guided by religious tenets in deciding whether to terminate or continue the pregnancy. This may be, in addition, a reflection of the long-held belief in Christian culture that sex is sinful and, therefore, must be punished by the bearing of unwanted children.

Pope John Paul II, in addressing some issues concerning sex and birth control, has not altered his opinion from that of Pope Paul VI's 1968 encyclical *Humanae Vitae*, which states that, "Each and every marriage act must remain open to the transmission of life" [5:p. 74]. The evidence is overwhelming that most Roman Catholics in the United States ignore the encyclical, but the official position will, according to most experts, remain as it has been. Many persons fear that official church doctrine may return to the view that all sexual pleasure is suspect even in marriage, although others believe that it may become more liberal [27]. Whatever the church's position, millions of Catholics and Protestants remain under the influence of Church laws that reflect the old idea of sex as sin unless for procreation.

Gametic engineering, which is an occupation of many scientists, is presently under attack as being an attempt to "play God" and, therefore, some say, should not be permitted. Gametic engineering is defined by David Rorvik as "the *in vitro* manipulation of germ cells, including such phenomena as test-tube babies and cloning" [19:p. 69]. The efforts of scientists in this new biological revolution, which also includes genetic engineering involving recombinant DNA and gene splicing, are seen as potentially dangerous, representing human intrusion into God's domain.

During the 1970s, the United States experienced a recrudescence of fundamentalist religious movements which permeated many social institutions. The appeal of a fairly concise anthropomorphic format as a frame of reverence and a basis for individual and group ethics is evidenced by the large numbers of adherents to fundamentalist doctrine, which has as its major thesis that the Bible is the inerrant word of God [8]. This religious revival has been augmented by modern technology, so that evangelists now command extremely large audiences by television media. This use of the media is also reflected in the ability to recruit financial support and thereby to organize indoctrination compaigns that were possible only by direct confrontation in previous centuries. Some of the leaders in this evangelical movement have encouraged the idea that they influence millions of voters and have used the religious podium to address political situations, on occasion endorsing or banning various political candidates for public office.

According to the November 3, 1980, issue of *Time*, some of the more fervant fundamentalists were circulating lists of the supposed Christian positions, and legislators who did not agree came under attack. The implication here seems to be that Christians who do not agree with the positions endorsed by their leaders are perhaps sub-Christian. The *Time* article specifies that some modern religious leaders are vocal on many issues whether they have "specific biblical underpinnings" or not [26].

Issues that have been addressed by the fundamentalist movement include leadership within the nation, the Equal Rights Amendment, the control of television, education, the role of women, and homosexuality [8,18]. By utilizing the Bible as an infallible source of validation for their positions, fundamentalists attempt to engender a sense of certainty into their world view by limiting their world to the old word world, which was quite prominent in ancient times.

Any format for organizing information about our world may be associated with extreme emotional fervor and a sense of awe and reverence that may, on occasion, lead its adherents to the point of fanaticism. Under stress we seem to gravitate to concepts that comfort us with a feeling of certainty.

For many of us "a still small voice" echoes our need to believe in something more than the practicality of politicoreligious movements or scientific reductionism. Perhaps this need is reflected in the vestiges of religion and magic that still subtly permeate our culture.

At the beginning of the decade of the eighties, more than 2500 saints were venerated in the Roman Catholic Church, and more than 1000 being considered for eventual canonization. The official Church position is that the saints can hear prayers and are able to intercede with God to work miracles. More than nine Americans are awaiting beatification. The Church has been revising its list of saints and has dropped many from the roll; only fifty-eight are now considered important to all Catholics in the world. The others are "optional," according to local loyalties [13].

Millions of Protestants still reverently recite a sacred rune called the Apostles' Creed during their services:

> I believe in God the Father Almighty, Maker of heaven and earth; And in Jesus Christ his only Son our Lord, Who was conceived by the Holy Ghost, Born of the Virgin Mary, Suffered under Pontius Pilate, Was crucified, dead, and buried: He descended into hell; The third day He rose again from the dead; He ascended into heaven, And sitteth on the right hand of God the Father Almighty; From thence He shall come to judge the quick and the dead. I believe in the Holy Ghost; The holy Catholic Church; The Communion of Saints; The Forgiveness of sins; The Resurrection of the body, and the life everlasting. Amen. [3:p. 28]

The words, "He descended into hell," as recited in the creed, are translated as meaning, "He went into the place of departed spirits" [3].

Belief in a spirit world is widespread, and speculation as to life after death still occupies our minds. Parapsychology is taught in a few major universities, and large sums of money are donated for the study of psychic phenomena. The occult sciences, as they are called, attract millions of people. Astrology, numerology, and the tarot, among others of the occult sciences, are thought by many to provide prophetic knowledge, and their practitioners are sought as guides. Almost every newspaper and periodical publishes a daily horoscope, which most readers scan along with the news and other features. "Basic astrological theory" is taught by correspondence courses to students from over 100 countries through The Mayo School of Astrology [14].

Zolar, one of America's foremost authorities on astrology, who is known as the Dean of Astrology, has an extensive background in business, sociology, and psychology. He casts charts and makes horoscopes and is instrumental in the effort to revive the ancient science of astrology. In his book *The Encyclopedia of Ancient and Forbidden Knowledge*, he writes:

> Not many years ago any claim about unknown forces from outside our world affecting the lives and behavior of human beings would have thrown scientists into an uproar. To acknowledge such a concept would have been to acknowledge a belief in Astrology. To the cynical scientist, believing in Astrology is like believing in ghosts or witchcraft. . . . Today, however, the climate is rapidly changing. There is evidence emerging which shows even the cynics that what goes on in the heavens may have cause-effect connections with all of us here on earth. [31:pp. 17–19]

Zolar's book also contains a chapter on the astral world, which presents the belief that there are supernatural entities that are not and never have been human. He believes that some of these astral entities are of the class that assisted ancient magicians and that still offer their assistance in India, Persia, China, and other Oriental lands:

> Some of these Astral entities are known as Nature Spirits, and inhabit the streams, rocks, mountains, and forests. . . . Various names have been given them, for instance: fairies, pixies, elves, brownies, peris, jdinns, trolls, satyrs, fauns, kobolds, imps, goblins, little folk, and tiny people. [31:p. 148]

We often think of ourselves as living in an age of science and technology, an age that has put superstition and magic aside. Anthropologist Bronislaw Malinowski spoke for many of us when he said:

> Looking from far and above, from our high places of safety in the developed civilization, it is easy to see all the crudity and irrelevance of magic. But without its power and guidance early man could not have mastered his practical difficulties as he has done, nor could man have advanced to the higher stages of civilization. [15:p. 285]

In spite of our "high places of safety" and our "higher stages of civilization," we continue to build an anthropomorphic world in our search for cause-and-effect sequences. The same need to control and to predict that drove us to explain events through recourse to spirits, gods, and demons exists today much as it did thousands of years ago. Magical thinking and the interpretation of symbols correlated to human behavior and activities is one of our predominant occupations. Magic and religion are now so intertwined that they are impossible to separate. Only a few of us are aware of our heritage. The rest of us adopt conceptual paradigms without questioning their origin or validity, feeling at times too small a part of the universe to question. As Sir Charles Sherrington expressed our plight:

> Rather, it would sometimes seem to him [man] he is merely a tragic detail in a manifold which goes its way without being even fully conscious of him. A lonely motive in a more than million-motivated construction whose whole

motive, if it have one, is unknown to him except as alien to his own and his to it. Master of his fate? Around him torrential oceans of energy; and his own energy by comparison a drop which trickles down the window-pane. [23:p. 285]

Rather than feeling merely "a tragic detail" we have tried to define ourselves as different from and more than other creatures. We have hinged our feelings of uniqueness on our possession of a self or soul. We have studied the self or soul in great detail, as we shall see in the next chapter. The concept of self, soul, or spirit that plays so prominent a part in Christian and Western history is the dominant feature of the word world.

References

1. Barraclough, G (Ed): *The Times Atlas of World History*. Maplewood, New Jersey: Hammond, 1978
2. Bible brouhaha. *Time*, June 22, 1981, p 69
3. *The Book of Common Prayer and Administration of the Sacraments*. Toronto, Canada: Oxford University Press
4. Broad, W: Louisiana puts God into biology lessons. *Science*, Vol. 213, August 7, 1981, pp 628–629
5. Contretemps over contraception. *Time*, October 13, 1980, p 74
6. Cunliffe, B: *Rome and Her Empire*. New York: McGraw-Hill, 1978
7. de Lys, C: *The Giant Book of Superstitions*. Secaucus, New Jersey: Citadel, 1979
8. Falwell, J: *Listen, America!* New York: Bantam, 1981
9. Frazer, J: *The Golden Bough*. New York: Macmillan, 1922
10. Gascoigne, B: *The Christians*. New York: William Morrow, 1977
11. Gould, S J: Evolution as fact and theory. *Discover*, May 1981, pp 34–37
12. Grimal, P (Ed): *Larousse World Mythology*. New York: Hamlyn, 1973
13. The long road to sainthood. *Time*, July 7, 1980, p 42
14. Mayo, J: *Astrology*. London: Hodder and Stoughton, 1964
15. Miner, H: Body ritual among the Nacirema. In Jennings, J, and Hoebel, E (eds): *Readings in Anthropology*. New York: McGraw-Hill, 1955, pp 282–285
16. Ostling, R N: Rivals to the King James throne. *Time*, April 20, 1981, pp 62–63
17. Pierce, K M: Putting Darwin back in the dock. *Time*, March 16, 1981, pp 80–82
18. Pingry, P: *Jerry Falwell: Man of Vision*. Milwaukee, Wisconsin: Ideals Publishing, 1980
19. Rorvik, D: Predestinations. *Omni*, October 1980, pp 68–72, 132
20. Russell, J B: *The Devil: Perceptions of Evil from Antiquity to Primitive Christianity*. Ithaca, New York: Cornell University Press, 1977
21. Scott, A, and Rohan, M C: *Fantastic People*. New York: Galahad Books, 1980
22. Seligmann, K: *Magic, Supernaturalism, and Religion*. London: Pantheon, 1971
23. Sherrington, C: *Man on His Nature*. London: Cambridge University Press, 1940
24. Simons, G: *Barbarian Europe*. New York: Time, Inc., 1968
25. Smith, H: *Man and His Gods*. New York: Grosset and Dunlap, 1952
26. Smiting the mighty right. *Time*, November 3, 1980, p 103
27. Tempest in a cappuccino cup? *Time*, October 27, 1980, p 106
28. Wells, H G: *The Outline of History: The Whole Story of Man*. Garden City, New York: Doubleday, 1971
29. Whitehead, A N: *Adventure of Ideas*. New York: Mentor, 1955
30. Wines, R, Pickett, R, Toborg, A, and Di Scala, S (Editorial Consultants): *Monarch Review Notes in World History, Part 1*. New York: Monarch, 1963
31. Zolar, *The Encyclopedia of Ancient and Forbidden Knowledge*. New York: Fawcett, 1970

Chapter 4

Self, Soul, and Psyche

In psychoanalytic treatment nothing happens but an exchange of words between the patient and his physician. . . . Words and magic were in the beginning one and the same thing, and even to-day words retain much of their magical power. . . . Words call forth emotions and are universally the means by which we influence our fellow-creatures. [17:pp. 21–22]

Sigmund Freud, 1915

Going inward—to find the self, or oneself, or the Self (in the case of Carl Jung), or the marvelous; or simply to express dissatisfaction with the external world dominated by science and reason—became a habit with many people, espccially as the psychoanalytical movement caught on. [3:p. 411]

Franklin L. Baumer, 1977

Who has ever been able to measure the libido, ego strength, the superego, the anima, individuation, and the like? The very existence of these entities has never been demonstrated. But to those psychiatrists who devote themselves exclusively to dealing with their patients in the immediate psychotherapeutic situation, these terms are not abstract conceptualizations; they are living realities whose existence is much more tangible than the statistics and computations of experimental researchers. [10:p. 896]

Henri F. Ellenberger, 1970

The Homunculus Within

As we have postulated in the previous three chapters, man used his skill in differentiation to divide the world into two major blocks—the me block, or internal world, and the not-me block, or external world. By use of his word tools he constructed concepts of the external world that reflected his internal world. He anthropomorphized the external world and populated it with spirits, demons, and gods. By a curious twist he then postulated that his internal world was a reflection of his concept of the external world—that he was a creature like the gods or created by God in God's image. It is a bit confusing as to whether God was manlike or man was godlike. This "image of God" concept was particularly prominent in the Christian paradigm that dominated Western thinking for several centuries.

The Christian world view as expressed in Saint Augustine's *City of God*, completed in 426, defines clearly the image of God ideology:

> When God made man according to His own image, He gave him a soul so endowed with reason and intelligence that it ranks man higher than all the other creatures of the earth, the sea, the air, because they lack intelligence. God, then, formed man out of the dust of the earth and, by His breath, gave man a soul such as I have described. It is not certain whether God's breathing imparted to man a soul previously created or whether God created the soul by the act of breathing, as though He wanted the soul of man to be the very breath of God. [26:p. 263]

Man's immortal soul was clothed in an earthly body. God's son had taken on the same form to redeem man from his sins. In the final event, man's body and soul were again reunited and appeared before their maker for judgment. The internal world was, therefore, manlike, perhaps ephemeral and ethereal, but recognizable in concepts as a person unique in creation in its likeness to God.

This anthropomorphic inside world was not new. Plato had speculated about the world of the psyche. Alfred North Whitehead suggested that the Christians adopted Plato's psyche as their model of the soul:

> Christianity rapidly assimilated the Platonic doctrine of the human soul. The philosophy and the religion were very congenial to each other in their respective teachings; although, as was natural, the religious version was much more specialized than the philosophic version. [29:p. 23]

Man's inner world as envisioned in the Platonic Christian concept became dominant in Western culture.

What was the psyche, soul, self, or I really like? During some periods of Western history, to speculate that the human soul varied from the concepts of Christian church dogma might result in an early death by fire and, for most, the eternal flames of damnation. Yet, there were a few who dared speculate, even during those periods of intellectual repression.

Those scholars who did attempt to organize a conceptual framework about the internal world used a homuncular model that depicted man's soul as being somewhat manlike, somewhat godlike, but, in any event, a self-contained, purposeful entity that participated in the linguistic operation of following rules and deciding along the binary paradigm of good and evil and right and wrong.

Alex Comfort describes homuncular vision as "discursive awareness of 'I' as an inner person, separate from 'my body,' and *a fortiori* from the extra-body environment: the 'dwarf sitting in the middle,' in the words of the *Katha Upanishad*" [6:p. 12]. He goes on to define homuncular identity as "the conviction or experience that there is 'someone inside,'" distinct from the outer world, the body and the brain, in whom the processes of experiencing, willing and so on are focused, and this 'someone' objectivizes both these processes and itself" [6:p. 12].

The homuncular model presupposes a tiny homunculus or manlike being, or perhaps two manlike creatures, the conscious and unconscious ones, shifting information inside the head to result in the final common pathway of a unified self. The homunculus organizes and sorts data and then makes decisions.

To those individuals immersed in the study of physics and the neurosciences, the complexity of the data processing activities of the human central nervous system seems much more awe inspiring than the simplistic model of a homunculus somewhere in the brain making decisions. The homuncular model seems to derive from the anthropomorphic word world and our concept of self and persists, even though we might ask the question, "Who tells the homunculus which decisions to make?" The response to this question, if we rely on the homuncular self theory, is another homunculus within the homunculus, and a homunculus within that homunculus, and on and on in an infinite regression of homunculi within homunculi.

The other answer, of course, is to evoke a superanthropomorphic being and an enormous homunculus somewhere in the cosmos, called a god, who directs the smaller homunculi that we call the selves or souls.

Sir James Frazer cites several examples of cultures that subscribe to the homuncular model for explaining the soul. He refers to this phenomenon as "the soul as a mannikin." Many people believe that animals have life because there is a little animal inside each one that makes it move around. When the animal sleeps, the little animal has gone for a while, just as when a man sleeps, the little man has gone elsewhere temporarily. It is this little mannikin that experiences life after death. Individuals in some cultures believe that the homunculus is exactly the same as the individual, including relative weight and height, a tiny replica of the person.

> The Hurons thought that the soul had a head and body, arms and legs; in short, that it was a complete little model of the man himself. The esquimaux believe that "the soul exhibits the same shape as the body it belongs to, but is of a more subtle and ethereal nature." According to the Nootkas the soul has the shape of a tiny man; its seat is the crown of the head. . . . Among the Indian tribes of the Lower Fraser River, man is held to have four souls, of which the principal one has the form of a mannikin, while the other three are shadows of it. The Malays conceive the human soul as a little man, mostly invisible and of the bigness of a thumb, who corresponds exactly in shape, proportion, and even in complexion to the man in whose body he resides. [13:pp. 207–208]

On our first encounter with the homuncular model specifically stated, it seems like a quaint and archaic concept, but it was and continues to be the predominant concept in Western cultures, although we pride ourselves upon objectivity. We do not at present specify the dimensions and attributes of the anthropomorphic *I*, but we still assume that there is a real entity within the body, whether we call it self, soul, ego, or personality, that guides and directs our operations "consciously or unconsciously." Speculations about this "person within" are well documented in Greek literature and continue to be the leading philosophic orientation of human behavior through the medieval religious period, the Age of Reason, and the Freudian revolution.

The first three intellectual geniuses who turned philosophic speculation from the external world of nature to the internal world of man were Socrates, Plato, and Aristotle, who epitomize the Golden era of Greek Philosophy, when the principal preoccupation was anthropocentrism. The fourth and fifth centuries B.C. are known as the anthropocentric, or metaphysical, period [21].

Socrates (470–399 B.C.) believed fervently that the only true philosophy was that in which the mind investigated itself, as is evidenced by his famous pronouncement, *"Ghothi seauton,"* or, "Know thyself." In this conviction we see a shift from the attention to the material world, which had fascinated the physical philosophers, such as Empedocles and Pythagoras, to an obsession with the mind of man. Socrates attracted a following of young men who, under his direction, began to examine the self, or soul.

Socrates is often credited with being the first philosopher to describe the soul in the form we have kept until today. Homer Smith reports that some scholars

> . . . argue that Socrates was the first to formulate the immortal soul which possesses consciousness, which is the seat of knowledge and error, and which is responsible for a man's thought and actions. . . . The Socratic soul, if it may be so designated, was a new spiritual entity which, far from being fragmentary and inferior in power to the animal body, was by virtue of its prerogative of domination entitled to a definitely superior status. [25:pp. 148–149]

The Socratic conception of an immortal soul was based on the belief that the soul was made of an indestructible substance that had always existed and would continue to exist. The spirit or self was unchangeable, being in essence divine [25].

The Sophists also appeared during the fifth century B.C. and proclaimed that the study of man was the only legitimate philosophic endeavor. They were led by Protagoras of Abdera (481–411 B.C.) and Gorgias of Leontini (483–375 B.C.). The byword for Protagoras was: "Man is the measure of all things." Gorgias was convinced that man can never know anything at all, because all reality consists of subjective experience, which cannot be taught [21].

Although man was the center of study for both the Sophists and Socrates, the prevailing difference was that the Sophists were convinced that certainty and truth were unavailable to anyone, and Socrates directed all his energies toward formulating concepts of truth. In his search for truth, Socrates led many of the young men of Athens away from the polytheistic beliefs of their fathers, a practice that resulted in his eventual condemnation and death by suicide. Socrates did believe in one god and held the idea that death was not the end of the self. This is suggested in the remark made to his sorrowing friends just before he died, "Be of good cheer and say that you are burying my body only" [9:p. 10].

Socrates himself wrote nothing, and we are aware of his teachings only through the work of Xenephon, Aristophanes, and Plato.

Plato believed that individual souls existed before they entered human bodies and that the soul was dragged down or debased by union with a body. Since the soul freely entered the body, it could also leave it and would continue its existence after the body had gone. Once the soul chose a body, it struggled to free itself and return to the star from which it came. If the soul failed in its attempts, it was destined to move from one body to another [18].

> The ultimate goal of life, according to Plato, is release of the soul from the body so that it may return to its star and there spend eternity contemplating the beautiful and pure world of ideas. But, whether or not the soul succeeds in becoming free from matter and its evils, it cannot be destroyed. The eternal pre-existence and immortality of the soul is a fundamental doctrine of Plato. [18:pp. 175–176]

Plato, as we have already stated, contributed his ideas of an immortal soul to Western thought and made the nature of man the object of much of his philosophic speculations. He conjectured at length about human knowledge, desire, and emotion and concluded that eros, or desire, is the force that motivates all human action and thought. He divided the human soul into three principles—the rational, which is located in the head; the irrascible, which is in the breast; and the concupiscible, or instinctive, which is located in the bowels.

Plato contended that the body is only a shadow of the soul and that the soul constitutes the true man. The *soma* (body) is the *sema* (sepulcher) of the *psyche* (soul). The soul exists before birth and after death. The soul forgets the ideas it had before joining with a body but can recollect these through the senses. Philosophy professor Nicholas A. Horvath gives an explanation of this phenomenon, which is reminiscent of the analytic process of making the unconscious conscious:

> Before entering its body, the soul forgets the Ideas it once saw face to face. Yet the imperfect copies of Ideas in the World of Sense suggest its own past to the soul, reminding the soul of what it has seen before. Hence all knowledge is reminiscence (anamnesis), and all learning is reawakening. Thus our concept of values—such as our notions of the true, of the beautiful, and of the good, as well as certain mathematical and logical notions, such as those of being and non-being, identity and difference, unity and plurality—is due to recollection. [21:p. 32]

Roback and Kiernan discuss the importance of Plato's doctrine of the soul to psychological thought, equating Plato's appetitive soul to Freud's id, his *thumos* to Freud's ego, and his pure reasoning soul to Freud's superego [24]. Alexander and Selesnick also suggest a comparison of Freudian concepts with Plato's idea of the soul. In their discourse on Platonic doctrine, they write:

> The whole body is ruled by the rational soul. The souls freely communicate by means of the bodily organs. The basic idea is that in the lower parts the psychological and physiological processes are chaotic and undirected, and they receive their organization and direction from the highest functions or reason. One cannot but be reminded of Freud's concept of the chaotic "id" that gradually comes more and more under the organizing power of the "ego." [1:p. 36]

These historians also compare Plato's and Freud's dream theories. They conclude that Freud might not have been directly influenced by Plato's writings but that the Greek philosopher's views had such profound effect upon

Western thinking that they were necessarily reflected in the subsequent development of psychological concepts.

Aristotle saw man as being endowed with creative reason, which is divine in origin. He taught that all living things have souls and placed them in a hierarchy of lowest to highest—from plant souls to human souls. Everything in the universe, including the soul, is composed of matter and form, the form realizing itself in the matter. The human soul, which is rated as superior to all other souls because of its ability to think and reason, is divided into creative reason (form) and passive reason (matter). Since only the creative reason is divine, it is the only part of the soul that survives death. Upon death, the creative reason rejoins God. There is no personal immortality for the individual.

Aristotle believed that the passions of man, his lower functions, are controlled by the mind. He described the senses and maintained that the heart receives all perceptions and is, therefore, the organ central to the senses. He was a major contributor to psychological theory concerning the content of consciousness. Alexander and Selesnick write:

> He (Aristotle) distinguished, obviously on the basis of introspective observation, between sensation, conation (striving), and affection. The affections are desire, anger, fear, courage, envy, joy, hatred, and pity, a list which hardly needs additions. The descriptions of these different affective states are as good as the modern ones, with the possible exception of Spinoza's descriptions, and in some respects more complete than those of modern psychologists. [1:p. 37]

Although Will Durant argues that Aristotle's god was not the simple anthropomorphic god of earlier philosophers, he also calls the divinity as represented by Aristotle a "self-conscious spirit." This god, being perfect and without desire, does nothing but think upon the essence of things. God, therefore, being himself the essence of everything, has nothing to do but contemplate his own nature. It would seem, then, that the god of Aristotle was without doubt an advocate of self-analysis, certainly an anthropomorphic endeavor.

Post-Aristotelian Greek philosophy is divided by Horvath into the Anthropocentric, or Ethical Period, and the Theocentric, or Religious Period. The major schools of thought in the Ethical Period include Stoicism, Epicureanism, Skepticism, and Eclecticism, all of which address the soul of man and advocate various ways in which he should lead his life. They hold differing views as to the immortality of the soul.

The homuncular model is of prime importance in the thinking of some of the great medieval philosophers, who saw the soul as leading a separate existence, created by God and immortal. Saint Augustine's belief that the soul is the essence of man and merely inhabits a human body for a short period of time is clearly a validation of the *I* as being separate from the body, an inner person directing the activities of the earthly body. There is a pronounced affiliation between Augustine's advocacy of right conduct as the key to eternal bliss and the teachings of Zeno the Stoic, which labeled all sensory pleasure as evil and considered the soul as the source of all judgment and perception. As the soul wills, so man acts. As the "person within" makes the decisions, so the fate of the individual is determined.

Augustine (354–430) believed that the soul is a substance, both spiritual and immortal. He also leaned toward the idea of Traducianism—that the soul emanates from the souls of the parents. This is in contrast with Creationism, which held that God created each soul separately. He believed that the union of the body and soul is of primary importance because the soul is the protector of the body and must guard over it constantly. Soul and body are two separate and different substances, and the body is clearly not equal to the soul. Man is a spiritual soul occupying an earthly body [21].

Augustine did not know how the soul came into being but did not believe that it existed before the body as did Plato. He did believe that, once the soul was born, it could not die. How it lived after death depended upon what kind of life the individual had lived during his earthly habitation. The body was a danger to the soul because it could lead the spirit into activities that would condemn it to eternal misery [18].

Throughout the Dark Ages, the prevalent belief was in a soul that was undoubtedly immortal and whose ultimate destiny was influenced by the activities it experienced while inhabiting a human body. Self-appraisal was essential in determining what was good and what was bad for each person. Saint Augustine spent much of his life in self-appraisal, and his writings reveal his lifelong struggle with his own passions, a struggle that eventuated in his attacking all his opponents as he attacked that which he abhorred within himself. Saint Augustine is important to the history of psychoanalytic thought because his *Confessions* are an excellent example of psychological thinking in order to construct and justify a belief system. He recounts vividly the experiences and subsequent mental machinations that arose from his conflict between love of pleasure and the desire for discipline. He believed that all men should study the inner being and be psychologically aware so that they can alter their behavior accordingly.

> In his *Confessions*, psychology becomes real and concrete; in contrast to the abstract descriptions of Plato and Aristotle, it assumes flesh and blood. St. Augustine's psychology tells about the feelings, conflicts, and anguish of an individual of greatest sincerity and introspective power, and can be justly considered as the earliest forerunner of psychoanalysis. [1:p. 59]

Saint Thomas Aquinas believed that body and soul are separate and that the soul lives apart from the body, continuing to exist after death of the body and continuing to act, forming for itself an eternal spiritual body. He did not acknowledge that the brain played any part in the activities of the soul.

Aquinas refined the early Christian beliefs concerning the soul into the one presently fundamental to Christianity. The human soul is added to the body at birth and is the creation of God. It is different from all other spirits because it has intelligence and can will. The soul continues to exist and to act after the body is destroyed. After death, it forms for itself a new spiritual body, and in that form, it functions throughout eternity [18].

The period of religious medieval philosophy is remarkable and important to any history of self concepts in its affirmation of the separation of soul and body, with the soul using the body, its declaration of the primacy of faith over intellect, and the assertion of a close relationship between theory and philosophy [21].

Science and the Soul

When we enter the Renaissance period of the fifteenth and sixteenth centuries, we notice an attempt to separate philosophy and theory and increasing interest in the scientific study of man and nature. Francis Bacon clearly wished to break with the past when he suggested that the human soul is composed of two souls, a divine, or rational, one and an irrational one. He taught that the divine soul was the province of religion but that the irrational soul, which he deemed the seat of memory, will, appetite, understanding, imagination, and reason, was a fit subject for scientific study. He also believed that this soul was located in the head and utilized nerve pathways to reach all parts of the body. It could not be seen but was, nonetheless, material [18].

In discussing the writings of Bacon, Durant notes:

> Nothing is beneath science, nor above it. Sorceries, dream predictions, telepathic communications, "psychical phenomena" in general must be subjected to scientific examination; "for it is not known in what cases, and how far, effects attributed to superstition participate of natural causes." [9:pp. 122–123]

Here we find clearly stated a mandate to examine the soul, or person within, using scientific methods.

Bacon was acutely aware of the influence upon the human mind of prejudices, preconceived opinions, and generalizations. He was also cognizant of the limitations of the individual. He wrote:

> For it is a false assertion that the sense of man is the measure of things. On the contrary, all perceptions, as well as the senses of the mind, are according to the measure of the individual and not according to the measure of the universe. And the human understanding is like a false mirror, which, receiving rays irregularly, distorts and discolors the nature of things by mingling its own nature with it. [2:p. 88]

Knowledge of human fallibility did not, however, diminish Bacon's belief in the sovereignty of man and in the power of the human mind to interpret nature:

> So assuredly the very contemplation of things as they are, without superstition or imposture, error or confusion, is in itself more worthy than all the fruit of invention. . . . Only let the human race recover the right over nature which belongs to it by divine bequest, and let power be given it; the exercise thereof will be governed by sound reason and true religion. . . . For interpretation is the true and natural work of the mind when freed from impediments. [2:pp. 157–158]

Thomas Hobbes went even further than Bacon in moving away from religious medieval philosophy by declaring that, since the universe is material in its entirety, nothing like the human soul as previously described by early philosophers could possibly exist after the destruction of the body.

Hobbes preferred to leave speculations about the soul to the theologians and tried to construct a materialistic system of explaining all phenomena. He included the mind by referring everything to the brain. He believed that all human emotions were a result of movements of the body and that sensory experiences produced all our ideas.

René Descartes was dissatisfied with the materialistic and mechanistic universe that seemed a logical result of scientific endeavor. He wanted to justify the existence of the human soul and, at the same time, take into consideration all the demands of science. In developing a theory that completely separated body and mind, he validated once again the homuncular model. Charles Furst explains:

> Descartes used the soul to explain intelligent brain function: there is something like an intelligent creature in your brain which sees what needs to be done and then pulls the right strings. Descartes did not concern himself with the question of just how intelligence works in a physical sense, since at that time intelligence was regarded as a purely spiritual property. [19:p. 17]

Essentially, Descartes' theory was that there was one absolute substance, God. In addition to God, there were two relative substances, mind and body. Descartes' originality was in his speculations about the nature of the union of the mind and body, which he believed to be conceptually separate. To explain the actions of the human being, he proclaimed that the mind and the body interacted in the pineal body at the base of the brain.

Descartes viewed the soul of the individual as being the thinking substance that, when confronted with sensory experiences, caused the body to react. This confrontation or interaction occurred in the pineal body. He wrote:

> Let us then conceive here that the soul has its principal seat in the little gland which exists in the middle of the brain, from whence it radiates forth through all the remainder of the body by means of the animal spirits, nerves, and even the blood, which, participating in the impressions of the spirits, can carry them by the arteries into all the members. [8:p. 93]

However successful or unsuccessful Descartes might have been in explaining the interaction of mind and body, he was, nonetheless, much preoccupied with the self concept and with the description of man as a thinking creature. In his *Discourse on Method*, he wrote:

> And as I observed that this truth, *I think, hence I am,* was so certain and of such evidence, that no ground of doubt, however extravagant, could be alleged by the skeptics capable of shaking it, I concluded that I might, without scruple, accept it as the first principle of the philosophy of which I was in search. [7:p. 186]

Durant indicates that, with Descartes and his theory of a machinelike body containing a spiritual soul (the ghost within the machine), philosophy entered into a period of 300 years' war, the principal war game being epistemology, the nature and origin of knowledge. This is total immersion in an anthropomorphic word world, notably that portion of the word world composing the me block, or inner world of man. What is the soul, self, or personality, and how can it know anything?

We see the ushering in of an age of contention between modern science and mystical medieval beliefs that necessarily required introspection, an examination of the self concept in relation to the world. Many philosophers saw the examination of human nature, the soul or person within, as supremely important to an understanding of the external world. [22] Alexander and Selesnick view this as a natural result of the debate between science and religion:

> This age of contradictions, the age of division between medieval mysticism and modern science—favored introspection. Doubt, leading to inner conflict, forces man to turn toward his own self in his attempt to resolve this puzzling contradiction in his mind. [1:p. 92]

Baruch Spinoza tried to solve the problem by "saving face" for both the adherents of natural science and the believers in a mystical soul within. He espoused the view that God is the only substance and the soul is part of this divine system. It is possible to study a human being from the side of the body or the side of the mind. Since the mind, or soul, is a mode of God, it is not regulated by the same laws as the body. The soul is subject to spiritual laws and the body to material or scientific laws [15]. Spinoza wrote:

> Our mind, insofar as it understands, is an eternal mode of thinking, which is determined by another mode of thinking, and this one again by another, and so on to infinity; so that they all constitute at the time the eternal and infinite intellect of God. . . . The human mind cannot be absolutely destroyed with the human body, but there is some part of it which remains eternal. [9:pp. 187–188]

Gottfried Wilhelm von Leibniz attempted to bring together in some sort of harmonic pattern all the past philosophic positions. He conceived the doctrine of monads, in which substance manifests itself in monads of individual forces, the highest of which is the human soul. The chief purpose of the soul monad is to systematize all the other monads of the organism into a unified whole. Since monads cannot influence each other, God has created them so that there is a preexistent harmony between all the other monads and the soul monad. All knowledge is implicit within the soul. Experiences serve the purpose of moving the soul to a realization of what it already knows [18,21].

Descartes, Spinoza, and Leibniz laid the foundation for modern philosophy. They were all Rationalists in that they believed reason to be the source of all knowledge. The other school of classic modern philosophy, Empiricism, is represented by Bacon, Hobbes, Locke, Berkeley, and Hume, who held to the conviction that all knowledge emanates from experience [21]. Locke, Berkeley, and Hume are considered the three patriarchs of British empiricism [24].

John Locke thought that two substances, bodies and souls, compose the universe. The body and the soul influence each other. The soul influences the body to move, and the body influences the soul to have ideas. Whether the soul is immortal is a matter of faith and has nothing to do with reason. There are no innate ideas within the soul. Ideas stem from internal experiences (reflections) and external experiences (sensations). The soul is spiritual and immaterial and is the thinking substance [18,21].

George Berkeley used the terms *mind* and *soul* interchangeably and took the position that nothing exists outside the mind. God is also mind and is the creator of all ideas not created by the individual mind. A thing does not exist unless it is perceived. His slogan was *"Esse est percipi"* (To be is to be perceived). A sound cannot exist unless it is heard. He also believed that the mind is immortal, as it is the alpha and omega of the universe [24].

David Hume was a skeptic who saw the self, or *I*, as being synonomous with sensations. He held the position that we can prove neither the existence of a soul or inner world nor the existence of an external world. All we can know is a succession of ideas or perceptions. It is useless to discuss the immortality of a soul because there can be no proof that one exists.

Immanuel Kant tried to create a system of thought that would unify Rationalism and Empiricism. Horvath is of the opinion that he failed in this endeavor, that he did not succeed in bringing together reason and experience. Frost believes that Kant did accomplish the task of giving us a system that drew the schools of thought together. About Kant's belief system, Frost writes:

> Since there can be no knowledge without a knower, it is legitimate for us to conclude that there is such a thing as a soul, and act as if it existed. Although we cannot prove the existence of an immortal soul, we may act as though one existed since there is real value in so doing. Kant held that this idea has regulative use in that it unifies many of our concepts, it systematizes many of our concepts or ideas. The idea of a soul serves as a focal point to which we may refer our conscious experiences. [18:p. 187]

Although Kant, with his "as if" paradigm, was condemned by his contemporaries for destroying both science and religion rather than unifying them, Durant sees his work as being influential to the point that all the "philosophic thought of the nineteenth century revolved around his speculations" [9:p. 291].

Kant argued that there is a real world of noumena (things in themselves), but we can be aware of this world only in causal, spatial, and temporal terms. The philosophers who followed immediately upon Kant scoffed at the noumena. Kant's ideas gained more credence in the later nineteenth and on into the twentieth centuries [28].

Three German philosophers, Johann Gottlieb Fichte, Friedrich Wilhelm von Schelling, and Georg Wilhelm Hegel developed Kant's teachings further in becoming the leaders of German Idealism. Fichte took as the beginning premise for his philosophy Kant's idea that one can act as if there is a world beyond science, basing this contention upon moral law. Fichte taught that the will, or ego, is the source and creator of the world. Each individual ego is immortal and lives after the body is destroyed. The universal ego is the creative principle of which each individual ego is a personification.

In *The Vocation of Man*, Fichte gives an eloquent defense of the premise that man must strive to know himself, that to achieve insight is commendable.

> But I shall open my eyes, shall learn thoroughly to know myself, shall recognize that constraint; this is my vocation. I shall thus—and, under that supposi-

tion, I shall necessarily—form my own mode of thought. . . . I am wholly my own creation. . . . My whole mode of thought, and the cultivation that my understanding receives, as well as the objects to which I direct it, depend entirely on myself. True insight is merit; the perversion of my capacity for knowledge—thoughtlessness, obscurity, error, and unbelief—guilt. [11:pp. 496–497]

Fichte, in picturing man as being part of the universal ego, maintained that two aspects emerge—the self of which the person is aware and the non-ego, or everything the person thinks of as other than himself [23].

Schelling espoused a pantheistic doctrine in which the universe, or God, is a living spirit that pervades all things. Inorganic nature is made of the same substance as the human mind. Man is conscious of himself through an awakened mind, and nature, as manifested in rocks, trees, and earth, is unconscious or asleep. Although he viewed all of nature as living and attempting to realize itself, only man achieves full self-consciousness. As Frost explains it, the difference between the living material world for Schelling and the human mind is one of degree only [18]. The world is directed by an all-pervasive will or universal force.

The Unconscious

This concept of a metaphysical universal ego, or will, underlying all phenomena is extremely momentous in the later development of the idea of an unconscious by the great philosophers of psychology. Alexander and Selesnick make the point:

> This extension of the concept of will to all phenomena of nature carried with it of necessity the concept of the unconscious. Indeed the term "unconscious" was used by several authors as an alternative for the "universal will" of the natural philosophers. [1:p. 169]

Another aspect of Schelling's philosophical thought that is worthy of comment is his attention to the binary paradigm, or split-level universe. He was very much aware of natural polarities, such as night and day, force and matter, and, especially, male and female, which he viewed as being a polarity of the utmost importance throughout all the natural world [10].

In discussing the influence of Schelling on modern dynamic psychiatry, Ellenberger quotes at least two authorities who have made comparisons of the philosophic approaches of Jung and Freud with the philosophy of Schelling.

> Leibbrand said that "C. G. Jung's teachings in the field of psychology are not intelligible if they are not connected with Schelling." . . . Jones has also observed that Freud's concepts of mental life were dominated by polarities (dualism of instincts, polarities of subject-object, pleasure-unpleasure, active-passive), and he adds that a peculiar feature of Freud's thinking, throughout his life, was "his constant proclivity to dualistic ideas." [10:p. 204]

Hegel, the third great leader of German Idealism, validated the importance of the idea of polar opposites by contending that the most significant universal relation is that of opposition, or contrast. He maintained that the purpose of the mind is to discover the unifying principles that are potential in all the diversities of nature [9,20].

Hegel taught that everything in the universe can be comprehended in terms of an objective, or absolute, mind, which is constantly attempting to reach some degree of synthesis. The evolution of the world can be explained as the absolute mind evolving to higher stages through a logical process, which Popkin and Stroll describe:

> The "logical" development is the famous Hegelian dialectic, wherein each attempt to formulate something about the universe (a thesis), is contradicted by another formulation (an antithesis), and the conflict between the two is resolved in a proposition which incorporates the partial truth of both of them (the synthesis). [23:p. 89]

We are aware of the manifestation of the Hegelian dialectic in his teachings concerning the evolution of the mind (as interpreted by Frost).

> For him [Hegel], mind passes through three stages of evolution: subjective mind, objective mind, and absolute mind. The subjective mind is dependent upon nature as soul, is opposed to nature as consciousness, and is reconciled with nature as spirit. At its highest, mind is creative of the world which it knows. [18:p. 273]

The same dialectical process occurs in the mind that occurs in nature. The human mind is replete with opposites, which it undertakes to reconcile by securing a synthesis. The resultant synthesis is superior to the presenting contradiction in that it is on a higher level. By the synthesizing process, man is able to realize more complex ideas because he retains the values of both the thesis and the antithesis [23].

Arthur Schopenhauer departed somewhat from the Kantian position that man can become aware of the phenomenal world as a thing in itself by differentiating between them. He defined the phenomenal world as one of representations and the world of the thing in itself as will. The entire universe is the result of a primal will. This will is supreme in man and directs all his actions. Man is a miniature of the universe, a reduced pattern of the primal creative will. As a result of this blind, driving force, man is irrational because, although he is conscious of will, he is unconscious of the internal forces or instincts of which he is a victim. The instincts are two in number—the sexual instinct and the instinct of conservation [10,18].

Durant credits Schopenhauer with the postulate that man is not the intellectual, thinking animal Kant had brought into focus but is the prey of dark and passionate forces that direct our thoughts according to desire. Although man may think that he is rational, he is but subject to the primal will. In no place is this more evident than in the sexual realm, where man repeatedly falls victim to desire and the ever-present wish to copulate. Schopenhauer wrote scathingly about women in this regard:

> It is only a man whose intellect is clouded by his sexual impulse that could give the name of the fair sex to that undersized, narrow-shouldered, broad-hipped, and short-legged race; for the whole beauty of sex is bound up with this impulse. Instead of calling them beautiful there would be more warrant for describing women as the unesthetic sex. Neither for music, nor for poetry, nor

for the fine arts, have they really and truly any sense of susceptibility; it is a mere mockery if they make a pretense of it in order to assist their endeavor to please. . . . They are incapable of taking a purely objective interest in anything. . . . The most distinguished intellect among the whole sex have never managed to produce a single achievement in the fine arts that is really genuine and original; or given to the world any work of permanent value in any sphere. [9:pp. 341–342]

Several scholars have remarked upon the similarities of the philosophical thought of Schopenhauer and Freud. Among these are Cassirer, Scheler, and Thomas Mann. Mann saw as essentially synonomous the Freudian description of the ego and the id and Schopenhauer's portrayal of the intellect and the will. Mann believed that Freud merely "translated from metaphysics into psychology" [10]. Ellenberger has also researched the writings of Luis S. Granjel and found that he

. . . says that Schopenhauer and Freud have three main points in common: an irrationalistic conception of man, the identification of the general life impulse with the sexual instinct, and their radical anthropological pessimism. These similarities, according to Granjel, cannot be explained only in terms of a direct influence of Schopenhauer upon Freud, but also in terms of the similarity in the personalities of these two thinkers: a reaction against the contemporary bourgeois society on the part of those men who, for different reasons, were permeated with resentment. [10:p. 209]

Eduard von Hartmann, in 1869, published *Philosophy of the Unconscious* in which he gave the label *the unconscious* to that phenomenon which Schelling and Schopenhauer had termed *the will*. Von Hartmann delineated between the absolute unconscious, the physiologic unconscious, and the psychological unconscious. Man's behaviors spring from the psychological unconscious.

From Soul to Psyche

The anthropomorphic word world reached a zenith in its speculations about "the unconscious" with the creative genius of Sigmund Freud. His philosophical brilliance is never more apparent than in his amalgamation of conceptual frames concerning the me block.

By using the word, we had developed a split universe and a divided world of the me and the not-me. The me, self, or soul was seen as a sacred given, or constant, and we focused our word tools in explaining how the outside world, or not-me, affected the me. We often projected the inside world, or me, block onto the external world, creating anthropomorphic selves, such as gods and demons, who ruled the external world and could affect the inside world of self, or psyche. In effect, we turned our word world inside out.

Freud developed a set of concepts that turned our word world outside in. He created a symbolic world inside the world of the psyche. With symbolic tools, or words, Freud first split the me block into the conscious and unconscious sectors. The conscious resembled the Christian concept of the soul, which the Christians had adopted from Plato's psyche. The unconscious contained the forces of evil, including sex, violence, avarice, death, and other manifestations of biologic drives.

As evidenced in the work of such thinkers as Kant, Fichte, Schopenhauer, and Schelling, philosophy, as a hypothetical study of the unknown, had fully adopted metaphysics as its domain. It was immersed in the attempt to discover the ultimate reality of everything, including "mind." Freeman and Small wrote of Freud's inclination toward philosophy:

> Philosophy was his deepest passion. He abandoned plans to study law at seventeen, changing to the field of physical science to study the mysteries of nature, inspired by Goethe's essay "Fragment upon Nature," which he heard read aloud at a popular lecture. This essay contains a spirited challenge to man to conquer nature.
>
> But though he became a physician, Freud never abandoned philosophy. When he started to write *The Interpretation of Dreams*, he commented to Fliess: "When I was young, the only thing I longed for was philosophical knowledge, and now that I am going over from medicine to psychology, I am in the process of attaining it. [14:p. 119]

Whatever Freud's proclivity for philosophic thought, the period during which he was formulating his hypotheses was one in which speculative philosophy had fallen into profound disrepute. The leading scientists of the latter part of the nineteenth century worked diligently to separate science from speculative philosophy and mysticism. Wittels explains the mood of these scientists:

> The ideal of that period was the famous Laplace man. Laplace [a mathematician] conceived of a man whose stock of knowledge should be so great that he would know at any given moment the position and the movement of all the atoms in the universe. This person would then necessarily be in the position to deduce from his knowledge the whole of the future and of the past according to the rules of mechanics; that is, of physics. . . . Laplace was a mathematician and the vision of his superman of the future is a mathematical one. [30:p. 48]

We are told that Freud consistently denied those qualities that we would term poetic and philosophical. He spoke of his own inability to understand philosophy. He was, of course, wholly aware of the scorn that the scientific world heaped upon those whom they labeled philosophers. He is reported to have often denounced fantasy and mysticism as without value and even as dangerous. He saw himself as working strictly within scientific boundaries. We may contrast the belief that Freud had a passion for philosophy with the following statement by Wittels:

> The young Freud either read philosophers not at all or with but little esteem. He says in 1925: "Even where I refrained from observation, I carefully avoided approach to actual philosophy. Constitutional incapacity rendered such self-restraint easy for me. . ." [30:p. 50]

Later on in the same chapter, Wittels asks the question, "Why not admit that Freud is also a great poet and that he could have been a great philosopher?" [30:p. 78] He speculates that perhaps Freud was afraid to pursue openly the pleasures of the philosopher or seer. He writes:

> I think that Freud, the fearless man who released the hell-hound out of Hades, is afraid of the song in his own heart. I wrote about Freud in 1923; thus: "All

great spirits are animated by the longing to look, once at least, into . . . the inner essence of things, instead of forever being content with the study of appearance. In Freud's mentality the mystical gift of the seer is continually at war with the need for mechanical description." [30:pp. 80–81]

The Viennese physicians who became aware of the cause-and-effect link that Freud made between the psychical experiences and the neuroses saw an analogy between the Freudian theories and devil possession of the Middle Ages. Their reaction was to label him a philosopher rather than a scientist.

Freud, seeing himself as a biologist and thinking in those terms, called the forces of the unconscious, drives. The sex instinct he called libidinal, and the death instinct he designated thanatos. The conscious part of the psyche was constantly buffeted by these forces from the unconscious. Freud borrowed from mythology to explore various patterns of behavior, which were later termed *complexes*. For example, the Oedipus complex was a pattern exhibited by all individuals in which the unconscious forces powered by libidinal energy urged the individual to kill the father and have sex with the mother. The similarity is evident between these concepts and the earlier medieval concepts of the soul being beset by incubi and succubi of the Devil. However, now the forces originate from inside, not outside. Some have criticized that Freud was not original but translated ancient concepts into modern terminology.

Although the scientific world was unwilling to accept the idea of psychical elements as causal agents in disease and did not even acknowledge psychogenic illness, this did not deter Freud from pursuing his course. And, even though he worked as a scientist, he did not abandon philosophy. Freeman and Small wrote:

Because of his intense wish to be a philosopher, Freud applied philosophically to mental life the concept of causality that scientists assume in investigating the physical world. He never stopped asking why. Nor, and this is perhaps his greatest quality, did he refuse to accept as answer a hunch that other men, lacking his intuition, would scorn, ignore or laugh at. His imagination, when unleashed, soared to the heights and the depths. He discarded nothing as a possibility. He considered seriously the ludicrous, the unreal. [14:pp. 120–121]

Freud continued to regard himself as an observer, whatever the opinions of the physicians of his time. He also regarded himself as having embarked upon a lonely pathway, as an innovative thinker who had chosen to devote a lifetime to a course of study that was suspect and not easily assimilated into the prevailing conceptual paradigms. He knew, for example, that psychoanalysis would never establish itself as a scientific doctrine if its creator were viewed as a philosopher only. His trials were sufficiently severe, even though he persistently denied the philosophic label and insisted that he was a scientist. In his first introductory lecture on psychoanalysis, given as one of a series at the University of Vienna in the winter sessions of 1915 and 1917, he said:

And further, if any one of you should feel dissatisfied with a merely cursory acquaintance with psychoanalysis and should wish to form a permanent connection with it, I shall not merely discourage him, but I shall actually warn him against it. For as things are at the present time, not only would the choice of such a career put an end to all chances of academic success, but, upon taking up work as a practitioner, such a man would find himself in a community which misunderstood his aims and intentions, regarded him with suspicion and hostility, and let loose upon him all the latent evil impulses harboured within it. [17:p. 20]

Freud was engaged in many struggles concerning the separation of psychoanalysis from biology and physiology. His differences with his scientific peers can be seen as a reflection of his own inner struggle between the poet-philosopher and the scientist. Wittels wrote:

Herein lies the explanation of Freud's acerbity, which has grown with the passing of the years. He is afraid of his own supreme talents, and throughout all his life as an investigator he has been imposing a curb upon himself. One who by temperament is a seer has been ardently devoting himself to the study of exact science by the ordinary methods of scientific investigation. That was why he heroically determined to study medicine, though his natural bent was toward the abstract sciences. [30:p. 80]

Today, philosophy has regained some degree of respectability in the scientific community, and such individuals as Bacon, Descartes, and Freud, among many others, are known as the philosophers of science. However, the tendency to want to defend Freud against those who would call him a philosopher, or to at least make sure we know otherwise, can be readily detected. Franklin L. Baumer, in discussing the theories of Bergson, Nietzsche, and Freud, wrote, in 1977:

He [Freud] was not, of course a philosopher, but a scientist, who, moreover, started out in the mechanist camp and tried to reduce psychology to neurophysiology. He soon discovered, however, that physiological psychology could not take him into the mysterious reaches of the mind he wanted to investigate. Freud was soon to say categorically, in a very different vein, that the unconscious, not in the least measurable or even directly observable, was "the true psychic reality." [3:p. 381]

It is true that Freud's background was in histopathology and neuropathology, that he definitely had a scientific orientation, and that he was meticulous in applying observation and stringent reasoning to the psychological phenomena he studied. It is equally correct that his theories in the field of personality were philosophic and speculative. We are not even sure why he originally entered the field of medicine. Perhaps it was through process of elimination—industry, business, medicine, or law [1].

Baumer emphasizes that, whatever Freud's problems with his peers, the climate of the times also furnished him with a support system. He points out that, by the 1870s, the idea of unconscious mental processes was commonly accepted throughout Europe. Evidently, Freud himself recognized the parallel thinking of the psychoanalysts and the intuitive insights of the philosophers. Baumer relates, too, that the world of art and literature contributed to psychoanalytic thinking, and he gives examples from Marcel Proust in literature and Odilon Redon in art.

By elaborating on the instinctual aspect of human behavior, Freud joined Copernicus and Charles Darwin in undermining the anthropocentric concepts of the not-me world. Man was placed on a continuum with other animals, dissolving the old belief that man was the center of the universe and totally unique. Freud compared himself with Copernicus and Darwin in this respect [5].

Although many of Copernicus' reasons for accepting the old Pythagorean heliocentrism were unsound, and although Darwin's theories about natural selection are not in themselves sufficient proof of biologic evolution, we must still credit both of them with revolutionizing our conceptual frameworks. J. A. C. Brown states:

> Yet inadequate, unsound, or downright wrong as some of their reasons may have been, we have regarded the world in a totally different light since we discovered our insignificant position in relation to the rest of the universe and our biological continuity with other living things, and it is not unreasonable to suggest that the transformation was completed by Freud, whose work implied that man's godlike intellect was, as H. G. Wells expressed it, "no more designed for discovering the truth than a pig's snout"! [5:p. 2]

Although Freud's brilliant intellectual theories of the mind did aid in forcing man to see himself as part of the animal kingdom and not as center of the universe, much of his terminology inadvertently reinforced the old anthropocentric model in that he focused most of his attention on the activities of the psyche. By separating the psyche from other processes, his theories allowed the continuation of a mind/body dichotomy. By developing a structural model of his psyche, that is, by division of the psyche into the ego, superego, and id, he allowed the continuation of an anthropomorphic or homunculouslike conceptual frame. His terminology led to a concretization or reification of functions. Freud cleverly reorganized concepts of our struggle with forces of the external world into a concept of our struggles with these same forces within the me block. His homuncular, or anthropomorphic, ego corresponded to the soul. The conflicts to be negotiated were within. In his paper "One of the Difficulties of Psycho-analysis" (1917), Freud wrote:

> The ego feels uneasy; it finds a limit to its power in its own house, the mind. Thoughts suddenly break in without the conscious mind knowing where they come from, nor can it do anything to drive them away. These unwelcome guests seem to be more powerful even than those which are at the ego's command; they resist all the well-proven measures instituted by the will, remain unmoved by logical rebuttal, and unaffected though reality refutes them. Or else impulses make themselves felt which seem like those of a stranger, so that the ego disowns them; yet it has to fear them and take precautions against them. The ego says to itself: "This is an illness, a foreign invasion"; it increases its vigilance, but cannot understand why it feels so strangely paralyzed. [15:p. 7]

This format can be readily identified with mythology, in which patterns of behavior are attributed to anthropomorphic entities in the realm of the psyche. Freud utilized the ancient model of personifying or reifying processes and functions. The superego, the ego, and the id struggled for dominance in the shadowy realm of the unconscious. Most of these concepts were in vogue in the Romantic period of Europe, as we have previously illustrated, but Freud's concepts resembled more those of the Greeks. He utilized mythology and mythological terminology, such as Eros, Oedipus, and narcissism, to move the gods from the outside world into the world of the soul.

Two other passages that clearly illustrate the mythological and anthropomorphic qualities of this paradigm can be found in *The Ego and the Id:*

> As a frontiers-creature, the ego tries to mediate between the world and the id, to make the id pliable to the world and, by means of its muscular activity, to make the world fall in with the wishes of the id. In point of fact it behaves like the physician during an analytic treatment: it offers itself, with the attention it pays to the real world, as a libidinal object to the id, and aims at attaching the id's libido to itself. It is not only a helper to the id: it is also a submissive slave who courts his master's love. [16:p. 56]
>
> The id, to which we finally come back, has no means of showing the ego either love or hate. It cannot say what it wants; it has achieved no unified will. Eros and the death instinct struggle within it; we have seen with what weapons the one group of instincts defends itself against the other. It would be possible to picture the id as being under the domination of the mute but powerful death instincts, which desire to be at peace and (prompted by the pleasure principle) to put Eros, the mischief-maker, to rest; but perhaps that might be to undervalue the part played by Eros. [16:p. 59]

Although Freud was careful to dissociate his theories from the ideas of demoniac possession that are a part of our conceptual heritage, the anthropomorphic nature of his concepts closely resembles demonology, even those he used to establish his paradigm as scientific. For example, he wrote:

> Psychiatry, it is true, denies that such things mean the intrusion into the mind of evil spirits from without; beyond this, however, it can only say with a shrug: "Degeneracy, hereditary disposition, constitutional inferiority!" Psycho-analysis sets out to explain these eerie disorders; it engages in scrupulous and laborious investigations, devises hypotheses and scientific expedients, until at length it can say to the ego: "Nothing has entered into you from without; a part of the activity of your own mind has been withdrawn from your knowledge and from the command of your will. . . . The blame, I must tell you, lies with yourself. You overestimated your strength when you thought you could do as you liked with your sexual instincts and could utterly ignore their aims. The result is that they have rebelled and have gone their own way in the dark to rid themselves of this oppression; they have extorted their rights in a manner you cannot sanction." . . . But these two discoveries—that the life of the sexual instincts cannot be totally restrained, and that mental processes are in themselves unconscious and only reach the ego and come under its control through incomplete and untrustworthy perceptions—amount to a statement that *the ego is not master in its own house.* [15:pp. 7–9]

In the unconscious lurked all the demoniac forces of myth and religion, forces as horrendous to some elements of the Victorian world as they had been to the Christian church because the driving force of evil was sex, or libidinal energy. The overwhelming drive for sexual expression powered the development of personality or characteristics of that fragile entity called the ego, which struggled to maintain its dignity and boundaries while buffeted by unconscious forces from the id and the punitive rule-making superego, derived from social or parental pressures. The ego, as a pilgrim, must contend with the demons of the id, chief of which was the desire to destroy one parent and have sex with the other. These concepts were as emotionally disturbing to individuals at the turn of the century as the Devil of the external world creating lust via demons had been during the Dark Ages.

Freud's emphasis on libidinal energy as flowing through the psychical apparatus and attaching itself to introjected objects, ideational patterns, or erogenous zones made an exceptionally functional, pragmatic model for clinical use. However, this type of energy was precluded from evaluation in scientific experiments because it could not be measured.

The "scrupulous and laborious investigations" Freud carried out used words as the instruments. Perhaps Freud's greatest contribution was his extraordinary studies of the human symbolic operation. With his work in dream studies and free association, he demonstrated the enormous fluidity of words and symbols and the tremendous variation in information contained in these symbols when used during human communication. Although his work has been used as an illustration of predictable patterns of human behavior motivated by instinctual drives, the same work indicates the relativity of words in any information exchange. In using the human symbolic operation to describe the human symbolic operation, one becomes aware of the potential for an infinite regression of meaning about meaning about meaning.

Using the binary system of conscious and unconscious, Freud developed a "word world within," in which symbols, fantasies, and dreams were used to construct word descriptions of the unconscious. In free association, which is a modified form of the trance, the subject is encouraged to say anything that comes into his "mind." Words and the association of words then became the central focus of study. Although Freud was a biologist and neurologist, his primary emphasis was on the symbols of the cultural system. For example, the vehicle of free association is used with the implication that anxiety is due to intrapsychic conflicts between biologic drives and social pressures.

It is not surprising that Freud chose the world of words as the focus of his scientific inquiry. He was known to be extremely gifted verbally. Ellenberger commented:

> Freud can also be understood as a man of letters. He possessed the attributes of a great writer to a supreme degree. First he had linguistic and verbal gifts, the love of his native language, a richness of vocabulary, the *Sprachgefühl* (feeling for the language) that infallibly led him to choose the appropriate word. Even his articles on histology are written in magnificent style. [10:p. 466]

Freud was familiar with many great literary works and believed that the great writers and poets had explored the human mind before the psychologists. He quoted from Shakespeare, the Greek tragedians, Goethe, Schiller, and others. Just as gifted writers can lead one through series of events fraught with meaning, Freud led his disciples through a world of words to build an anthropomorphic theory in which every slip of the tongue, any chance word or garbled dream, had symbolic meaning reflecting deep currents in the unconscious.

In Search of the Psyche

Freud's use of words and symbols as instruments of investigation of the human psyche led to the arduous system of therapy known as *psychoanalysis*. In this system, the analyst is endowed with the knowledge and technique required to interpret the meanings of the symbolic world. He functions in somewhat the same capacity as the astrologers, shamen, and priests who interpreted the meanings of the stars, read the intestines of animals, and prophesied according to events in nature. Just as the seeker after prophetic knowledge had to believe in the power of the priest or shaman, the seeker after self-knowledge has to believe in the ability of the analyst to lead him through the dark caverns of the unconscious and to control the intense relationship (transference) that evolves between him and the analyst. The success of the analyst, as that of any shaman or healer, is in large part dependent on the patient's perception of him as being possessed of the knowledge necessary to effect healing.

In order to ensure that the analyst be properly trained in the accepted beliefs and techniques, a program of intensive indoctrination is required. The trainee or candidate must himself undergo the process of psychoanalysis and must enter a program that is expensive, very long, and extremely difficult. Because of the length of time required for the analysis and the program of study, most candidates must go into debt and must devote a great deal of their time to the institute in which they are enrolled [12]. Psychoanalysis involves months or years of frequent sessions in which the analysand (candidate) "is in duty bound 'to tell everything which passes through his mind, even if it is unpleasant to him, even though it seems to him to be unimportant, irrelevant, or absurd' [Freud]. . . . A unity is created in the form of participation called by Freud transference, out of the group of two in which psychoanalysis takes place, a unity that is first felt and afterward becomes understood" [30:pp. 322–323].

Several scholars have noted the similarity between the training analysis and thought reform. This has resulted in labeling the analysis a very powerful indoctrination method. The candidate, or analysand, is put through exactly the same process as the patient's experience. All of the teaching staff and all of the other trainees are consistent in their viewpoints and may be called "true believers." The candidate permits a complete review and interpretation of his life, with his thoughts and feelings undergoing the interpretation of the analyst. All interpretation will, of course, reflect the prevailing doctrines of the institute.

Jerome Frank, author of *Persuasion and Healing*, notes that the entire process of the training analysis encourages, over a period of several years, improvisation, participation, and repetition, three factors he claims are necessary to produce changes in attitude. The analysis, or training phase, is not considered successful or complete until the analysand can satisfy the analyst that he is now a sufficient believer in the institute's doctrines to carry on the tradition [12]. Wittels also remarks upon the importance of this process. He calls psychoanalysis an artistic science rather than a pure science and emphasizes that it cannot be learned from books but must be experienced or "felt" [30].

Any tendency on the part of a candidate to disagree with the tenets of the institute is labeled resistance. Any criticism of the interpretations of the teaching analyst can be dismissed as being based on transference. The trainees tend to spend their time with the training staff and with each other and, in so doing, reinforce their beliefs and their investment in the entire training process. This promotes a type of conviction analogous to that achieved through religious conversion [12].

Frank is most emphatic in his suggestion of a similarity between religious conversion and the training analysis:

> The founders of institutional psychotherapeutic training must ask themselves whether the demand for a training analysis does not sometimes hide something like a demand for a declaration of faith and the vindication of something that pertains more to the preservation of a sect than to a public form of therapy. [12:p. 173]

Perhaps this type of indoctrination is necessary to ensure the belief of the therapist in his own powers of persuasion. Whether or not one conceptualizes psychoanalysis as a religious format, it becomes obvious that anyone electing to remain within the training program must emerge fully convinced of his own powers of interpretation and of the validity of the theories upon which psychoanalysis is based. The theoretical validity of these theories cannot, as a matter of fact, be disproved. This in itself gives tremendous impetus to the candidate to continue his belief in the entire system.

In addition to having at his disposal a theoretical set that cannot be disproved, the analyst can always gather from his patients the material necessary to validate his views. Patients may be selected according to their suitability for analysis. If they do not respond well, that is, fail to improve, the failure may be excused because of the unsuitability of the patient. Any criticism of the tenets of psychoanalysis may be viewed as the ignorance of the untrained individual. Analytic theory can always be made to fit the situation. Regarding this phenomenon, Frank says:

> The validity of analytic hypotheses cannot be tested by making predictions from them and determining whether the predictions are confirmed. For no matter how the test comes out, analytic theory can explain the results. Freud's handling of the discovery that traumatic experiences in infancy, which formed a cornerstone of psychoanalytic theory, were often fabrications, illustrates this point. [12:p. 178]

When Freud was confronted with the fact that some of his patients had confabulated their infantile memories, he refused to let it undermine his faith in the analysis or to discredit the patient. He said that "these phantasies possess *psychological* reality in contrast to *physical* reality" and "*in the realm of neurosis the psychological reality is the determining factor*" [12:p. 174].

Ellenberger stresses that psychoanalytic theory has not yet achieved scientific status. He compares Freud's situation with that of Mesmer, explaining that while Mesmer's theories were being debated, discoveries made in the field of physics at the same time were accepted. Although discoveries made in such fields as endocrinology and bacteriology during Freud's time are treated as scientific doctrine today, Freud's theories are questioned by many epistemologists and experimental psychologists. He says, "This paradox has brought many Freudians to view psychoanalysis as a discipline that stands outside the field of experimental science and more akin to history, philosophy, linguistics, or as a variety of hermeneutics" [10:p. 549].

Ellenberger believes the three foremost contributions of Freud to be the psychoanalytic organization, the psychoanalytic theory, and the psychoanalytic method:

> But Freud's most striking novelty was probably the founding of a "school" according to a pattern that had no parallel in modern times but is a revival of the old philosophical schools of Greco-Roman antiquity. . . . The similarity between the psychoanalytic and the Greco-Roman philosophical schools was reinforced after the imposition of an initiation in the form of the training analysis. Not only does the training analysis demand a heavy financial sacrifice, but also a surrender of privacy and of the whole self. By this means a follower is integrated into the Society more indissolubly than ever was a Pythagorian, Stoic, or Epicurean in his own organization. . . . We are thus led to view Freud's most striking achievement in the revival of the Greco-Roman type of philosophical schools, and this is no doubt a noteworthy event in the history of modern culture. [10:p. 550]

The psychoanalytic theories concerning the nature of the human soul or psyche had an enormous impact upon the world of philosophical thought and changed our ideas of ourselves. These theories are still being debated and continue to be controversial with regard both to their scientific validity and to their use as a treatment paradigm in the form of psychoanalysis and related therapies. In regard to these questions, Ellenberger answers:

> To undergo a successful psychoanalysis thus amounts to a journey through the unconscious, a journey from which a man necessarily emerges with a modified personality. But this in turn leads to a dilemma. Psychoanalysts proclaim that their method is superior to any other kind of therapy, being the only one able to restructure personality. On the other hand, an increasing number of limitations, contra-indications, dangers, have been pointed out by Freud and his successors. Could it be that psychoanalysis, as a therapy, will come to be replaced by other less laborious and more effective therapies, whereas a few privileged men will afford it as a unique experience apt to change their outlook upon the world, their fellowmen, and themselves? [10:pp. 524–525]

Dr. Jeffrey Moussiaeff Masson is a Berkeley psychoanalyst selected by Anna Freud as director of the project to publish for the first time her father's complete letters to his closest confidante, Wilhelm Fliess, and to others. In addressing a meeting of the Western New England Psychoanalytic Society at Yale University in June 1981, he declared:

> By shifting the emphasis from a real world of sadness, misery and cruelty, to an internal stage on which actors performed invented dramas for an invisible audience of their own creation, Freud began a trend away from the real world that, it seems to me, has come to a dead halt in the present-day sterility of psychoanalysis throughout the world. [4:p. F3]

Robert J. Trotter, in an article titled "Psychiatry for the 80's" in the May 30, 1981, issue of *Science News*, wrote an account of the 1981 meeting of the American Psychiatric Association in New Orleans which contains the following:

> And it seemed obvious that the legacy of Freud—the myth of psychoanalysis—is being abandoned for the potential precision of biology, as Freud predicted it would. The talk at the meeting was not of psychodynamic theory and

Oedipal complexes but of psychopharmacology and brain chemicals. Strict diagnostic techniques and procedures are being combined with increasingly sophisticated and selective drug treatments to bring about more effective therapies. [27:p. 348]

Freud's work does join that of Copernicus and Darwin in deemphasizing man as a unique entity and allowing him to rejoin the animal kingdom. His work has also been used to concretize an anthropomorphic symbolic operation. Freud's studies emphasized that a great deal of information, if not most of the information, processed within the human central nervous system is not in the cognitive or conscious operation. He called these processes "unconscious" and hoped that some of them could be explored and translated to the cognitive frame of reference and symbolized in words. Unfortunately, some of his devotees have inadvertently implied that the unconscious is an entity that has a word language, that is, a purposeful symbolic operation that often threatens the conscious symbolic operation. This gives a homuncular or anthropomorphic nature to the unconscious by implying that it is a discrete entity with its own conscious, purposeful processes.

If one takes the anthropomorphic reification approach to Freud's theories, his work becomes the apex of the old word world in which symbols and meanings are dominant. If one accepts the fluidity and relativity of the symbolic operation, implied throughout Freud's studies, this work heralds the new world of information processing. We can, therefore, consider the philosophic speculations of Sigmund Freud as the watershed between the anthropomorphic word world and the world of information processing.

Throughout Freud's theories there seems to be a recurrent attempt to present a mechanical or cause-and-effect sequence of psychical events. Libidinal energy is portrayed as one of the major forces driving the psychical machinery. This mechanistic approach, though subtle with Freud, reflects a major trend of the times, as we will elaborate in the next chapter.

References

1. Alexander, F, and Selesnick, S: *The History of Psychiatry: An Evaluation of Psychiatric Thought and Practice from Prehistoric Times to the Present.* New York: Harper & Row, 1966

2. Bacon, F: Novum organum (Book 1). In Commins, S, and Linscott, R (Eds): *Man and the Universe: The Philosophers of Science.* New York: Washington Square Press, 1954, pp 75–158

3. Baumer, F L: *Modern European Thought: Continuity and Change in Ideas, 1600–1950.* New York: Macmillan, 1977

4. Blumenthal, R: How important was Freud's theory reversal? *The Daily Progress,* Charlottesville, Virginia, August 30, 1981, p F3 (from New York Times News Services)

5. Brown, J A C: *Freud and the Post-Freudians.* Baltimore, Maryland: Penguin Books, 1961

6. Comfort, A: *I and That: Notes on the Biology of Religion.* New York: Crown, 1979

7. Descartes, R: Discourse on method. In Commins, S, and Linscott, R, (Eds): *Man and the Universe: The Philosophers of Science.* New York: Washington Square Press, 1954, pp 163–220

8. Descartes, R: Supplementary passages from *The Passions of the Soul*. In Beardsley, M (Ed): *The European Philosophers from Descartes to Nietzsche*. New York: Random House, 1960, pp 25–96

9. Durant, W: *The Story of Philosophy: The Lives and Opinions of the Greater Philosophers*. New York: Washington Square Press, 1953

10. Ellenberger, H F: *The Discovery of the Unconscious*. New York: Basic Books, 1970

11. Fichte, J G: The vocation of man. In Beardsley, M (Ed): *The European Philosophers from Descartes to Nietsche*. New York: Random House, 1960, pp 490–531

12. Frank, J: *Persuasion and Healing*. Baltimore, Maryland: Johns Hopkins University Press, 1961

13. Frazer, J: *The Golden Bough*. New York: Macmillan, 1922

14. Freeman, L, and Small, M: *The Story of Psychoanalysis*. New York: Pocket Books, 1960

15. Freud, S: *On Creativity and the Unconscious: Papers on the Psychology of Art, Literature, Love, Religion*. New York: Harper & Brothers, 1958

16. Freud, S.: *The Ego and the Id*, Strackey, J (Translator and Editor). New York: W. W. Norton, 1960

17. Freud, S: *A General Introduction to Psychoanalysis*. New York: Washington Square Press, 1952

18. Frost, S: *Ideas of the Great Philosophers: A Survey of Their Basic Teachings*. New York: Barnes and Noble, 1942

19. Furst, C: *Origins of the Mind: Mind-Brain Connections*. Englewood Cliffs, New Jersey: Prentice-Hall, 1979

20. Hegel, G H F: Supplementary passage from the phenomenology of spirit. In Beardsley, M (Ed): *The European Philosophers from Descartes to Nietzsche*. New York: Random House, 1960, pp 636–639

21. Horvath, N A: *Essentials of Philosophy: Hellenes to Heidegger*. Woodbury, New York: Barron's Educational Series, 1974

22. Hyde, W: *The Five Great Philosophies of Life*. Toronto, Canada: Collier Books, 1962

23. Popkin, R, and Stroll, A: *Philosophy Made Simple*. Garden City, New York: Doubleday, 1956

24. Roback, A, and Kiernan, T: *Pictorial History of Psychology and Psychiatry*. New York: Philosophical Library, 1969

25. Smith, H: *Man and His Gods*. New York: Grosset and Dunlap, 1952

26. St. Augustine: *City of God*. Garden City, New York: Image Books, 1958

27. Trotter, R J: Psychiatry for the 80's. *Science News, Volume 119*, May 30, 1981, pp 348–349

28. Wertheimer, M: *A Brief History of Psychology*. New York: Holt, Rinehart and Winston, 1970

29. Whitehead, A N: *Adventures of Ideas*. New York: Mentor, 1955

30. Wittels, F: *Freud and His Time*. New York: Grossett and Dunlap, 1931

The Anthropomorphic World of Words

Benediction

And now, my Brothers and Sisters in Christ, I must tell you that as sure as God makes the sun to rise each morning, and as sure as He created each and every insect, every plant, every animal to be of service to man, whom He created in His likeness, no sparrow shall fall, no flower will wither without His consent. The spirits of the rocks, trees, and rivers all obey Him. Since those seven days in the Beginning, His movement can be seen in all things. And, if we depart from His way, if we fail to give Him the glory, Satan, the Fallen Angel, the King of Darkness, will bind our hearts and chain our souls in the everlasting torment of hellfire. Let us not revel in the vain glory of those ever-present temptations to separate ourselves from God in the service of man's knowledge. Call it science, philosophy, or what you will, it is the same path, that path taken by Eve in the Beginning in search of knowledge, that led to man's fall from grace and all the evils that now befall us. Let us turn away from the broad and atheistic road and scientific self-conceit and deceit, to that straight and narrow path of simple faith that led the saints to sing in God's presence forever.

I bid you peace.

Amen

*The Mechanical World
of
Form and Function*

Chapter 5

Knowledge in Numbers

Most remarkable among archaeoastronomy's revelations is the universality of this intellectual awakening in mankind. Both interest in the sky and skills in astronomy seem to have developed independently and naturally on different continents in different eras among peoples as unrelated in time and character as the builders of Stonehenge and the cliff dwellers of the American Southwest. Some attempts at astronomy dead-ended, others flowered into sophisticated cosmologies, and still others borrowed concepts and techniques from contemporary cultures. But all seem intended as a response to the human desire to fix man's place in the universe, to control the vast and frightening environment by understanding it. [12:pp. 11–12]

James Cornell, 1981

A sense of strong personal aesthetic delight derives from the phenomenon that can be termed order out of chaos. To some extent the whole object of mathematics is to create order where previously chaos seemed to reign, to extract structure and invariance from the midst of disarray and turmoil. [13:p. 172]

Philip J. Davis and Reuben Hersh, 1981

The Language of Numbers

Using our ability to differentiate became one of our great passions. By using word tools, we began to differentiate or interrupt the continuum of being into discrete units. We dissected our world into blocks and then attempted to put the blocks back together again. The inclination to analyze, synthesize, to interrupt the continuum, is so pronounced that we might term it an innate human property. We see small children dissecting their new toys, sometimes with disastrous consequences, attempting to reduce them to the smallest possible units and then rebuilding them so that the parts at least resemble the original wholes.

But as we progressed in our skill of differentiation and dissection, resynthesizing or integrating the parts back to the whole became a major problem. Some argued that reductionism must precede holism and that if the reductionism, or analysis, is performed with precision, the parts fit as they should back into the whole. The synthesis is accomplished easily if the analysis is done correctly.

In order to dissect accurately, we developed a new type of language, the language of measurement, or numbers. With this language we found comfort, because the units were discrete and differentiated and at the same time fit neatly into harmonic wholes. If the world could be translated into these units, we could comfortably analyze phenomena into minute packages that could then be realigned or synthesized into well-fitting patterns, with the whole always equal to the sum of its parts. To some extent this new language resembled the phenomenon of music, in that separate notes harmonized with other notes into pleasing patterns.

The world of words was constantly refined by the language of numbers. Discrete blocks could be aligned in a cause-and-effect sequence, with the blocks and sequences measured by mathematics. As we became more aware of dynamic processes within our internal and external environments, we conceptualized the construction of both the internal world and the external world as precise organizations of well-defined forms functioning in a matrix of space and time governed by the immutable laws of nature.

Mathematics was more than a tool for quantitating, differentiating, and integrating—it was the language of relationships, and not just random relationships, but periodic or harmonic relationships. Mathematics provided the format for ordering and appreciating patterns or systems. Our need for certainty led to our assumption that all relationships could be organized by using periodic patterns of wholes validated by repeated observation.

If, at times, the whole did not resemble the sum of its parts, the measurer or observer reasoned that the measurements and/or observations were in error and so set about measuring again. The language of measurement progressed from comparing the units in the external world with the number of fingers on a hand, steps from the cave to the watering place, and times between full moons, to light years of distance and microseconds of time measured by instruments. Our models were ever more complex and expansive until we learned to address even the ultrasmall and the ultralarge.

Many individuals became dissatisfied with the simplistic approach to the internal and external environments afforded by the anthropomorphic models of philosophy and religion. Their frame of reference moved away from man as the ultimate in the universe to numbers and pointer readings as the basic denominators of knowing.

We were still using our imagination to describe events, but with numbers, we could conceive relationships that seemed to prove cause and effect and sequential alignment of phenomena that, otherwise, could not be understood in any rational way. Alfred North Whitehead said, "The originality of mathematics consists in the fact that in mathematical science connections between things are exhibited which, apart from the agency of human reason, are extremely unobvious." [31:p. 25]. Using the language of numbers, we could perform experiments that, when repeated, sometimes gave the same results, lending credibility to our speculations. We found new sources of power in the complex and seemingly infallible world of mathematical proof.

> The symbol is the tool which gives man his power, and it is the same tool whether the symbols are images or words, mathematical signs or mesons. And the symbols have a reach and a roundness that goes beyond their literal and practical meaning. They are the rich concepts under which the mind gathers

many particulars into one name, and many instances into one general induction. . . . . When a man counts "one, two, three," he is not only doing mathematics; he is on the path of the mysticism of numbers in Pythagoras and Vitruvius and Kepler, to the Trinity and the signs of the zodiac. [8:pp. 28–29]

The evolution of numbers and mathematics allowed a much more predictable unitization of our symbolic operation than was possible in the world of those immeasurable word symbols used in religion, mythology, and philosophy. The standard unitization as reflected in numerical relationships, influences, and entities was destined to become our most refined attempt to modulate or further refine our symbolic operation.

Words were modulated by numbers. Numbers helped to quantify relationships into standardized frequencies. They also gave a certain exactness or implicitness to thoughts that were otherwise rather abstract. As Whitehead wrote, "By comparison with language, we can now see what is the function in thought which is performed by pure mathematics. It is a resolute attempt to go the whole way in the direction of complete analysis, so as to separate the elements of mere matter of fact from the purely abstract conditions which they exemplify" [31:p. 30].

At first, numbers were used to reify and modify entities. Instead of stating "wheat" or "large amounts of wheat," one could say "one bushel of wheat" or "ten bushels of wheat." Being able to count made relationships appear more logical. By using numerical instruments, our power of reason was augmented so that we might say definitively that two bushels of wheat plus two bushels of wheat equals four bushels of wheat. This statement could be validated by anyone who had learned to use the numerical language.

In Western civilizations, reliance on measurement, unitization, and cause-and-effect sequencing culminated in the conviction that everything would yield to standardized measurements and that, by using this language tool of mathematics, the laws of nature could be translated into our word world. This philosophic attitude was enormously enhanced by the work of physicists and astronomers, as well as by mathematicians.

It is impossible to set a single date for the time when people began counting. Evidence suggests that we have counted in every culture, just as we have talked in every culture. Every language has given some suggestion of numbers, and even the most primitive languages provide evidence of at least an acquaintance with the concept of numbers. Although historians and archeologists have pursued the question of the origin of numbers with great diligence, no general agreement has been reached. Many mathematicians express perplexity as to the controversy that has occasionally arisen concerning the origin of numbers, feeling that such argument is of little practical value. Levi Conant has said, "The origin of number would in itself, then, appear to be beyond the proper limits of inquiry; and the primitive conception of number to be fundamental with human thought" [10:p. 433].

Historians do agree that the propensity to count goes back very, very far, so far that it seems futile to attempt to pinpoint the origin of numbers to any particular time in prehistory. The futility of this effort has not discouraged individuals from attempting to discover its origins, however. Although the question of the origin of numbers will probably remain forever unsolved, we do have evidence that counting has been of prime importance to us for thousands of years. H. G. Wells took his account back in prehistory to at least the time of Neolithic man.

> And Neolithic man was counting, and falling under the spell of numbers. There are savage languages that have no word for any number above five. Some people cannot go above two. But Neolithic man in the lands of his origin in Asia and Africa even more than in Europe was already counting his accumulating possessions. He was beginning to use tallies, and wondering at the triangularity of three, and the squareness of four, and why some quantities like twelve were easy to divide in all sorts of ways, and others, like thirteen, impossible. Twelve became a noble, generous, and familiar number to him, and thirteen rather an outcast and disreputable one. [30:p. 105]

Alexander Marshack of Harvard University's Peabody Museum is a journalist who has spent some fifteen years looking for examples of how prehistoric man measured time. Although his findings are controversial, he believes that he has evidence that systems for marking time were in use more than 30,000 years ago, 25,000 years before the hieroglyphics of Egypt and the cuneiform of Mesopotamia. Marshack also claims that an engraved bone tool found in Ishango in the Congo and believed to be 8500 years old is carved with lines representing lunar phases. The discoverer of the tool has interpreted the lines as a type of arithmetical game [12]. Although we will probably never be certain of the exact interpretation of the markings on the engraved bone, we can surmise that they represent either some recognition of periodicity or some primitive method of counting.

The earliest counting must have been accomplished through the use of sign language, which is always the precursor of intelligible speech. Conant writes, "It may, indeed, be stated as a universal law, that some practical method of numeration has, in the childhood of every nation or tribe, preceded the formation of numeral words" [10:pp. 434–435].

We can also speculate with some degree of certainty that the number 1 was represented by a finger and that finger counting was the foremost method used by all primitive peoples. All research up to the present time has validated this belief. In addition to using the fingers to count, it has been common to number events or items by representing them with notches on a stick, kernels of corn, heaps of grain, pebbles, seashells, or whatever object is easily available. Such methods of keeping track of events or numbering items is still in use today all over the world: The gunfighters of the Old American West are reputed to have carved notches on their guns, and German students are reported to count the number of beers they drink by chalk marks on the wall or table [10].

Just as individuals learn to speak words before they learn to write them, we learned first to count by using the words before we learned to write symbols. The word sound *three* was in use long before the written numeral *3*. The first civilization to leave any record of a numeral system was the Sumerian of Mesopotamia. We can surmise that they had a system of numerals in use 5000 years ago, about 3000 B.C. The Sumerians are credited with the invention of number symbols, and histories of arithmetic begin with that era. They, as all ancient peoples, used the numeral 1 just as we do today, a basic numeral that probably originated in that form as representative of one finger [26].

Scholars differ about the origin of mathematics, although the difference may be in the realm of semantics. Louis J. Halle regards the Mesopotamians as the founders of mathematics. His definition of mathematics includes the statement:

> Mathematics defines relationships among quantities abstractly conceived, and in so doing provides logical procedures for determining those relationships—as when it defines the relationships between the length of a right-angle triangle's longest side and that of its remaining perimeter, thereby providing a procedure for determining the one, in the case of any particular triangle, on the basis of knowing the other. [17:p. 349]

He emphasizes that the Mesopotamians were able to deal with numbers as abstract concepts rather than as adjectives needing word symbols of tangible objects for completion.

Jacob Bronowski implies a difference between the origin of arithmetic and of mathematics, saying, "Arithmetic, like language, begins in legend" [7:p. 155]. He views Pythagoras as the originator of mathematics, which he defines as "reasoning with numbers" [7:p. 155].

Eric Bell defines arithmetic as a field of mathematics, so he might, therefore, view the Sumerian numeral system as the origin of mathematics [4]. Philip Davis and Reuben Hersh claim, "The mainstream of western mathematics as a systematic pursuit has its origin in Egypt and Mesopotamia" [13:p. 9].

The earliest accounts of Sumerian numbers on record are those dealing with amounts of produce passing in and out of the temple storerooms. Before 2500 B.C., the Sumerians were using multiplication tables for determining areas of fields. They did this by multiplying a field's breadth by its length. They also estimated volumes of things by multiplying the height, breadth, and length of the container. They could roughly calculate the area of a circle and the volume of a cylinder, taking the value of pi as 3 [20].

The Sumerians developed a sexagesimal (rather than decimal) system. They also solved linear equations and laid the foundations of algebra. By 2000 B.C., the Sumerians had been conquered and the ruling power in Mesopotamia was the Semitic Hammurabi dynasty of Babylon. In the temple schools set up to train priestly administrators, mathematics was developed even further. Fractions were now represented in the same way as the Sumerians had designated integers. The Babylonians could divide and drew up tables of reciprocals, the squares of numbers, their square roots, and cube roots. They solved problems involving cubic and quadratic equations. Babylonian geometry had a distinctively algebraic character. The Babylonians antedated Pythagoras in their knowledge of right-angled triangles, and they were aware that all triangles inscribed in a semicircle were right-angled [17,20].

The Egyptians of the same time contributed a better value for pi, 256/81, but their mathematics in general was not as sophisticated as that of the Babylonians. The Egyptians were not familiar with the properties of right-angled triangles. They also lacked knowledge of some of the procedures that were inherent in the numerical system of the Babylonians. From about 3000 B.C., the Egyptians used a numeral system based upon the number 10.

Our main source of information concerning Egyptian mathematics is the Rhind papyrus, purchased in Egypt in 1858 by A. Henry Rhind. It is a scroll written by a scribe named Ahmes, and it contains a collection of mathematical exercises. "The Rhind Papyrus," writes James R. Newman, "though it demonstrates the inability of the Egyptians to generalize and their penchant for clinging to cumbersome calculating processes, proves that they were remarkably pertinacious in solving everyday problems of arithmetic and mensuration, that they were not devoid of imagination in contriving algebraic puzzles, and that they were uncommonly skillful in making do with the awkward methods they employed" [21:p. 178].

In our exploration of the world of mathematics and the development of the language of numbers, we will now make a leap in time from over 2000 B.C. to the years between 600 and 400 B.C. We will also make a geographical jump from Mesopotamia to Ionia, which is often considered the birthplace of science as we know it today.

The first scholar to make major contributions in the field of mathematics was Thales of Miletus, ca. 625–545 B.C., who was familiar with geometric theorems and astronomy. He is credited with presenting us with the first proof in the history of mathematics, the proof that a circle is bisected by its diameter. According to Davis and Hersh, "The genius of the act was to understand that a proof is possible and necessary. What makes mathematical proof more than mere pendantry is its application in situations where the statements made are far less transparent. In the opinion of some, the name of the mathematics game is proof; no proof, no mathematics" [13:p. 147].

If this be so, then we must certainly credit Thales with being the founder of mathematics.

Thales also learned how to measure the height of a pyramid from the length of its shadow and the angle of the sun above the horizon and to prove that the angles at the base of an isosceles triangle are equal. These types of calculations led some scholars to become increasingly obsessed with numbers, observations, measurements, and speculations.

Thales assumes a particular importance to our brief history of the evolution of our self concept because of the attitude with which he observed and measured the world around him. Thales removed the gods from nature, viewing natural events as impersonal and subject to objective measurement and prediction. From this time on, many of the Greeks continued to speculate upon the world in a much more mechanistic and impersonal way than was possible when the gods were considered to be powerful beings who, at any whim, could alter the course of nature.

The Greek credited with having the profoundest influence upon Western scientific thought is Pythagoras, a pupil of Thales, who first applied the word *cosmos* as a descriptive term denoting harmony and order. Pythagoras was a mathematician and mystic who believed that there were definite laws of nature that one could discover by thought. The language he used was the language of numbers, numbers being the language of nature. All the universe could be explained through mathematics.

The enthusiastic followers of Pythagoras formed a society or brotherhood called the Order of the Pythagoreans. Its influence was felt far beyond the borders of Ionia. They were not experimenters, but in the tradition of their master, they were mathematical mystics who were certain that, with the language of numbers, they could discover the only true reality, which was composed of mathematical relationships not easily discernible to our perception, but there nonetheless. The Pythagoreans were fanatic in their allegiance to their founder and justified their pronouncements by the phrase, "The Master said so."

Harmony in Form and Function

The basic relationship between mathematics and musical harmony that Pythagoras determined to exist convinced the Pythagoreans that all of nature was composed of simple harmonic numbers. The movement of the planets was the music of the spheres.

> [Pythagoras] surmised that one way of explaining reality was by measurable relationships, relationships of proportion, that accorded with logically definable natural laws and could be expressed in numerical terms. Every aspect of music, for example, can be described in such terms, for music does obey mathematical laws and may therefore be regarded as simply one expression of the mathematics that govern and explain the universe. . . . The order that stands opposed to chaos is a mathematical order. [17:p. 417]

Philolaus of Tarentum, a Pythagorean, is reputed to have said, "You can see the power of number exercising itself not only in the affairs of demons and of gods, but in all the acts and thoughts of men, in all handicrafts, and in music" [20:p. 28].

To the Pythagoreans, all nature was filled with music, whose component parts are rhythm and harmony. Plato, who was greatly influenced by Pythagoras, believed that classical music was imitative of the principles of nature [23].

These simple harmonic numbers had, for the Pythagoreans, a geometrical shape as well as a quantitative size. Numbers, therefore, were the images and forms of natural objects. Pythagoras saw the numerical relations in the shapes of nature, such as waves and animal and human bodies. He combined what we now call geometry and numbers to prove that the world of vision is ruled by exact numbers just as is the world of sound. This effort was of incalculable importance in validating the exalted position of space or form in the natural order. Numbers assume form. Numbers compose the stuff of nature. The forms of nature are, therefore, subject to the exact laws of mathematics. Bronowski explains the visual method Pythagoras must have used to prove the Pythagorean theorem:

> To this day, the theorem of Pythagoras remains the most important single theorem in the whole of mathematics. That seems a bold and extraordinary thing to say, yet it is not extravagant; because what Pythagoras established is a fundamental characterization of the space in which we move, and it is the first time that is translated into numbers. And the exact fit of the numbers describes the exact laws that bind the universe.
>
> The point is that the theorem of Pythagoras in the form in which I have proved it is an elucidation of the symmetry of plane space. . . . And space is just as crucial a part of nature as matter is, even if like the air—it is invisible;

that is what the science of geometry is about. Symmetry is not merely a descriptive nicety; like other thoughts in Pythagoras, it penetrates to the harmony in nature. [7:pp. 160–161]

The Pythagorean doctrine that numbers, which assumed shapes, lie at the base of the real world, has had far-reaching consequences. According to Whitehead:

Owing to the Greek mode of representing numbers by patterns of dots, the notions of number and of geometrical configuration are less separated than with us. Also, Pythagoras, without doubt, included the shape-iness of shape, which is an impure mathematical entity. So to-day, when Einstein and his followers proclaim that physical facts, such as gravitation, are to be construed as exhibitions of local peculiarities of spatio-temporal properties, they are following the pure Pythagorean tradition. [31:p. 28]

In discussing the influence of mathematics upon general thought, Whitehead claims that the 200-year period from Pythagoras to Plato has had the most profound effect. It was during this time that the Greeks set the stage for science and outlined the shape or character of scientific thought. John Burnet concurs with this opinion: "It is an adequate description of science to say that it is thinking about the world in the Greek way. That is why science has never existed except among peoples who came under the influence of Greece" [25:p. 102].

Those philosophers who had been troubled by the metaphysical nature of religious speculation concerning how the universe is organized now had the certainty of the language of numbers. As Erwin Schrödinger wrote in a discussion of the impact of Greek thought upon our scientific world picture, "About one of these fundamental features there can be no doubt. It is the hypothesis that *the display of Nature can be understood*. . . . It is the non-spiritistic, the non-superstitious, the non-magical outlook" [25:p. 103].

The world of words was quickly augmented by the world of relationships for many of those engaged in the search for certainty. Plato believed that mathematics was the ultimate form of all knowledge. It is the Greek influence, primarily through Plato, that has led to the widespread and commonly held belief that, unless knowledge assumes mathematical form, it may not be classified as knowledge at all [22].

Through the use of mathematics, we reified the relationships between the absolutes of mass, energy, space, and time. We were able to use the language of numbers to describe events in a linear sequence of cause and effect. We were able to unequivocally divide the world into form and function and to prove the existence of mathematical, harmonic relationships that reified our theories concerning form and function.

Scientific scholars became engulfed in a spiral of logic and increasing certainty about the quantification of relationships among absolute entities that lead to concepts of truths that could be validated. These truths were termed *laws*. We could, with the use of observation, measurement, and logical reasoning, know the laws of nature. This belief in the infallibility of mathematical proof reified the ever-present hope that the whole world was indeed the sum of its parts. All the entities that composed the whole of nature could be reduced to their smallest parts, studied and understood, and rebuilt.

We had within our grasp the number tools necessary for total comprehension.

The idea of a god or gods responsible for form and function was, to Plato, the idea of a god who realized an intellectual, rational design for the universe. The world is composed of numbers and is under the sovereignty of mathematical regularities. Supposedly, Plato's reply to the question, "What does God do?", was "God always geometrizes" [28,15]. The universe, to Plato, was essentially mathematical, and the philosophy of mathematics was the philosophy of geometry.

> For Plato, the mission of philosophy was to discover true knowledge behind the veil of opinion and appearance, the change and illusion of the temporal world. In this task, mathematics had a central place, for mathematical knowledge was the outstanding example of knowledge independent of sense experience, knowledge of eternal and necessary truths. [13:p. 325]

We can extrapolate from this reasoning the implication that mathematical proofs and truth are synonomous, that the world of the senses can be realized and understood by means of mathematics.

Euclid, one of the finest of analysts, wrote thirteen books on mathematics, the eighth book proving "the constructions for the five regular solids of Pythagoras, extolled by Plato; and it ends with the dodecahedron, the symbol of the Universe itself" [28:p. 101]. The appearance of these volumes and their corresponding acclaim gave us the Euclid myth, which is defined by Davis and Hersh:

> It is the belief that the books of Euclid contain truths about the universe which are clear and indubitable. Starting from self-evident truths, and proceeding by rigorous proof, Euclid arrives at knowledge which is certain, objective, and eternal. Even now, it seems that most educated people believe in the Euclid myth. . . . It has been the major support for metaphysical philosophy, that is, for philosophy which sought to establish some a priori certainty about the nature of the universe. [13:p. 325]

The world of mathematics rested on the foundation of geometrical certainty, and geometry was considered an area of unassailable knowledge. Geometry, the study of the properties of space, supplied proof that these properties "existed absolutely and independently, were objectively given, and were the supreme example of properties of the universe which were exact, eternal, and knowable with certainty by the human mind" [13:p. 330].

Johannnes Kepler (1571–1630) was to reify this point of view in his belief that the geometry of the Greeks was synonomous with mathematics and that the theorems of Euclid were infallible. In his *Harmonice Mundi* (*Harmony of the World*), he wrote, "Geometry existed before the Creation, is co-eternal with the mind of God, is God himself" [5:p. 15]. He also wrote, "Thus God himself was too kind to remain idle and began to play the game of signatures signing his likeness unto the world; therefore I chance to think all nature and the graceful sky are symbolised in the art of Geometria" [5:p. 28].

Carl F. von Weizsacker credits Kepler and Galileo with the initiation of modern mathematical science and its "belief in the strict validity of the mathematical laws of nature" [29:p. 317].

René Descartes (1596–1650), Galileo's greatest contemporary, made considerable advancement in mathematical technique with the invention of coordinate geometry. He applied geometry to the measurement of matter, velocity, and time, developing the idea that time and mass are the basic dimensions of the world. He apparently altered this concept, however, and concentrated on extension and motion. He said, "Give me motion and extension and I will construct the world" [20:p. 169].

Descartes presented a mechanical world view, with man seen as a machine ruled by the same laws as all of nature. "For Descartes, the physical and organic world was a homogeneous mechanical system composed of qualitatively similar entities, each following the quantitative mechanical laws revealed by the analysis of the mathematical method" [20:p. 171]. He espoused a belief in absolute certainty and saw mathematical knowledge as the prime example of certainty and universality. "The rules of nature," he wrote, "are the rules of mechanics" [20:p. 172]. Descartes is credited with being the first to be a consistent believer in the idea of natural laws and the first to consistently use the phrase *laws of nature*.

Sir Isaac Newton (1642–1727), considered by many to be the monarch of the Age of Reason, gave tremendous impetus to the idea of a world that could be revealed to us through the use of mathematical tools. He believed that the universe was a riddle whose clues were to be found in the constitution of the elements and the evidence of the heavens. John Maynard Keynes, in "Newton, the Man," wrote:

> He regarded the universe as a cryptogram set by the Almighty—just as he himself wrapt the discovery of the calculus in a cryptogram when he communicated with Leibnitz. By pure thought, by concentration of mind, the riddle, he believed, would be revealed to the initiate. . . . And he believed that by the same powers of his introspective imagination he would read the riddle of the Godhead, the riddle of past and future events divinely fore-ordained, the riddle of the elements and their constitution from an original undifferentiated first matter, the riddle of health and of immortality. [19:p. 278]

The mechanical world view, the idea that all natural phenomena can be described in terms of simple forces between unalterable objects is, according to Albert Einstein and Leopold Infeld, evident in all scientific endeavors. Hermann von Helmholtz clearly formulated the mechanical view:

> Finally, therefore, we discover the problem of physical material science to be to refer natural phenomena back to unchangeable attractive and repulsive forces whose intensity depends wholly upon distance. The solubility of this problem is the condition of the complete comprehensibility of nature. [16:p. 54]

The idea of a comprehensible universe of mathematical design composed of the absolute quantities of mass, energy, space, and time has persisted to the twentieth century and is reflected in our world picture. The measurers and the calculators, in their search for certainty, used the language of numbers to build a world subject to reductionism and open to experiment and proof.

The mathematicians were joined in their efforts to explain the universe by those observers known as astronomers. They also searched for cause and effect and a linear sequencing of events in the study of the heavens.

Bronowski says, "It is natural to come to astronomy straight from mathematics; after all, astronomy was developed first, and became a model for all the other sciences, just because it could be turned into exact numbers" [7:p. 189].

Natural Periodicities

Astronomy, which can be defined as the scientific study of the universe beyond the earth, was a very natural field of inquiry. It must have had its beginnings long before the time of recorded history, those beginnings rooted in our curiosity as to our place in the vastness of the universe. Fred Hoyle wrote, in discussing Stonehenge, "The intellectual activity of mankind during prehistory is a vast almost uncharted ocean. . . . There have been only about 200 generations of history (but) upwards of 10,000 generations of prehistory. . . . Among the great throng, it seems to me likely that some must have gazed up at the sky and wondered earnestly about the sun, moon, and the stars. They would have done so with a basic intelligence equal to our own" [12:p. 1]."

We in the modern world, especially those of us living in urban areas, probably have no real understanding of the fascination of the stars for early people. The artificial light in our cities prevents us from experiencing darkness in the totality with which it engulfs an individual in the forest or desert away from the more heavily populated centers. Light pollution is a man-made phenomenon most of us accept without protest. It is a problem for today's astronomers, so much so that they have difficulty finding a place for their telescopes where the atmosphere is not affected by waves of neon and mercury vapor light.

We have little need to study the heavens, even though we may be compelled to remark upon the beauty of the starry night if we are fortunate enough to be in a dark place where the stars are visible. We have ready access to calendars, clocks, watches, and compasses. Even if we do not refer to these inventions ourselves, we are reminded by the media and those around us what day it is, what time it is, what season it is, and what holiday we are currently looking forward to celebrating.

In earlier times we did not have the benefit of advanced technology. We needed the sky in a way difficult to imagine today. From cyclic celestial phenomena, we developed our clock, our calendar, and our sense of direction. It is probable that we charted or marked time by the clock of the full and new moons. From the phases of the moon, we were able to develop some understanding of the seasons. The earliest recorded reckoning of time was probably by moons and by passing generations [30].

Knowledge of the heavens was obtained by careful and prolonged observation. The viewing of celestial events had to be accompanied by a system of counting or keeping record. Early counting systems were probably very simple, consisting of lines on a cave wall or piles of stones or sticks. Some people believe that the necessity for keeping track of lunar phases is the very basis of the power of mathematics. Davis and Hersh write:

> The universe expresses itself naturally in the language of mathematics. The force of gravity diminishes as the second power of the distance; the planets go around the sun in ellipses; light travels in a straight line, or so it was thought

before Einstein. Mathematics, in this view, has evolved precisely as a symbolic counterpart of the universe. It is no wonder, then, that mathematics works; that is exactly its reason for existence. The universe has imposed mathematics upon humanity. [13:p. 68]

The observers, of necessity, used the language of numbers to record what they saw when they studied the sky. The heavens seemed to cooperate very nicely in adding to our belief that everything is subject to the laws of mathematics as evidenced in the natural periodicities of the sun, the moon, the stars, and the planets.

Homer Smith dates the origins of modern astronomy to more than 3000 years B.C., claiming for the Egyptian priests who were guardians of the temple the designation of our first astronomers [27]. In order to be aware of the flood dates for the Nile, the priests had to study the stars. Normal flooding time for the Nile began when Sothis or Sirius, the Dog Star, rose above the horizon just before dawn. The priest was quick to learn that the observation of uniformities in nature gave him power over the people who worshipped the heavenly bodies.

He [the priest] had in his possession knowledge never before available to any human being, for he could tell the people when to prepare the ground and plant the seed, when the flood would begin and when it would subside. He could measure the annual circle of the winds, the reproduction of animals, the bleeding of women, the germination of the seed, the birth of men. [27:p. 23]

Although we have no actual records of observational Egyptian astronomy, we know from the inscriptions and pictures on coffin lids what they saw in the heavens. They divided the stars of the equatorial belt into thirty-six groups and the year into thirty-six 10-day periods, each period beginning when its star group rose above the horizon just before dawn. In order to make the year come out to 365 days, they added five days to the thirty-six 10-day groups. They regulated their calendar by the rising of the star Sothis [20].

The Babylonians of the same period accomplished more in the realm of astronomy than did the Egyptians. They were very close observers of the heavens and left numerous astronomical records. They had a 360-day year divided into twelve 30-day months. The astronomers of Babylonia also left us the legacy of the 7-day week, naming the days after the sun, moon, and five planets. In addition, they divided the day into twelve double hours and the hour into sexigesimal minutes and seconds. We have also inherited, from the Babylonians, the names of the constellations of the stars and the zodiac, which they determined by mapping the constellations in the equatorial belt through which the sun passes into the twelve groups corresponding to the months [20].

Extremely accurate astronomical observations concerning the motions of the planets were made in Mesopotamia. That Venus returned to the same position five times in eight years was noted as early as 2000 B.C. From 700 B.C., these observations were systematically recorded. The Mesopotamians could predict astronomical events and could, according to world historian Stephen F. Mason, "calculate the correct average values of the main periodic phenomena of the heavens, such as the periods of the planetary revolutions" [20:p. 19]. Mason gives us good indication of the importance of astronomy in Mesopotamia to our own history.

The Mesopotamians found, for example, that lunar eclipses occur every eighteen years, the so-termed Saronic cycle. Moreover, in the fourth century B.C. they developed an algebraic method of analysing the complex periodic phenomena of the heavens into a number of simple periodic effects. They found, for example, that on the average the lunar month was twenty-nine and a quarter days, and that the deviations from this average were regular and periodic too. This method, when put into a geometrical form by the Greeks, served as the main method of analysing the motions of the heavenly bodies down to modern times. [20:p. 20]

Astronomical observations were not confined to the civilizations of Egypt and Mesopotamia. All over the world, early people gazed at the stars and noted their natural periodicities. Stonehenge, in England, was built in three phases, the first of which was estimated to have begun around 2800 B.C. [12]. The second stage of building began around 2300 B.C., and the third and final stage between 1900 and 1600 B.C. [12]. Most scholars are now willing to accept that the first phase, at least, had an astronomical orientation. In noting the importance of astronomy to our prehistoric ancestors, James Cornell writes:

Astronomy played an important, indeed central, part in their lives but it was fully integrated, not a specialized activity such as we associate with today's academic pursuit of science; preliterate astronomy was practical, immediate, and direct; and perhaps most important, . . . the experience of watching, recording, measuring, and predicting led to the development of cognitive abilities that may have laid the foundation for the development of other technologies [12:p. 82]

Astronomy appeared in all early cultures. Its importance was based upon the need for knowledge of the cycle of the seasons, so that early civilizations could fix a time for planting, harvesting, and moving their herds. Although Bronowski believes astronomy to be the first modern science to develop in the Mediterranean, he begins his discussion of astronomy with the observations made in the New World, especially by the Mayans [7]. Although the Mayans had a system of arithmetic that was ahead of the European, their observations concerning the motions of the planets were quite simple and they were chiefly concerned with the passage of time. They were not, as were the navigators of the Mediterranean, to use their knowledge of the movement of the stars as an aid in making land and ocean voyages.

We note the developments in astronomy by early people to stress the obvious human preoccupation with the appearance of periodicities in nature and the desire to construct a mathematical world that could be validated by the marking of celestial events. Although the very earliest astronomical observations of prehistoric people might not be as scientifically significant as those beginning with the Greeks, they give us some indication of our propensity to strive for predictability in the linear sequencing of events in time and space.

The influence of early cultures in the field of astronomy is clearly evident. Thales, for example, is reported to have visited Egypt and Mesopotamia, studying Egyptian geometry and Mesopotamian astronomy. Carl Sagan states, "There is a clear continuity of intellectual effort from Thales to Euclid to Isaac Newton's purchase of the *Elements of Geometry* at Stourbridge Fair in

1663 . . . the event that precipitated modern science and technology" [24:p. 176].

In their search for a knowable universe, Pythagoras and his followers developed the hypothesis of a uniform and circular motion for the sun, moon, and planets. They considered the sphere to be the most perfect geometrical solid and determined that the universe was, therefore, spherical. Since the circle was the perfect geometrical figure, the movements of all the heavenly bodies must be circular. The idea of circular and uniform motion for the celestial bodies has dominated astronomy down to the present century.

The early Greeks also assumed that the Earth was the center of the universe. A notable exception among Greek scientists was Aristarchus, who deviated from the anthropocentric model. He postulated, and was the first individual to do so, a planetary system with the sun at the center and all the planets revolving around the sun. His idea was not well received by many of his colleagues and was considered to be heretical. Mason writes:

> The views of Aristarchus were not accepted because the Greeks, in general, found it difficult to rid themselves of the conception that the earth and the heavens were entirely different in regard both to their material constitutions, and to the laws they obeyed. Such a conception entailed the view that the base earth was stationary at the centre of the universe, whilst the more perfect heavenly bodies moved uniformly in circles through the purer regions above. [20:p. 53]

Although the Greeks took the position that the earth is at the center of the planetary system, it was the theory developed by Claudius Ptolemy (85–165 A.D.) of an earth-centered universe that became the dominant theory for the next 1500 years. The Ptolemaic theory is contrasted in history with the Copernican theory of a heliocentric universe. Although Aristarchus is considered the first to formally hypothesize a sun-centered planetary system, it is Nicholas Copernicus whose name is associated with this revolutionary departure from anthropocentric thinking. It is interesting to note that the early Greek and Ptolemaic influences are still present in what Carl Sagan refers to as "a kind of geocentrism." We do not speak of the earth rising and setting but as the sun rising and setting [24].

Copernicus, explaining and defending his theory in "On the Revolutions of Celestial Spheres," wrote, "Although there are so many authorities for saying that the earth rests in the center of the world that people think the contrary supposition is ridiculous and inopinable; if, however, we consider the thing attentively, we will see that the question has not yet been decided and is by no means to be scorned" [11:p. 53]. We hear the voice of a master observer who dared to confront the anthropocentrism of his day with an opinion that was politically unacceptable but scientifically unassailable.

One of the greatest of the observers and measurers was Tycho Brahe (1546–1601), who, along with Copernicus, Kepler, Galileo, and Newton, is one of the architects of the New Astronomy [5]. Brahe's major discovery, and the one that earned him the title of Father of Modern Observational Astronomy, is that the science of astronomy must have continuous and precise data.

Today, we would not find that bit of information particularly surprising, but Brahe's attention to the minutest detail and to the concept of accuracy and objectivity were a revelation in the sixteenth century. Johannes Kepler is reported to have said that Brahe's accurate data "took such a hold of me that I nearly went out of my mind" [5:p. 22]. We should also note that Brahe's precise observations were made without the aid of a telescope. It is thought that he observed as much with the naked eye as is possible.

Kepler's famous *Rudolphine Tables*, concerning the motions of the planets, published in 1627, were based on Brahe's observations plus a new geometry that Kepler had evolved from the observations. The *Rudolphine Tables* were, for the next century, the standard charts for astronomy. Kepler also postulated three laws that were to become the fundamental building blocks upon which Newton's theories were based. We begin to see the development of our dependence upon accurate and precise data and our reliance upon proof, as Kepler noticed astronomical periodicities and used these to validate his theory that the universe is comprehensible and subject to mathematical laws.

Although the scientific method was rapidly developing, insistence by some upon the reliability of theological dogma was clearly evident. When Kepler introduced his first law in *A New Astronomy*, published in 1609, it did not win easy acceptance. The law states that all the planets move in elliptical, not circular, orbits around the sun and that the sun is not in the center of the planetary ellipses but at their foci. According to Koestler, Kepler received a letter from a clergyman and amateur astronomer named David Fabricius that said, in part, "With your ellipse you abolish the circularity and uniformity of the motions, which appears to me the more absurd the more profoundly I think about it. . . . If you could only preserve the perfect circular orbit, and justify your elliptic orbit by another little epicycle, it would be much better" [5:p. 23].

Eventually, the idea of altering data to suit the needs of the observer became almost criminal, but to Fabricius, the priority was the preservation of the old Greek notion of the perfect circular orbit. One might extrapolate that, in the seventeenth century, as evidenced by events in the lives of both Kepler and Galileo, the religious establishment took the position that the observer and not the observed was in error, if the data did not produce results consistent with preconceived opinions.

Galileo Galilei (1564–1642) is considered the creator of the modern scientific method. He built his own apparatus, the telescope (which he derived from a type of spyglass developed by Johannes Lippershey, a Dutch spectacles maker), performed his experiment, and then published the results. His results, as we have touched upon in previous chapters, were so threatening to the religious establishment that he was condemned for heresy and forced to recant his beliefs [18]. Urban VIII insisted that Galileo's position, that the ultimate test of a theory must be found in nature, was in error. As Bronowski points out, Urban VIII "blocked Galileo from stating any definite conclusion (even the negative conclusion that Ptolemy was wrong), because it would infringe the right of God to run the universe by miracle, rather than natural law" [7:p. 209]. Again, we confront the question of the old world of words and theological dogma versus the new world of relationships and natural laws. Galileo wrote, in a letter to the Grand Duchess Christina in 1615:

Some years ago as Your Serene Highness well knows, I discovered in the heavens many things that had not been seen before our own age. The novelty of these things, as well as some consequences which followed from them in contradiction to the physical notions commonly held among academic philosophers, stirred up against me no small number of professors (many of them ecclesiastics)—as if I had placed these things in the sky with my own hands in order to upset Nature and overturn the sciences. They seemed to forget that the increase of known truths stimulates the investigation, establishment, and growth of the arts. [24:p. 142]

The discovery of "known truths" was to be the primary concern of the scientific world, and despite the efforts of many to insist that the only pathway to truth was theological, the discoveries would be made as modeled by Galileo—the building of the apparatus, the actual performance of the experiment, and the publication of the results.

Galileo's trial and imprisonment did halt the scientific revolution in the Mediterranean, which then moved to Northern Europe. Belief in the scientific method, in a known universe of absolute entities, was to continue and to fluorish. The mathematicians, with their language of numbers and the astronomers, also using the tools of mathematics in making their celestial observations, continued to construct a scientifically oriented world.

Science as Master—The Reign of Certainty

Francis Bacon (1561–1626), in *The New Atlantis*, which was published in 1627 and was his unfinished last work, defined the concept of scientific progress as it was to achieve dominance in the seventeenth, eighteenth, and nineteenth centuries. In this book he told of a ship's crew that was lost at sea and found a previously unknown land where the people were supremely happy because there were no politicians and little government. Only those of a scientific bent, such as astronomers, biologists, chemists, physicists, and geologists, lived there, and they were wholly occupied in controlling nature. "The End of Our Foundation is the Knowledge of Causes and secret motions of things; and the enlargement of the bounds of human empire, to the effecting of all things possible" [27:p. 430].

Bacon foresaw a utopia in which science assumed its rightful place as the master of all things. He believed that science should be in control, that through science we could find the forms of things. By *form* Bacon meant the secret nature and inner essence of any phenomenon. He wrote, "When we speak of forms we mean nothing else than those laws and regulations of simple action which arrange and constitute any simple nature. . . . The form of heat or the form of light, therefore, means no more than the law of heat or the law of light" [15:p. 134].

Bacon advocated the accumulation of an enormous body of facts from which he would be able to collect enough information to explain all natural phenomena [2]. He felt that it was the duty of the scientist to ferret out whatever is behind the visible world of nature in the structures and processes not accessible to our sense organs. These he termed the "Latent Configurations" (those of an atomic nature) and the "Latent Processes" (the motions of the atoms or particles). From his collection of facts, he hoped to construct hypotheses and, from these, to obtain axioms of wider generality. When tested experimentally at each stage of the process, "a pyramid of scientific theory would be built up inductively, solidly based on an encyclopedia of factual information, with applications stemming off at every stage" [20:p. 145].

Hans Reichenbach says, "It was Bacon who clearly saw the indispensability of inductive inferences for scientific method, and his place in the history of philosophy is that of a prophet of induction" [22:p. 229]. The scientific method, to Bacon, was inductive, experimental, and qualitative. According to Mason, he "distrusted mathematics and the art of deductive logic that went with it" [20:pp. 146–147].

It was Descartes who was to elaborate the mathematical-deductive method that was to dominate scientific progress during the seventeenth century. He is considered by many to be the person who initiated modern science. Bacon and Descartes complemented each other, in that Descartes disregarded the role of experimentation and Bacon was not as appreciative of the role of mathematics in the scientific method. Descartes was familiar with the writings of Bacon and disagreed with the inductive method as being the best way to comprehend the world. He felt, instead, that one must begin with general principles, using these as a basis for deductive investigation. In his *Discourse on Method*, Descartes advanced four precepts as composing his system of logic:

> The first was never to accept anything for true which I did not clearly know to be such; that is to say, carefully to avoid precipitancy and prejudice, and to comprise nothing more in my judgment than what was presented to my mind so clearly and distinctly as to exclude all ground of doubt.
> The second, to divide each of the difficulties under examination into as many parts as possible, and as might be necessary for its adequate solution.
> The third, to conduct my thoughts in such order that, by commencing with objects the simplest and easiest to know, I might ascend by little and little, and, as it were, step by step, to the knowledge of the more complex; assigning in thought a certain order even to those subjects which in their own nature do not stand in a relation of antecedence and sequence.
> And the last, in every case to make enumerations so complete, and reviews so general, that I might be assured that nothing was omitted. [14:pp. 175–176]

Descartes believed that God had set the universe in motion at the creation and that it operated according to rules or laws of nature that were constant and eternal. Celestial phenomena, such as supernovae, were scientific problems subject to scientific investigation. God never interfered with the cosmic order. All natural phenomena could be explained using the deductive method of investigation. The universe is a clockwork mechanism that has been wound up by the Creator and is running according to mechanical laws.

Thomas Hobbes (1588–1679) was also a believer in sequential reasoning and the power of deductive thought. The laws of nature dictate the sequence of events, so that the end follows inexorably from the beginning. Cause must always lead to effect, and this must be without alteration along a very predictable path. If we are aware of a sufficient number of details, we can formulate exact laws that will predict in every detail. Natural phenomena can be divided indefinitely. Nature is continuous, and her mechanisms are discernible if we can divide into small enough units.

We owe to Newton the rigorous scientific method that made it possible to explore a world of absolutes and discern its eternal and unchanging laws.

The genius of Newton as a theorist and an experimenter is evidenced in the work he did in the three fields with which he is most closely associated—the nature of white light, calculus, and universal gravitation and its consequences. His work lifted science to heights never before achieved and assured science a preeminent position in the minds of almost all individuals. Ernst Mach said, in 1901, "All that has been accomplished in mechanics since his [Newton's] day has been a deductive, formal and mathematical development of mechanics on the basis of Newton's laws" [1:p. 275]. Einstein said, of Newton, "Nature to him was an open book, whose letters he could read without effort. In one person he combined the experimenter, the theorist, the mechanic and, not least, the artist in expression" [1:p. 275].

Newton's contributions to a mechanistic world view were unmistakable, "Newton stabilized the unity of mechanics," writes Carl F. von Weizsacker, "The hope of basing upon such a science the full unity of physics, indeed a universal ontology, was referred to as the mechanistic world view" [29:p. 149]. He explains further that, at times, it has seemed that the period from Newton until the end of the nineteenth century was one of "an incorporation into the mechanistic world view of ever new areas" [29:p. 149].

To Newton, space and time were absolutes, and believing that, he constructed a world system contained in a single set of laws. His theories concerning time plus the effort by mariners to make use of them at sea prompted many inventors to concentrate on building a clock that would keep accurate time on a ship. This preoccupation with time, which began with Newton, has dominated science ever since. Newton's universe was also to dominate our thinking for the next 200 years.

Newton was a solitary and lonely man, as well as a genius who knew that, even with his unparalleled accomplishments, much was yet to be done. In one of his most poignant statements, he said, "I do not know what I may appear to the world; but to myself I seem to have been only like a boy playing on the sea-shore, and diverting myself in now and then finding a smoother pebble or a prettier shell than ordinary, while the great ocean of truth lay all undiscovered before me" [7:p. 236].

Many great experimenters continued to play upon the seashores of scientific inquiry, using the deductive method to discover the laws of nature. The world of the very small fell under their scrutiny, just as the universe had come under the discriminating gaze of the astronomers. A revolution began to take place in chemistry that was to overthrow the old phlogiston theory and the ancient Greek doctrine, discussed in Chapter 2, that the four elements, earth, water, air, and fire, formed the composition of all natural substances.

It was the German iatrochemical school that produced the phlogiston theory, and it was Georg Ernst Stahl (1660–1734) who introduced the term *phlogiston* to mean the motion of heat or the motion of fire. Phlogiston can be defined as the "essential element of all combustible bodies, oils, fats, wood, charcoal, and other fuels containing particularly large amounts. The phlogis-

ton escaped when those bodies were burnt and entered either into the atmosphere or into a substance which would combine with it, like a calx which
formed a metal" [20:p. 303].

The phlogiston theory, which was purported to explain combustion and
calcination, was to meet its demise in the work of many chemists, but most
notably through the efforts of Joseph Black (1728–1799), Henry Cavendish
(1731–1810), Joseph Priestly (1733–1804), and Antoine Lavoisier (1743–
1794). Black proved the existence of carbon dioxide, "fixed air" he called it,
which had weight and which could be isolated and studied. Black's work
attracted the attention of several other chemists, including Cavendish and
Priestly, to the study of the chemical nature of gases. Cavendish wrote a
description of the preparation of "inflammable air," or hydrogen, and developed the pneumatic trough. Priestly, using the pneumatic trough, discovered
and isolated several gases, including oxygen, nitrogen, carbon monoxide,
sulfur dioxide, ammonia, nitrous oxide, nitric oxide, nitrogen dioxide, and
hydrochloric acid gas. The discovery, by Priestly and by Carl Scheele (1742–
1786), a Swedish apothecary, of oxygen was momentous, but it was Lavoisier who gave it meaning.

Lavoisier had long been searching for the active constituent of the atmosphere, and now he had it in Priestly's oxygen or "dephlogisticated air."
Lavoisier had been planning a revolution in chemistry since 1773, and in
1783, he announced the complete renovation of chemical theory. Madame
Lavoisier "ceremonially marked the beginning of the new chemistry by burning the books of Stahl and the phlogiston theorists, just as Paracelsus had
opened the iatrochemical era some two and a half centuries before by burning
the books of the medieval medical authorities" [20:p. 309].

Lavoisier's new theories concerning the composition of the elements explained the known facts of chemistry much more completely than the old
phlogiston theory, but Cavendish never gave up the phlogiston theory and
Priestly ended up writing a treatise in its defense. Cavendish was so upset by
the new chemistry that he gave up chemical work in 1785.

The work of Lavoisier, the chemical revolutionary, which owed so much
to the discoveries of Cavendish and Priestly, heralded the complete abandonment of the theory that earth, water, air, and fire were the basic elements.
Water was composed of hydrogen and oxygen, air was composed of oxygen
and nitrogen, fire could be decompounded into heat, light, and smoke, and it
was already known that there were many kinds of earth. In *Elements of
Chemistry*, published in 1789, Lavoisier listed twenty-three authentic elementary substances.

The expression of the notion of the chemical elements in atomic terms was
made by John Dalton (1766–1844). In 1803, Dalton, a Quaker scientist,
published his atomic theory for the first time, and he published a preliminary
outline from a full account in 1808 entitled *New System of Chemical Philosophy*.
In this work, concerning the arithmetic of the atoms, Dalton laid the foundation of modern atomic theory. Dalton proposed that the elements are distinguished each by only one basic property: a characteristic atomic weight.

Dmitri Ivanovich Mendeleev (1834–1907) concentrated his attention upon
the problem of how the properties that make the elements alike or different
derive from that one single basic constant, atomic weight. He systematically

and carefully arranged the elements according to their atomic weights in a *Periodic Table of the Elements*, finding, in the process, evidence for a mathematical key among them. When he came to a difficulty, he interpreted it as a "gap" and left a blank in the table. The gaps were eventually filled, as Mendeleev predicted, and the practical predictions he made were done through the process of induction as introduced by Bacon many years before. Mendeleev proved that the underlying pattern of the atoms is numerical [7].

The idea that the weight of an atom might hide some internal structure was inconceivable until the discovery of the electron by Sir Joseph John Thomson in 1897. This discovery was to mark the beginning of modern physics, for as Bronowski explains, "The place in the table that an element occupies is called its atomic number, and now that turned out to stand for a physical reality within its atom—the number of electrons there. The picture has shifted from atomic weight to atomic number, and that means, essentially, to atomic structure" [7:p. 330].

But we are getting ahead of our story. By the late 1800s, we had constructed a universe of absolutes in the world of the very large and the world of the very small, a mechanistic universe governed by the immutable and unchanging laws of nature and waiting for further discoveries to validate its existence. Science did indeed become the master and was reputed to have the answers to all problems, an idea accepted as a feature of modern times to this very day. Reichenbach says:

> The belief in science has replaced in large measure the belief in God. Even where religion was regarded as compatible with science, it was modified by the mentality of the believer in scientific truth. The period of Enlightenment, into which Kant's lifework falls, did not abandon religion; but it transformed religion into a creed of reason, it made God a mathematical scientist who knew everything because he had a perfect insight into the laws of reason. No wonder the mathematical scientist appeared as a sort of little god, whose teachings had to be accepted as exempt from doubt. All the dangers of theology, its dogmatism and its control of thought through the guaranty of certainty, reappear in a philosophy that regards science as infallible. [22:p. 44]

Scientific Discovery and Technology

Belief in scientific infallibility has been supported by the enormous technological advances that have been made using the language of numbers and the accompanying scientific discoveries [3,6]. We have always been inclined to invention and to finding some practical use for our theoretical knowledge. Although it would not be possible to list all the inventions science has allowed, a brief discussion of the progression in technology makes quite understandable the widespread belief in the world of science and its present preeminence.

The earlier scientists found it necessary to rely on their sensory impressions. Although some of them were extremely perceptive and intuitive, their sensory impressions did not allow the accurate measurement later instruments would provide. Certainly, research and rapid technological progress would rest upon the development of tools that would allow us to explore areas beyond those accessible to our senses alone.

An example of an instrument that added immeasureably to our data base is the telescope. Lippershey, as we noted earlier, is credited with being the first person to make and sell the telescope, but Galileo is the one who stepped up the magnification to thirty and began to use the telescope as a research instrument. Because of Galileo's experiences with the building of telescopes and with the subsequent research and publication of the results, he is credited with being the first "practical scientist."

The use of scientific instruments would soon realize rapid expansion. Zacharias Jansen, a Dutchman, had constructed a compound microscope before 1600. In 1648, Blaise Pascal, a French mathematician, developed a mercury barometer to measure air pressure. In 1721, a German scientist, Gabriel Daniel Fahrenheit, developed the temperature scale that bears his name. In 1742, Anders Celsius, a Swede, began to use a temperature scale of 100 degrees, the centigrade scale.

As important to the advancement of technology as the invention of various instruments was the means of disseminating the information and deciding upon what projects would be supported. The seventeenth century saw the establishment of scientific academies, which were designed as institutions to provide scientists with a forum for the exchange of ideas, publication of journals, raising of money for research, and the attempt to apply the results of the research to practical problems. Several small academies in Italy began in the early years of the seventeenth century. The two most important were the Royal Society of England (1645) and the French Academy of Sciences (1631). Both these organizations exist today, but the Royal Society of England was renamed by Charles II in 1662, when he granted it a charter as The Royal Society of London for Promoting Natural Knowledge.

Chemistry and physics were to advance rapidly, and the study of electricity became particularly important. William Gilbert (1540–1603) first used the word *electric* for the phenomenon of attraction that occurred when he rubbed amber on fur, causing the fur to attract such objects as hair and straw. He took the word *electric* from the Greek word for amber, *elektron*. Although many individuals were to experiment with electricity in the seventeenth century, little progress was made in the field until 1729, when Stephen Gray discovered that some substances would conduct electricity and others would not.

In 1745, the Leyden jar was devised, providing an electric charge for experiments. In 1752, Benjamin Franklin made his famous kite demonstration showing that lightning was electricity. With this information, he devised the lightning rod. In 1799, Count Alessandro Volta invented the battery. This was a most important development, as it allowed the steady flow of electricity for experimentation and practical use, something that had not been possible before. By the early 1800s, technological instruments were available to large numbers of researchers and inventors.

Instruments of Change

There had been a steady progression of technological advancement from the Middle Ages until the early modern period, when that advancement suddenly accelerated with tremendous speed in the Industrial Revolution. Technological development was essential to the growth of industry, and industrial requirements spurred the growth of technology in a cybernetic, or feedback, fashion. (It is common to speak of the Industrial Revolution, but this period is often divided into two periods—the first, from 1815 to 1870, the revolution of coal and iron, and the second, from 1870 to 1914, the revolution of steel and electricity.)

England was the first country to industrialize and was the foremost leader in the development of technological skills necessary for industrialization. Even before 1815, several mechanical devices were invented that revolutionized industry. John Kay invented the flying shuttle for weaving cloth. James Hargreaves devised the spinning jenny in 1767 to supply the yarn needed for the flying shuttle. In 1779, Samuel Crompton invented the spinning mule, which could spin 400 threads of fiber-type yarn and could be run by either water power or steam. In 1785, Edmund Cartwright developed the power loom, which wove cloth more efficiently than did the earlier models. Eli Whitney supplied American cotton in large quantities to the English mills through his invention of the cotton gin in 1793.

All these machines were used in the manufacture of cotton cloth. Machines had been used before this time, but machine development now escalated phenomenally. The cotton cloth industry, which doubled its output between 1700 and 1750, is only one example of the many uses that would be found for machines in the industrial nations, with their growing emphasis on mechanics. The reliability of machinery also validated the belief that anything could be done through technology if enough research was done to find the missing pieces. A growing number of individuals subscribed to the idea that everything was a type of machine, with its own form and function. The more mechanistic our approach to problems, the more likely we would find answers that could be put in a true cause-and-effect sequence.

The steam engine soon replaced water power in the textile and iron industries and provided a cost-efficient source of power that escalated industrial production. The steam engine also heralded a revolution in the development of transportation. James Rumsey, in 1785, and John Fitch, in 1790, operated steam-powered vessels, and the first steamships crossed the Atlantic in 1838. The first steam-powered locomotive was developed by Richard Trevithick (1771–1833), and upon its improvement by George Stephenson (1781–1848), the great era of railroad construction began.

Although it was Great Britian that had enjoyed supremacy in the first revolution of coal and iron, it was Germany that gained industrial sovereignty during the second revolution of steel and electricity. Germany was the primary site for the development of the internal combustion engine, the diesel engine, the automobile, the electric dynamo, and electric traction. The electrical industry was to provide the world with a new source of energy dynamos and hydroelectric power stations. The internal combustion engine provided the masses with rapid transportation, and the petroleum industry grew out of this demand. The internal combustion engine and the electric generating stations made possible the rapid industrial expansion of the United States and Europe after 1870.

With the development of the airplane, radio, the telephone, and television, the transportation and communication industries began to make significant changes in public awareness of the world of science and technology. The exchange of ideas was both more rapid and more public. Whereas the communication industry allowed contact between people of different cultures, the airplane, and the jet in particular, put those cultures within physical proximity in a matter of hours. James Burke says, "The jet aircraft has probably done more than any other modern product of science and technology to bring change to the global community" [9:p. 185].

Burke, in his book *Connections*, credits eight inventions with ushering in the modern technological age—the computer, the production line, telecommunications, the airplane, the atomic bomb, plastics, the guided rocket, and television. He traces the development of each of these and discusses their relative importance. Whether we agree with Burke as to the magnitude of the inventions he chooses to emphasize, he vividly illustrates the enormous leaps in technology that have brought us to our present dependency upon mechanical devices.

From the invention of the wheel to the first supersonic flight in 1947, the landing of Neil Armstrong on the moon in 1969, and the almost unimaginable orbits in space of our satellites, with their accompanying pictures of planets vast distances away, we have seen our faith in science rewarded. Science, the master, has indeed provided the answers. Where once we fantasied about trips to the moon, we can now make them. We have convinced ourselves that the combination of scientific research and technological invention has no limits in what it can accomplish. Bacon's dream of a scientific Utopia that reveals to man the secret nature and inner essence of all phenomena would seem to be within our realization.

The power of science to change the world in which we live has been demonstrated in its inexorable march through time to our present mechanistic world of form and function, linear sequencing, and cause-and-effect thinking. Belief in the infallibility of science has also had an enormous effect upon our concepts concerning self, mind, and body, as we shall illustrate in our next chapter concerning the development of scientific thought as it has affected our concept of living systems.

References

1. Andrade, E: Isaac Newton. In Newman, J (Ed): *The World of Mathematics*, Volume One. New York: Simon and Schuster, 1956, pp 255–276

2. Bacon, F: Novum organum, Book I. In Commins, S, and Linscott, R (Eds): *Man and the Universe: The Philosophers of Science*. New York: Washington Square Press, 1954, pp 73–158

3. Barraclough, G (Ed): *The Times Atlas of World History*. Maplewood, New Jersey: Hammond, 1978

4. Bell, E: The queen of mathematics. In Newman, J (Ed): *The World of Mathematics*, Volume One. New York: Simon and Schuster, 1956, pp 498–520

5. Bernstein, J: *Experiencing Science: Profiles in Discovery*. New York: E. P. Dutton, 1978

6. Bernstein, P, and Green, R: *History of Civilization*, Volume II: *Since 1648*. Totowa, New Jersey: Littlefield, Adams, 1976

7. Bronowski, J: *The Ascent of Man*. Boston: Little, Brown, 1973

8. Bronowski, J: *A Sense of the Future*. Cambridge, Massachusetts: MIT Press, 1977

9. Burke, J: *Connections*. Boston: Little, Brown, 1978

10. Conant, L: Counting. In Newman, J (Ed): *The World of Mathematics*, Volume One. New York: Simon and Schuster, 1956, pp 432–441

11. Copernicus, N: On the revolutions of the celestial spheres. In Commins, S, and Linscott, R (Eds): *Man and the Universe: The Philosophers of Science*. New York: Washington Square Press, 1954, pp 43–72

12. Cornell, J: *The First Stargazers: An Introduction to the Origins of Astronomy*. New York: Charles Scribner's Sons, 1981

13. Davis, P J, and Hersh, R: *The Mathematical Experience*. Boston: Birkhauser, 1981

14. Descartes, R: Discourse on method. In Commins, S, and Linscott, R (Eds): *Man and the Universe: The Philosophers of Science*. New York: Washington Square Press, 1954, pp 159–220

15. Durant, W: *The Story of Philosophy: The Lives and Opinions of the Greater Philosophers*. New York: Washington Square Press, 1953

16. Einstein, A, and Infeld, L: *The Evolution of Physics from Early Concepts to Relativity and Quanta*, New York: Simon and Schuster, 1938

17. Halle, L J: *Out of Chaos*. Boston: Houghton Mifflin, 1977

18. Hensen, J: The crime of Galileo. *Science 81*, Volume 2, Number 2, March 1981, pp 14–19

19. Keynes, J M: Newton, the man. In Newman, J (Ed): *The World of Mathematics*, Volume One. New York: Simon and Schuster, 1956, pp 277–285

20. Mason, S F: *A History of the Sciences*. New York: Collier Books, 1962

21. Newman, J R: The Rhind papyrus. In Newman, J (Ed): *The World of Mathematics*, Volume One. New York: Simon and Schuster, 1956, pp 170–179

22. Reichenbach, H: *The Rise of Scientific Philosophy*. Berkeley, California: University of California Press, 1951

23. Robertson, A, and Stevens, D (Eds): *The Pelican History of Music*, Volume 1: *Ancient Forms to Polyphony*. London, Penguin Books, 1960

24. Sagan, C: *Cosmos*. New York: Random House, 1980

25. Schrödinger, E: *What Is Life? and Other Scientific Essays*. Garden City, New York: Doubleday, 1956

26. Smith, D, and Ginsburg, J: From numbers to numerals and from numerals to computation. In Newman, J (Ed): *The World of Mathematics*, Volume One. New York: Simon and Schuster, 1956, pp 432–441

27. Smith, H: *Man and His Gods*. New York: Grosset and Dunlap, 1952

28. Turnbull, H: The great mathematicians. In Newman, J (Ed): *The World of Mathematics*, Volume One. New York: Simon and Schuster, 1956, pp 75–168

29. von Weizsacker, C F: *The Unity of Nature*. New York: Farrar, Straus, Giroux, 1980

30. Wells, H: *The Outline of History*. Garden City, New York: Doubleday, 1971

31. Whitehead, A N: *Science and the Modern World*. New York: Mentor, 1948

Chapter 6

Living Machines

I venture to repeat what I have said before, that so far as the animal world is concerned, evolution is no longer a speculation, but a statement of historical fact. It takes its place alongside of those accepted truths which must be reckoned with by philosophers of all schools. [28:p. 434]

Thomas Henry Huxley, 1889

This DNA structure is so special for each of us that it will never be repeated and it has never existed in any human of the past or present, except if you have an identical twin. It is our evolutionary inheritance. It embodies in fact the entire creative endowment generated by the evolutionary process in the long line of contingency that led to each one of us. It contains the basic instructions for building our bodies and our brains. [15:p. 124]

John C. Eccles, 1979

We have come a long way in our technologic capacity to put death off, and it is imaginable that we might learn to stall it for even longer periods, perhaps matching the life-spans of the Abkhasian Russians, who are said to go on, springily, for a century and a half. If we can rid ourselves of some of our chronic degenerative diseases, and cancer, strokes, and coronaries, we might go on and on. [41:p. 56]

Lewis J. Thomas, 1974

Early Views of Man as a Biologic Organism

Just as many early observers were interested in natural periodicities as evidenced in the movements of the celestial bodies and the elements of chemistry, there were those who used a reductionistic approach to focus upon the mechanical aspects of human form and function. It is to ancient Egypt that we are indebted for the beginnings of medical science [9]. Since much of the medicine of ancient Egypt was connected with belief in the demon theory of disease, most early Egyptian physicians served as a combination of doctor and magician. However, there were some doctors in Egypt who can be said to have practiced "rational medicine" as we might define it today.

Evidence of medical practice in ancient Egypt is found in the Edwin Smith Surgical Papyrus, which dates from about 1700 B.C. and is named after the American Egyptologist who acquired it. This papyrus lists forty-eight descriptions of injuries in a systematic order, starting from the head and moving downward. It is a medical textbook that describes injury, treatment, and prognosis (favorable, uncertain, and unfavorable). It contains no magical formulas or incantations but a rational, logical diagnostic and treatment approach.

The Ebers Medical Papyrus, dating from about 1600 B.C., is actually a teaching manual for general practitioners. It contains a section on the heart and its vessels, a surgical section, and essays on pharmacy and speculative medical philosophy. What is striking about early Egyptian medical practice is its practical approach, its attention to cause and effect, and the logical sequencing of steps to treatment. Because of their practical approach, Egyptian doctors and their herbal prescriptions and treatments were in demand throughout much of the ancient world, far beyond the Nile Valley, to Persia, Assyria, Syria, and into the Mediterranean area. Egyptian medicine is considered to be basic to modern Western medicine.

Although the Egyptians left a considerable legacy of practical approaches to the study of physical man, it is to Greece that we look for the earliest known concept of man as an organism like other animals [6]. Anaximander (611–547 B.C.) anticipated Darwin in some respects when he postulated that life originated spontaneously in mud, fish being the first animals, and other life forms evolving from those fish who left the water and moved to dry land. He is quoted as saying, "Living creatures rose from the moist element as it was evaporated by the sun. Man was like another animal, namely a fish, in the beginning" [30:pp. 26–27]. Because of Anaximander's belief that man developed through progressive adjustment to the environment, he is credited with being the first to advocate a theory of organic evolution.

Other early Greeks also speculated about man's origin. Alcmeon (ca. 500 B.C.) believed that man was a smaller copy of the same plan or blueprint that was used to construct the universe. He was an anatomist who dissected animals, locating the Eustachian tubes and the optic nerves. He postulated that the brain was the organ in which thought originated.

Empedocles (ca. 500–430 B.C.), who was influenced by the Pythagoreans, offered a theory of organic evolution in which, originally, various parts of human and animal bodies (arms, legs, heads, and others) wandered around by themselves until, through some kind of attraction or love, they came together in forms of different kinds. His theory of man's origin may seem rather strange, but he did concentrate on more practical matters and is credited with discovering that the blood flows to and from the heart.

The Atomists also subscribed to the idea that man originated from primeval slime just as did plants and animals. They believed that everything in the universe was composed of atoms, and man, being a microcosm of the universe, contained all the different kinds of atoms.

The development of medicine into a science in Greece is associated with Hippocrates (ca. 460–377 B.C.), the most outstanding of a group of physicians responsible for the earliest Greek medical writings. The Hippocratic physicians were loyal to a common medical doctrine, followed similar practices, exchanged ideas, and shared a common knowledge base. They followed scientific principles in developing new theories and stressed the importance of being careful observers and classifiers. The Hippocratic doctrine adopted diagnosis as its central point. Hippocrates took the position that diseases originated from natural rather than supernatural causes. His prescribed treatments included exercise, proper diet, and rest. Hippocrates wrote, "Men think epilepsy divine, merely because they do not understand it. But if they called everything divine which they do not understand, why, there would be no end of divine things" [38:p. 179].

Aristotle (384–322 B.C.) laid the foundations of biology and emphasized classification, an emphasis that was to characterize the biologic sciences. He classified 540 animal species. He engaged in the study of anatomic structures and dissected fifty different species of animals, noting the differences and similarities among them. He postulated a hierarchy of living things from plants to man, with man the most perfect. He saw correlations between complexity of structure and intelligence and believed that the nervous system and the brain were slowly created by life as it grew in complexity and power. He did not, however, even with the most careful observations and detailed classifications, reach the theory of evolution. Will Durant wrote, "The remarkable fact here is that with all these gradations and similarities leaping to Aristotle's eyes, he does not come to the theory of evolution" [14:p. 67].

Although Aristotle made many errors in his biologic studies, such as attributing brain activity to the heart, he asked questions that would be addressed by many great men of science in their search for answers to how living systems can be analyzed. He established the science of embryology by performing experiments that gave him enough data to describe the development of a chick. He addressed the problems of heredity and performed experiments in genetics.

Although the biologic sciences are indebted to Aristotle for the collection and classification of vast amounts of data, in some ways he can be held responsible for impeding the progress of biology and related studies. Alfred North Whitehead explains:

> The practical counsel to be derived from Pythagoras, is to measure, and thus to express quality in terms of numerically determined quantity. But the biological sciences, then and till our own time, have been overwhelmingly classificatory. Accordingly, Aristotle by his Logic throws the emphasis on classification. The popularity of Aristotelian Logic retarded the advance of physical science throughout the Middle Ages. . . . Classification is necessary. But unless you can progress from classification to mathematics, your reasoning will not take you very far. [42:pp. 33–34]

From the time of Aristotle to the third century A.D., medical science continued to advance, as is evidenced in the work of three individuals, Herophilus (ca. 300 B.C.), Erasistratus (300–260 B.C.), and Galen (ca. 129–199 A.D.). Herophilus is considered the foremost anatomist of his time. He made a distinction between the veins and the arteries, correlated the brain with intelligence, made a connection between the functions of sensation and motion and the nerves, and described the cerebrum, cerebellum, retina, optic nerve, uterus, ovaries, and prostate. He was the first medical teacher to perform dissections in public. Erasistratus traced the pathway through the body of the nerves, veins, and arteries, and explained the functions of the aortic and pulmonary valves of the heart. He believed the nervous system to be centered in the brain and also correlated human intelligence with the complex convolutions of man's brain. Erasistratus, who was a pupil of Herophilus, is thought to be the founder of physiology.

Our need to know "how" things work is clearly illustrated in the endeavors of these early medical scientists, who were not satisfied with metaphysical and religious explanations. Without the benefit of modern instruments, such as the microscope, they made enormous advances in the study of the physical bodies of animals, including man. The works of Galen, which are considered to be among the classics of Greek scientific writing, are indicative of our inclination to seek logical cause-and-effect explanations for living systems and to note the similarities between man and other animals.

Galen, a Greek physician who traveled to Rome and became physician to the emperors Marcus Aurelius Antoninus and Lucius Aurelius Verus, produced 131 medical writings, 83 of which have been preserved. The great medical encyclopedia he compiled was used until the sixteenth century. Although he may not have been aware of the impetus his work gave toward negating the anthropocentric view of man as the center of creation, through his observations and the records Galen validated the biologic position that man is similar to other animals. Before 200 A.D. and over sixteen centuries before Darwin was to postulate the theory of evolution through natural selection, Galen noted the similarities between man and the Barbary ape. He studied the forearm of the ape and compared it to that of man. He studied the brains of both ape and man and was particularly impressed by their large, hollow chambers.

Galen's work was acceptable to the religious establishment of his day and beyond because he made religious interpretations of what he saw. For example, he saw the chambers of the brain as being the place where the animal spirits of the soul assembled. The brain movements he observed he interpreted as being the movements of the spirits within the chambers. Stephen F. Mason, in discussing Galen's acceptance by the medieval church, writes, "Like Plato and Aristotle, Galen was much concerned with the cosmic purposes for which objects and organisms were intended, though, in keeping with the spirit of the age, his religion was more mystical and less intellectual than that of the Athenians" [30:p. 60].

In keeping with their concern with practicality, the Romans saw the study of medicine as necessary to the training of their army surgeons. [4] They adopted Greek medical science, and a Greek, Asclepiades, organized the first medical school in Rome during the first century. Celsus, who was one of his students, wrote a series of volumes on surgery called *De medicina*, which was copied largely from Greek sources. Celsus also described operations involving the removal of the tonsils, goiter, and cataracts.

After Rome was invaded by the barbarians, Roman medicine began to decline. Vesalius remarked upon this phenomenon by writing, in 1543:

> The more fashionable doctors, first in Italy, in imitation of the old Romans, despising the work of the hand, began to delegate to slaves the manual attentions they judged needful for their patients, and themselves merely to stand

over them, like architects. Then, when all the rest who practised the true art of healing gradually declined the unpleasant duties of their profession, without however abating any of their claim to money, or to honour, they quickly fell away from the standard of the doctors of old. Methods of cooking, and all the preparation of food for the sick, they left to nurses; compounding of drugs they left to the apothecaries; manual operations to the barbers. [30:p. 63]

The Moslem civilization was to bestow tremendous respectability upon the science of medicine. Hynayn ibn-Ishaq (808–877) wrote an impressive study of diseases of the eye entitled *The Ten Dissertations on the Eye* and translated the works of Hippocrates and Galen into Arabic. Rhazes (ca. 860–925) was a Persian physician who wrote more than 200 texts on medicine, philosophy, and other subjects, his most important medical text being a book entitled *On the Smallpox and the Measles*, which noted the differences between them. His medical encyclopedia, which was translated into Latin as *Liber continens*, along with his other texts, was used for over 500 years in the medical universities of Europe.

The greatest authority on medicine after 1100 was Avicenna (980–1037), an Arab whose *Canon of Medicine*, five books concerning the treatment of disease, the making of drugs, and theoretical medicine, was widely used throughout Western Europe. The Arabs were the first to recognize the contagious quality of certain diseases.

From ancient Egypt of 2000 B.C. to the Middle Ages, many scholars concentrated upon the discovery of the mechanism of the human body. Considering the superstitious and magical thinking that permeated the early word world, their contributions to many fields, including medicine, physiology, anatomy, and embryology, were enormous. Rather than focusing entirely on the question, "Why is man the way he is?", they asked, "How does man function in the form in which he is found?", and "What similarities are there between the form and function of man and the forms and functions of the rest of the animal kingdom?"

The Biologic Sciences from the Medievalists to Darwin

Certainly, few individuals have added more to the study of form and function in man than the artist-engineer named Leonardo da Vinci (1452–1519). He was a pioneer in the field of anatomy, sketching human bones, muscles, nerves, and veins in minute and exquisite detail. He was fascinated by form and structure, dissecting more than thirty cadavers to make the observations necessary for his exceedingly accurate anatomic studies. His analysis of the similarities in structure between the human leg and the leg of a horse is one of the earliest studies in comparative anatomy. He was fascinated by the science of mechanics and applied it to the study of living organisms, showing that the joints and bones of animals are lever systems operated by the forces of their muscles [27].

Medieval physicians looked to the Greeks for their medical knowledge, relying upon the works of Hippocrates and Galen. Those few physicians who dared to challenge the ancient authorities ran the risk of losing their reputations, but a few in the sixteenth century did dare, paving the way for the advances that were to come in the seventeenth and eighteenth centuries.

Philippus Aureolus Paracelsus (1493–1541), a Swiss physician, was one who challenged the work of Galen. He emphasized the close relationship between chemistry and medicine, introducing a new field called iatrochemistry. His real name was von Hohenheim, but he renamed himself Paracelsus because he considered himself to be greater than Celsus. His exalted view of himself is indicated in his remark, "For even as Avicenna was the best physician of the Arabs, and Galen of the men of Pergamum, so also most fortunate Germany has chosen me as her indispensable physician" [30:p. 231]. He accompanied his words with acts, one of those being the public burning of an ancient medical textbook by Avicenna, the Arab physician whose works had dominated the medicine of Western Europe since 1100.

Iatrochemistry became popular in Germany, and Paracelsus was given the title "the Luther of Chemistry." Paracelsus was very mystical in his thinking and believed that "all things in nature were autonomous living beings" [30:p. 230]. He believed that every living thing contains within itself or its seed a predetermined form and function, and he wrote, "For God has carefully differentiated all His Creation from the beginning, and has never given to different things the same shape and form" [30:p. 230].

Another sixteenth century physician who questioned Galen was Andreas Vesalius (1514–1564), a Dutchman who taught medicine in the Italian university of Padua. His 1543 text, *On the Structure of the Human Anatomy*, was a landmark in the history of medicine. As he dissected bodies, he noted the various errors in the works of Galen and chose to rely on his own observations. One example of his disagreement with Galen concerned Galen's theory that the blood flowed from the right to the left chamber of the heart through the septum. Vesalius wrote, "Not long ago, I would not have dared to diverge a hair's breadth from Galen's opinion. But the septum is as thick, dense, and compact as the rest of the heart. I do not see, therefore, how even the smallest particle can be transferred from the right to the left ventricle through it" [30:pp. 216–217].

Vesalius, who had won his degree in medicine at the age of twenty-three and was appointed Professor of Surgery one day later, lectured and dissected in three universities. He collected bones for his studies from mortuaries, public gallows, and graveyards. When he published his findings, he illustrated them with more than 270 detailed woodcuts. Although some of Vesalius' contemporaries were outraged at his refutation of Galen's work, his teachings made the University of Padua so famous that people from all over Europe went there to be treated.

Paracelsus and Vesalius smoothed the pathway for William Harvey (1578–1657), an English physician who continued the argument with the long-revered Galen. Galen's teachings concerning blood flow as it was reflected in the brain through the rhythmic movements of the spirits were firmly ensconced in medical science. Sir Charles Sherrington comments:

> Galen's eminence and the subsequent conspiracy of the ages to maintain and exalt it, carried this teaching not only unchallenged but hardened into dogma century after century, down to and beyond Descartes and Harvey. For Descartes however the spirits of the anima were not incorporeal—they were a kind of "flame", travelling with incredible velocity. Harvey was more objective. His

observations had engaged him for sixteen years, but he said in all that time he had met no evidence of the spirits. The negation fell with the force of a positive blow. [39:p. 194]

In 1628, Harvey published a book entitled *Anatomical Exercise on the Motion of the Heart and Blood in Animals*, which was widely opposed. It refuted Galen's theories about the spirits causing the blood's motion, the heart a passive organ serving the spirits. Not only did he refute Galen, but he gave a mechanical explanation for blood circulation. He described the heart as a muscle, its contractions responsible for the transport of the blood through the veins and arteries. In presenting his mechanical philosophy of the circulatory system, he joined da Vinci in applying the science of mechanics to the study of living systems.

Marcello Malpighi (1628–1694) confirmed Harvey's theory of blood circulation by using the new compound microscopes to discover capillary circulation of the blood, explaining how the blood traveled from the arteries to the veins. Microscopic study also allowed Malpighi to concentrate on human nerve tissue and human skin, one layer of which is today known as the Malpighian layer. From his study of respiratory organs, particularly their size, Malpighi devised a way to vertically classify all living creatures, placing plants at the bottom, then insects and fishes, and finally man and the higher animals.

Many scientists continued to focus their studies upon the functioning of the human body. Robert Whytt (1714–1766) discovered reflex action and initiated the study of neurology [5]. Johannes Muller (1801–1858) wrote a handbook on human physiology, explaining, among other things, his law of specific energies, which demonstrates that a definite sensation results upon the stimulation of a sensory nerve. Claude Bernard (1813–1878), a French physiologist, discovered the vasomotor system and studied the digestive processes, especially internal secretions and glands.

As the eighteenth century progressed, many thinkers, especially the determinists and materialists, propounded the idea of man as a machine. In 1748, in his book *L'Homme machine*, Julian Offray de la Mettrie wrote, "Let us then conclude boldly that man is a machine, and that there is in the whole universe only a single substance differently modified" [3:p. 167]. la Mettrie saw the body as an automatically functioning machine, and of the soul he wrote, "The diverse states of the soul are always correlative with those of the body. . . . From animals to man, the transition is not violent" [3:p. 167].

The transition from animal to man was to become a subject of intense study. Theories concerning evolution were developing rapidly and would dominate the thinking of much of the scientific world. Stephen J. Gould writes:

> Evolution is one of the half dozen "great ideas" developed by science. It speaks to the profound issues of genealogy that fascinate all of us—the "roots" phenomenon writ large. Where did we come from? Where did life arise? How did it develop? How are organisms related? [24:p. 37]

Comtes Georges Louis Leclerc de Buffon (1707–1788), the author of *Natural History*, consisting of more than forty volumes, suggested that it was through the process of degeneration that organic species changed. In this respect, he was different from the modern evolutionists, who subscribe to the theory that the more complex living systems develop from simpler and more primitive ones. Buffon's theories were unpopular at the time he proposed them because it was thought that any evolutionary process, degeneration being only one, would detract from the idea of a constant and perfect creation. Although Buffon discussed a hypothesis of evolution, he subsequently rejected its application to biologic species, insisting instead that they were eternal and unchanging. Species did not change, but individuals might. Buffon wrote:

> Minister of God's irrevocable orders, depository of his immutable decrees, Nature never separates herself from the laws which have been prescribed for her; she alters not at all the plans which have been made for her, and in all her works she presents the seal of the Eternal: this divine imprint, unalterable prototype of existences, is the model on which she operates, model all of whose traits are expressed in ineffaceable characters, and pronounced forever. [3:p. 214]

Charles Bonnet (1720–1793) developed a theory of evolution that incorporated the process of ontogenesis, the idea that each single organism develops from germs fixed by the Creator for all time. Organic change came about only as the result of catastrophes, such as the great flood of Biblical description. Although all individuals might be destroyed, they would live on in germ form, moving up in the hierarchy toward greater complexity. Baumer writes, "Though Bonnet and his friends were experimental scientists, they had their metaphysical reasons for refusing to accept the idea of a 'living matter,' having the power of creation and adaptation. As both Christians and mechanists, they began with the assumption that nature had the power to function only as a machine created by God" [3:p. 213].

The writings of both Buffon and Bonnet carry the unmistakable imprint of the anthropocentric thinking prevalent at that time. The "truth" about the world as evidenced by many thinkers during the eighteenth century was a combination of Christianity and Platonism, in which everything existed as it was formed in the beginning by the Creator. The Abbé Pluche stated, in 1752, in one of his science books, "Nothing new under the sun: no new production; no species whatever that existed not from the beginning" [3:p. 202]. This was in keeping with the teachings of Newton, that the whole mechanistic world had been created by a supreme being in a cause-and-effect sequence governed by immutable laws.

Jean Baptiste de Lamarck (1744–1829) upset the whole of the scientific world with the publication of his *Natural History of Invertebrate Animals*, in which he proposed that evolution proceeded from simpler to more complicated forms and that new organs could be developed if the need was continually there over a long enough period of time. In addition, he believed that any new organs acquired by a body would be transmitted to the next generation. Environmentally induced changes in the habits of animals would lead to greater or lesser use of certain organs, thus determining which would be inherited and cause a permanent change in the species. Lamarck's theory is credited with being the first important modern theory of organic evolution.

Although Lamarck's general laws of evolution were controversial, it was the publication in 1859 of *The Origin of Species* by Charles Darwin (1809–1882) that ultimately destroyed the anthropocentric view of the world created expressly for man. Darwin, in *The Origin of Species* and in *The Descent of Man*, published in 1871, emphasized the idea of evolution through the process of natural selection. Gould writes, "Darwin did two very separate things: he convinced the scientific world that evolution had occurred and he proposed the theory of natural selection as its mechanism" [23:p. 44]. Even Darwin himself noted many times that he had accomplished two separate and different things. He also declared that he had both these objectives clearly in mind.

Darwin acknowledged the influence of Sir Charles Lyell, the geologist, on his thinking. Darwin had taken Lyell's *Principles of Geology* (1830) with him on the Beagle. Lyell's doctrine of "uniformitarianism," which proposed that geologic changes occurred very slowly and uniformly throughout time, gave Darwin the suggestion of steady and irreversible change throughout a vastly extended period of time. Darwin wrote in his *Autobiography:*

> The investigation of the geology of all the places visited was far more important, as reasoning here comes into play. On first examining a new district nothing can appear more hopeless than the chaos of rocks; but by recording the stratification and nature of the rocks and fossils at many points, always reasoning and predicting what will be found elsewhere, light soon begins to dawn on the district, and the structure of the whole becomes more or less intelligible. I had brought with me the first volume of Lyell's "Principles of Geology," which I studied attentively; and the book was of the highest service to me in many ways. [10:p. 71]

Lyell, who had influenced Darwin so profoundly, never did wholly accept Darwin's theory. He reluctantly acknowledged the "probability" of natural selection, but not as an explanation of man, whom he thought to be separate from the rest of the animal kingdom. Baumer writes, "The great geologist had concluded that man must have been elevated to his proud estate by a cause outside the usual course of nature. Man was the one great exception to his own 'uniformitarian' law of nature" [3:p. 349].

Darwin had also read and been influenced by Thomas R. Malthus' *Essay on the Principles of Population* (1789), in which Malthus theorized that the fight for existence was the result of the population outgrowing the food supply. Malthus had observed that two things seem necessary to the existence of man, food and "passion between the sexes." Based upon these two postulates, his conclusion was that the food supply would never be enough. He wrote, "I say that the power of the population is indefinitely greater than the power of the earth to produce subsistence for man . . . (for) population when unchecked increases in geometrical ratios, subsistence only increases in an arithmetic ratio. A slight acquaintance with numbers will show the immensity of the first power in comparison with the second" [30:p. 413].

Malthus' observation, that nature was very liberal in allowing species to propagate but she was very sparing in the resources necessary for survival, causing a tremendous struggle to exist, provided Darwin with the mechanism of evolution. In the competition for food, only those organisms with favorable variations would survive and continue to reproduce. Darwin wrote, in *The Origin of Species:*

If under changing conditions of life organic beings present individual differences in almost every part of their structure, and this cannot be disputed; if
there be, owing to their geometrical rate of increase, a severe struggle for life at
some age, season, or year, and this certainly cannot be disputed; then, considering the infinite complexity of the relations of all organic beings to each other
and to their conditions of life, causing an infinite diversity in structure, constitution, and habits, to be advantageous to them, it would be a most extraordinary fact if no variations had ever occurred useful to each being's own welfare,
in the same manner as so many variations have occurred useful to man. But if
variations useful to any organic being ever do occur, assuredly individuals thus
characterised will have the best chance of being preserved in the struggle for
life; and from the strong principle of inheritance, these will tend to produce
offspring similarly characterised. This principle of preservation, or the survival
of the fittest, I have called Natural Selection. [11:pp. 218–219]

Although it is Darwin whose name is linked for all time with the modern
theory of evolution through natural selection, Alfred Russel Wallace (1823–
1913) arrived independently at the same conclusion. Wallace had also been
influenced by Malthus, and while ill and feverish in February 1858 on the
island of Ternate in the Spice Islands, he remembered the Malthus theory
and came up with the same explanation as had Darwin. Wallace wrote:

It occurred to me to ask the question, Why do some die and some live? And
the answer was clearly, that on the whole the best fitted lived. From the effects
of disease the most healthy escaped; from enemies, the strongest, the swiftest,
or the most cunning; from famine, the best hunters or those with the best
digestion; and so on.

Then I at once saw, that the ever present variability of all living things
would furnish the material from which, by the mere weeding out of those less
adapted to the actual conditions, the fittest alone would continue the race.

There suddenly flashed upon me the idea of the survival of the fittest.

The more I thought over it, the more I became convinced that I had at
length found the long-sought-for law of nature that solved the problem of the
Origin of Species. [7:pp. 306–308]

Wallace subsequently wrote a paper presenting his ideas and sent it to
Darwin with the suggestion that he might wish to give it to Lyell. This must
have produced tremendous confusion in Darwin, who had been looking for
ways to validate his own theories for twenty years. He said, after he received
Wallace's paper, "I never saw a more striking coincidence; if Wallace had my
MS sketch written out in 1842, he could not have made a better short
abstract!" [7:p. 308].

Lyell helped to arrange the presentation of Wallace's paper plus one by
Darwin at a meeting of the Linnean Society in London. Although the papers
did not make any particular impact, Darwin now felt compelled to publish
his findings and subsequently wrote *The Origin of Species*.

The theory of evolution is said by many scholars to be the single most
important scientific theory of the nineteenth century. Its impact upon the
anthropocentric world view that prevailed at that time was crunching, and
the debates it engendered are still going on with almost as much vigor as
when it originated. Gould writes, "The Western world has yet to make its

peace with Darwin and the implications of evolutionary theory. The hippocampus debate merely illustrates, in light relief, the greatest impediment to this reconciliation—our unwillingness to accept continuity between ourselves and nature, our ardent search for a criterion to assert our uniqueness" [23:p. 50].

The proponents of Darwin's theories, and they would continue to increase in number, were most emphatic in their support. Germany's Ernst Heinrich Haeckel (1834–1919) became one of the most vocal and succeeded in popularizing Darwin. He applied Darwinian principles to embryology, invoking what he called the biogenetic law of recapitulation. He coined the phrase, "Ontogeny recapitulates phylogeny" and used it against those people who thought themselves to have special status. Although Haeckel's ideas on recapitulation were not accepted in the form which he preferred, he did give impetus to embryological research. Mason says, "However, Haeckel, among others, performed a valuable service in assimilating the German work on morphology, embryology, and the cell theory into the Darwinian system" [30:p. 428].

The acceptance by the scientific community of natural selection as a mechanism for evolution spurred enthusiasm to uncover other mechanisms associated with life. Reductionism, cause and effect, and form and function were the major emphases in the search for scientific truth. In order to understand anything it was necessary to dissect it, to find the basic building blocks, and then to determine how these blocks fit together and how they functioned separately as a system. All life was supposed to have a lowest common denominator, which, when understood, would yield a true picture of the whole.

The Building Blocks of Life

The Greek philosophic theory of atomism, which stated that the basic components of the entire universe are simple, indivisible, and indestructible atoms, had an influence upon the field of biology as evidenced in the growing interest in cell theory. The cell was to the science of biology what the atom was to the science of chemistry. At the same time that John Dalton was working with weights of atoms in different elements, biologic scientists were delving into the mysteries of the living cell.

In the seventeenth century, Anton van Leeuwenhoek (1632–1723) had viewed a plant cell with a microscope. In 1797, Xavier Bichat (1771–1802) elaborated a tissue theory, differentiating twenty-one different kinds of tissue, each, he conjectured, having a life of its own. In 1831, Robert Brown (1773–1858), with the aid of the new achromatic microscope, discovered the nuclear body of the plant cell. It was Mathias Schleiden (1804–1881), however, who in 1838 proposed the theory that the fundamental entity of all plants was the cell, the basic living unit of any plant structure. Up to this time botanists had been more interested in classification than in plant anatomy. Schleiden hypothesized that much more could be learned about a plant by observing the cells of which it was composed than by classification and examination of the structure at full growth. He also proposed that each cell had two lives, one of its own as a single unit and one as part of the structure.

The first was the primary life, and the second, the secondary life. He believed that each cell originated from the nucleus of an old cell, starting its life as part of the old cell and then splitting off and creating a new cell.

Theodore Schwann (1810–1882), in 1839, applied the cell theory to the animal kingdom, theorizing that fertilized eggs are single cells and, therefore, all organisms start as single cells. He also suggested, as had Schleiden, that "new cells were formed by the crystallization of organic matter inside or outside of the old cells" [30:p. 390]. Schwann also reviewed Bichat's tissue theory and applied his cell theory, making a cellular differentiation of five different classes of tissue. By 1840, with the work of Dalton, Schleiden, and Schwann, an atomic basis had been suggested for both biology and chemistry.

In 1858, Rudolph Virchow (1821–1902), who had also studied Bichat's tissue theory, proposed that a single cell was responsible for the development of disease within tissue. Mason explains, "Adopting the view of Schwann that the cells were autonomous living entities, Virchow regarded the human body as a 'state in which every cell is a citizen', and a disease as a kind of revolt or civil war" [30:p. 391]

The search for the smallest component of living systems was continued by Louis Pasteur (1822–1895), the founder of microbiology. Pasteur was able to prove the existence of small yeast organisms in fermenting liquors, and in 1863, he discovered that a microorganism was responsible for the souring of wine. He also demonstrated a way to destroy the microorganism by heating the wine.

Pasteur progressed from the microorganisms in liquors to those responsible for diseases in silkworms, chickens, and cattle, until in 1880 he began to look at disease-producing microorganisms in humans.

Pasteur continued the work of the cell theorists by extending the concept of atomicity still further into the region of biology. Whitehead comments:

> The cell theory and Pasteur's work were in some respects more revolutionary than that of Dalton. For they introduced the notion of *organism* into the world of minute beings. There had been a tendency to treat the atom as an ultimate entity, capable only of external relations. This attitude of mind was breaking down under the influence of Mendeleef's periodic law. But Pasteur showed the decisive importance of the idea of organism at the stage of infinitesimal magnitude. The astronomers had shown us how big is the universe. The chemists and biologists teach us how small it is. There is in modern scientific practice a famous standard of length. It is rather small: to obtain it, you must divide a centimetre into one hundred million parts, and take one of them. Pasteur's organisms are a good deal bigger than this length. In connection with atoms, we now know that there are organisms for which such distances are uncomfortably great. [42:p. 95]

Pasteur performed another great service for the scientific community. There was a widespread belief that such creatures as the maggots in apples or the bluebottles in meat came to life spontaneously, without parents. Pasteur, in his experiments with microscopic lives, could find no case in which the germs arose de novo from the material he used and thus abolished the idea of spontaneous generation. Sherrington commented:

It is impossible to prove a negative, but he challenged the world to show a positive contradicting his negative. The world has been trying to do so ever since on a colossal scale, for instance, through the fermented-liquor industries of the united world. But Pasteur's negative stands unshaken. [39:pp. 85–86]

Through his work with bacteria, Pasteur was able to link the evolutionary process of natural selection with chemistry, suggesting that organic molecules evolved through the process of chemical evolution. Jacob Bronowski wrote, "For the first time Pasteur had linked all the forms of life with one kind of chemical structure. From that powerful thought it follows that we must be able to link evolution with chemistry" [7:p. 313].

The cell became an entity of even more intensive study, with attention directed to its reproductive aspects. The asexual reproduction of the organic cell by fission was known before 1850 [26]. Between 1850 and 1900, several individuals began to study the reproductive behavior of sexual cells, becoming interested in the questions of inheritance and mutation. Hugo De Vries (1848–1935) began, in 1885, to look for mutative changes in organisms in order to reconcile the short estimates physicists had made about the age of the earth with the time required for organic evolution. He found such changes in the American evening primrose, but he wanted more material than he had and began to look for evidence from the work of other individuals. He discovered the papers of Gregor Johann Mendel (1822–1884).

Mendel, an Austrian botanist who was a monk, had published papers in 1866 and 1869 that laid the foundation for a simple mathematical procedure to be utilized in predicting the inheritance of certain simply determined traits. Mendel's work was ignored, even though he sent it to Karl Nageli (1817–1891), a professor of botany, who, because of his work with plant and animal cells, suggested that evolution occurred in a series of mutations and was not a gradual and continuous process.

Nageli had also published a theory that all creatures evolve from micelles, smaller units that make up the composition of cells. He coined the term *idioplasm* to describe the part of the egg that determined heredity. The idioplasm was composed of micelles and linked together in chains. It was the idioplasm that was solely responsible for the form the adult organism would take. Evolution occurred as the inner force within each organism operated to bring about discontinuous changes in the idioplasm, with natural selection a factor in eliminating the nonviable forms. Although Mendel's work supported Nageli's particle theory of inheritance, Nageli chose to disregard it. Mason states that Nageli ignored Mendel because he found his work "empirical rather than rational" [30:p. 430], but Bronowski claims that Nageli "had no notion what Mendel was talking about" [7:p. 385].

Classical, or Mendelian, genetics was finally recognized as one of the great accomplishments in the field of genetics through the work of de Vries and other scientists beginning around the turn of this century. Mendel had guessed that species produce individual shape, color, and behavior through the coupling of genes. He clearly, through the use of statistics and algebraic equations, proved that heredity occurs in an all-or-none fashion and not by averaging, as was commonly believed. He gave the scientific world the genetic mechanism. "To the question of what is transmitted by way of the genetic mechanism," state Lyons and Barrell, "we may now answer, 'Parents pass on to the next generation of their species some molecules located in specific arrangements within the chromosomes of the children, and this in turn leads to, although it may not completely determine, a set of active, functioning structures'" [29:p. 19].

In 1953, the question of how the message of inheritance is transmitted from one generation to the next was answered through the work of James Watson and Francis Crick. Together, Watson and Crick deciphered the structure of DNA, or deoxyribonucleic acid. Researchers had already proven that chemical messages of inheritance are carried by nucleic acids. DNA is a nucleic acid located in the central part of cells, the nucleus [22]. Watson and Crick were able to determine that the structure of the DNA molecule is a double helix, or spiral.

The importance of the discovery by Watson and Crick is described by Jacques Monod of the Salk Institute:

> The fundamental biological invariant is DNA. That is why Mendel's defining of the gene as the unvarying bearer of hereditary traits, its chemical identification by Avery (confirmed by Hershey), and the elucidation by Watson and Crick of the structural basis of its replicative invariance, without any doubt constitute the most important discoveries ever made in biology. To which of course must be added the theory of natural selection, whose certainty and full significance were established only by those later discoveries. [7:p. 393]

The search for the building blocks of life made an unprecedented leap in the discovery of the DNA spiral. Bronowski wrote:

> The DNA spiral is not a monument. It is an instruction, a living mobile to tell the cell how to carry out the processes of life step by step. Life follows a time-table, and the treads of the DNA spiral encode and signal the sequence in which the time-table must go. The machinery of the cell reads off the treads in order, one after another. A sequence of three treads acts as a signal to the cell to make one amino acid. As the amino acids are formed in order, they line up and assemble in the cell as proteins. And the proteins are the agents and building blocks of life in the cell. [7:p. 395]

The language used by Bronowski to describe the DNA spiral is indicative of its importance to a mechanical view of life—instruction, timetable, machinery of the cell, sequence, order, and the building blocks of life.

Molecular biology, the study of the molecular machinery of life, has continued to escalate and has resulted in even newer fields, such as genetic engineering, which validate further the possibility of a blueprint for the building of living structures. In November 1981, in an article entitled "Tinkering with Life," Boyce Rensberger wrote, "The more molecular biologists learn about the ultimate nature of life, about the nuts and bolts, the cogs and wheels of our genetic apparatus, the more we reduce living organisms to machines" [36:p. 45]. He goes on to point out that, "Some new geneticists now talk not just of engineering the genes of bacteria; they want to redesign the genetic core of higher organisms including those of human beings" [36:p. 45].

Technology is also playing an important part in the increasing sophistication of genetic engineering. Several important advancements were made in

1981. Genetic engineering was mechanized by the introduction of "gene machines," which can assemble DNA segments automatically. Interferon, a natural animal protein that combats invading viruses and that can be assembled by genetically engineered bacteria, was injected into a cancer patient. Other patients began to receive a human growth hormone, which is another product of recombinant DNA technology. Experiments progressed in the transfer of genes from one animal or plant species to another. Advancements were made in cloning, which is the creation from a single parent of genetically identical individuals. Several researchers learned how to turn off and turn on segments of DNA molecules, which are sometimes dormant and sometimes active. These and other discoveries have aroused speculation that, "The day may come when scientists are able to design their own chemical keys to fit genetic locks, and thereby regulate genetic activity and attack diseases that are caused by failures in the machinery of cells" [25:p. 79].

What Controls the Machinery of the Body?

Just as numerous measurers and observers concentrated on the mechanism of the human body, others were concerned with what controlled that mechanism. What machine ran the machine? It was long thought that something called "mind" ran this beautiful mechanistic apparatus. If one could know the mind, then, one could have all the secrets of the mechanical universe, including those of the body. Marquis Pierre Simon de Laplace, the French mathematician, said:

> "An intellect which at a given instant knew all the forces acting in nature, and the position of all things of which the world consists—supposing the said intellect were vast enough to subject these data to analysis—would embrace in the same formula the motions of the greatest bodies in the universe and those of the slightest atoms; nothing would be uncertain for it, and the future, like the past, would be present to its eyes. [8:p. 57]

How could one examine the nature of the intellect? Of what was the mind composed? René Descartes (1596–1650) had discussed at length the relationship of mind to body. In explaining the operation of sensation, he wrote:

> We must know, therefore, that although the mind of man informs the whole body, it yet has its principal seat in the brain, and it is there that it not only understands and imagines, but also perceives; and this by means of the nerves which are extended like filaments from the brain to all the other members, with which they are so connected that we can hardly touch any part of the human body without causing the extremities of some of the nerves spread over it to be moved; and this motion passes to the other extremities of those nerves which are collected in the brain round the seat of the soul. [13:p. 135]

In discussing the way in which the soul perceives, he wrote:

> It is however easily proved that the soul feels those things that affect the body not in so far as it is in each member of the body, but only in so far as it is in the brain, where the nerves by their movements convey to it the diverse actions of the external objects which touch the parts of the body (in which they are inserted). [13:p. 135]

The brain was part of the human body, the seat of the soul. As you may recall from Chapter 5, Descartes believed that the human body, being a machine, was ruled by the same mechanical laws that ruled all material beings. He declared the entire organic and physical world to be a mechanical system open to analysis through the use of mathematical methods. He proposed that, for man, there existed another world, the spiritual one, but that world was not open to scientific inquiry. The role of science is to investigate the objective or physical world, which lends itself to the use of scientific methodology, and to separate out the subjective aspects. The physical mechanical world, of which man was a part, could be studied objectively with no attention paid to the human observer. This Cartesian dualism became the scientific ideal.

Even though advances in science destroyed the anthropocentric world, our differentiation of self from nature was enhanced subtly by heavy emphasis on objectivity. We, the observers, were separated from what we observed, including our world and the various parts of our bodies, including our brains and perceptive organs. Our observations were enhanced by technological equipment, but our mind was still the final point of observation, the entity that assigned the meaning to the data collected by measurement and observation. We became even more certain that mind is a function of the brain.

We had speculated about the brain for some time, arguing over its function. The early Egyptians knew about some of the results of head wounds. Hippocrates, after observing patients with head wounds, wrote, "Men ought to know that from the brain and from the brain only arise our pleasures, joys, laughter, and jests as well as our sorrow, pains, griefs and tears" [2:pp. 9–10]. Plato had ascribed the faculty of reason to the head. Aristotle rejected the idea of the brain as the source of feelings because brain tissue is insensitive to pain, claiming that the function of the brain was to cool the blood.

The idea of the brain as a machine developed during the sixteenth and seventeenth centuries as experimental scientists were discovering the functions of various body organs. The brain became the object of reductionistic analysis. If we could determine the form and function of the smallest elements or basic units of the brain, we could fully comprehend the machine that ran the machine.

"For Descartes," writes Steven Rose, "the brain and nerves were a sort of hydraulic system, an elaborate arrangement of canals, pistons and pumps through which vital spirits infused, invigorating muscles and tissues with their energizing content" [37:pp. 39–40]. In their search for basic units, Descartes and his followers established the notion that ideas are the basic units of thought processes and are located in the mind. These ideas or elementary mental events can be ordered sequentially. If the mind could be treated as a machine it could be taken apart and each part assigned to some bit of behavior. "Some of the Cartesians," according to Karl R. Popper and John C. Eccles, "then assumed that to each elementary mental event there corresponds a definite brain event" [35:p. 89].

The notion that acts of behavior could be correlated with different parts of the brain became a major doctrine in brain research and is termed *localization*. During the first part of the nineteenth century, a heated debate took place between the localizers and those who claimed that the localization of incorporeal functions was not possible. At times, the debate was tinged with bitterness. The anatomist who took localization to absurdity was Franz Joseph Gall, who maintained that bulging eyes indicated the presence of highly developed gray matter exerting enough pressure on the eyes to push them forward, and from this observation went on to develop the pseudoscience of phrenology. The phrenologists, who became extremely popular during the first half of the nineteenth century, purported to be able to ascribe specific traits and powers to protuberant areas of the skull. Thousands of people, including Queen Victoria and Karl Marx, consulted phrenologists.

Gall was correct in his hypothesis that specific areas of the brain have specific functions. It was his idea of protuberances on the skull being matched with particular traits and talents that earned him the scorn of much of the academic community. It was not Gall, therefore, who gave respectability to localization.

During the second half of the nineteenth century, the French surgeon, Paul Broca, located the region of the brain that controls speech. It was in the 1860s, while performing autopsies on patients with speech disorders, that he noted many of their brains to be damaged in the same area. In 1874, Carl Wernicke discovered the area of the brain that acts as a word selector and retriever. It was later postulated that Broca's area and Wernicke's area were connected by the angular gyrus, which served as a linking station between those two main speech centers. It was also thought that the angular gyrus was involved only when language depended on vision.

Through experimentation with dogs, two German physicians, Eduard Hitzig and Gustav Fritsch, located the area of the brain that controlled voluntary movements. Dr. Hitzig had become interested in performing such experiments after noticing that the soldiers with head wounds he treated during the Prussian-Danish war twitched their muscles if their brains were touched.

Such discoveries of localization of function gave a rational basis to this type of research and to the idea of the control of different body functions by different parts of the brain. Rose states:

> By the end of the century brain would be accommodated at last into that certain Victorian universe of Lord Kelvin, archetypal technologist and physicist, who refused to accept any scientific theory or datum for which he could not design a mechanical model or analogy. To T. H. Huxley, the great champion of Darwinism, the relationship of mind and brain could be summed up in the most classic of Victorian analogies, as the whistle to the steam train. [37:p. 42]

It is interesting to note that the idea of the brain as a machine developed at the same time as the Industrial Revolution, with its emphasis on mechanical models. In the eighteenth century, the brain was compared to clocks, cogs, gears, and pulleys. In the nineteenth century, the comparison was to be with the newly invented telegraph and telephone after it was discovered that the brain utilizes electrical signals. The wiring of the brain became a subject of intense research and speculation.

Brain researchers determined the brain's smallest working units were microscopic nerve cells called *neurons*. The neurons and their tentacles, called *axons* and *dendrites*, were interconnected to compose millions of circuits. Behavior was controlled through this complex electrical and chemical maze. It was estimated that each individual had 10,000,000,000 neurons in his brain, so small that 100,000,000 neurons might be found in a cubic inch of brain matter. The neurons did not touch but were separated by tiny spaces eight millionths of an inch in length. The brain was not wired in a continuous fashion but with minute breaks known as *synapses*. The story behind the discovery of the synaptic gap is one of the most famous in brain research.

At the end of the nineteenth century, Camillo Golgi, an Italian physician, invented a stain for studying brain tissue under the microscope. He claimed that continuous electrical circuits were formed by the neurons. Santiago Ramon y Cajal, a Spanish histologist, used Golgi's staining technique and suggested the synaptic gap. This precipitated an intense debate. In 1906, Cajal and Golgi shared the Nobel Prize. The bitterness of their dispute was evident in the fact that they chose not to speak to each other when they went forward to accept their awards [2]. Their joint endeavors, however, gave tremendous thrust to brain research.

Cajal, who Sherrington described as "the greatest anatomist the nervous system has ever known" [16:p. 203], worked with Sherrington on the theory that the basic unit of brain activity was the neuron, a specialized cell that received information through its dendrites and sent out information through its axon. This meant that the cell always moved information in one direction. Sherrington, who spent two weeks hosting Cajal on a visit to London, was, according to Eccles and William C. Gibson, extremely impressed with the Spanish scientist. "To find, especially in far-off Spain, a peasant genius who had for fifteen years been unravelling the secrets of nerve cells under the microscope, was something to celebrate, thought Sherrington" [16:p. 10]. Sherrington seemed, however, a little baffled by Cajal's anthropomorphic approach, and wrote:

> The intense anthropomorphism of his descriptions of what the preparations showed was at first startling to accept. He treated the microscopic scene as though it were alive and were inhabited by beings which felt and did and hoped and tried even as we do. It was personification of natural forces as unlimited as that of Goethe's *Faust*, Part 2. A nerve-cell by its emergent fibre "groped to find another"! We must, if we would enter adequately into Cajal's thought in this field, suppose his entrance, through his microscope, into a world populated by tiny beings actuated by motives and strivings and satisfactions not very remotely different from our own. He would envisage the sperm-cells as activated by a sort of passionate urge in their rivalry for penetration into the ovum-cell. Listening to him I asked myself how far this capacity for anthropomorphizing might not contribute to his success as an investigator. I never met anyone else in whom it was so marked. [16:pp. 204–205]

Once the determination was made that the neuron was the brain's smallest working unit, researchers continued their analyses, working upon the mechanism of the neuron itself. They ascertained that these microscopic nerve cells could be dissected into four components, the cell body, dendrites, axon, and synapses. Each cell had many dendrites and synapses but only one axon and one cell body. Once the form of the neuron was analyzed, scientists ascertained the function of each of the component parts.

The reductionistic approach to the machinery of the brain proved most successful, but mechanical models were also needed for the brain as a system. How could one tie the parts together to make a functioning whole? Many individuals were to compare the brain to the telegraph and then to the telephone, using such phrases as "the central telephone exchange of the brain" to describe electrical activity in the reception and transmission of messages. These attempts to describe the working system of the brain were also influenced by other manifestations of the machine age, such as factory management. "In this model," explains Rose, "the whole human body was a factory with inputs and outputs, control centres, distribution points and so forth. The brain was the management of the factory, the administrator, receiving information about the state of progress and rapidly and efficiently taking the appropriate actions" [37:p. 43].

Sherrington has given us perhaps the most poetically beautiful description of the system of the brain, comparing it to the loom. He wrote:

> In the great head-end which has been mostly darkness spring up myriads of twinkling stationary lights and myriads of trains of moving lights of many different directions. It is as though activity from one of those local places which continued restless in the darkened main-mass suddenly spread far and wide and invaded all. The great topmost sheet of the mass, that where hardly a light had twinkled or moved, becomes now a sparkling field of rhythmic flashing points with trains of travelling sparks hurrying hither and thither. The brain is waking and with it the mind is returning. It is as if the Milky Way entered upon some cosmic dance. Swiftly the head-mass becomes an enchanted loom where millions of flashing shuttles weave a dissolving pattern, always a meaningful pattern though never an abiding one; a shifting harmony of subpatterns. Now as the waking body rouses, subpatterns of this great harmony of activity stretch down into the unlit tracks of the stalk-piece of the scheme. Strings of flashing and travelling sparks engage the lengths of it. This means that the body is up and rises to meet its waking day. [39:pp. 177–178]

It was argued that the brain could not be studied as an integrated system until it was defined in terms of its parts and their functional relationships. Equally, brain-cell functions could not be comprehended except with respect to the entire system of which they were only units. Recent study of the brain system has indicated that there are actually two brains, which assume different roles. The left and right cerebral hemispheres share the work of the brain and are ordinarily interconnected. Each hemisphere can learn, think, and remember, and each has the capacity to feel strong emotions.

The two hemispheres in man are specialized, with the left responsible for language skills, reasoning, and mathematics, and the right responsible for spatial perception and intuition. Localization of language in the left brain (and this is so of ninety-seven percent of the population) has caused scientists to call it the major, or dominant, hemisphere. Only recently has research begun to reveal the importance of the right, or minor, hemisphere.

Roger W. Sperry is one of the chief researchers concerned with the split brain. He has demonstrated clearly the influence of the right hemisphere on significant aspects of behavior and has demonstrated that man does not have one brain, but two. After Ronald Myers, a student of Sperry's, discovered that a split-brain cat could use either brain independently, Sperry and

Michael Gazzaniga began an investigation of behavior in humans with split brains. Their research, plus that of numerous others, has succeeded in giving us detailed clinical pictures of the two hemispheres and a new appreciation of the importance of the right brain.

Split-brain research has also presented man with some interesting questions concerning awareness and consciousness. "It has been asked," writes Jose Delgado, "whether patients with surgically disconnected cerebral hemispheres have two consciousnesses; whether they are one or two persons; who is who; who is the original individual; and even whether they should have two votes!" [12:p. 386].

Gazzaniga comments:

> All the evidence indicates that separation of the hemispheres creates two independent spheres of consciousness within a single cranium, that is to say, within a single organism. This conclusion is disturbing to some people who view consciousness as an indivisible property of the human brain. It seems premature to others, who insist that the capacities revealed thus far for the right hemisphere are at the level of an automaton. There is, to be sure, hemispheric inequality in the present cases, but it may well be a characteristic of the individuals we have studied. It is entirely possible that if a human brain were divided in a very young person, both hemispheres could as a result separately and independently develop mental functions of a high order at the level attained only in the left hemisphere of normal individuals. [20:p. 100]

A group of scientists have concentrated on memory, both visual and verbal. They are also studying another division of memory—short-term and long-term. Karl Lashley, an American neuropsychologist, was one of the first to try to localize memory within the brain. His experiments seemed to suggest that memory was everywhere and could not be localized. Just as he was coming to this conclusion, Wilder Penfield, a Canadian neurosurgeon, began to examine phenomena that suggested a physical existence for memory. Penfield's conclusion was that at least a part of the memory circuitry is located in the temporal lobe. Work on visual memory by a Princeton psychologist, Charles Gross, and a Stanford psychologist, K. L. Chow, supports Penfield's premise [2].

There is general agreement among brain researchers that the production of protein is involved in the storage of long-term memory. Others go even further and theorize that the storage containers for long-term memory are protein molecules. This idea has led to the suggestion that a single protein molecule might contain a complex memory, such as a symphonic score. Why, then, ask some scientists, would it not be possible to graft pieces of brain in order to transfer memory?

Two scientists, James McConnell at the University of Michigan, and Allan Jacobson, a colleague, performed different memory molecule experiments on flatworms and rats, respectively, and reported successful results. McConnell fed some of his flatworms to others, and Jacobson injected RNA from the brains of trained rats into the brains of untrained ones. These experiments were extremely controversial, and many individuals felt compelled to dispute them, claiming that they could not be duplicated. The McConnell and Jacobson experiments were performed in the early 1960s, and the skepticism surrounding their work caused them to abandon them. Since then, a pharmacology professor at Baylor College of Medicine, Georges Ungar, has claimed the successful transfer of learned behavior in the brains of mice through the extraction of a protein molecule. Ungar's experiments are being received with even more skepticism than the previous ones [2].

Technology is playing a primary role in brain research, allowing much more advanced experimentation than was possible even ten years ago. The electrical activity of the human brain was first recorded by Hans Berger, a German psychiatrist, almost sixty years ago, with the aid of the electroencephalograph. The EEG (electroencephalogram) reveals the varying voltages and frequencies of brain waves. Today, neuroscientists are using sophisticated graphics and high-speed computers to monitor brain activity. The BEAM (brain electrical activity mapping) machine being utilized by Dr. Frank Duffy, Harvard Medical School, is able to convert "the output of an ordinary 20-channel electroencephalograph into a color-contour map of the electrical activity at the surface of the brain" [33:p. 31]. As Duffy explains BEAM, it is a visual aid of the topographical display of the brain, giving a "movie" of the brain's response.

Other techniques available for monitoring the brain's activity include the CT (computed tomography) scan, which uses penetrating x-rays, and the PET (position emission tomography), scan which requires the injection of a radioactive substance into the bloodstream as well as the use of x-rays. Kevin McKean explains that the advantage of the BEAM technique is that it is noninvasive; "it involves only the passive monitoring of brain waves" [33:p. 32]. McKean reports that plans are being made to connect the BEAM machine with other instruments and to combine the data of BEAM and PET. "Using these machines in tandem," McKean says, "should help scientists learn more about what is still one of nature's greatest mysteries: the human brain" [33:p. 33].

Scalp-recorded electrical activity of the brain was a major area of study for investigators during the 1970s. The neuroscientists of the eighties are hoping to develop even more sophisticated methods of creating images of the functional electrical activity of the brain by using advanced cybernetic tools. According to Kathleen Stein, researchers at the EEG Systems Laboratory at Langley Porter Neuropsychiatric Institute in California are using a sixty-four–channel EEG scalp-recording helmet that will allow brain activity to be monitored through computerized signal processing. Stein writes:

> The long-term results of their lines of research could virtually open a door into the brain, admitting its user for the first time to look in on his own "wiring." With this kind of knowledge, a person just might be able to enhance his learning capabilities, his memory, his hand-eye coordination. One may even be able to employ his own brain in a biocybernetic capacity, be able to link his brain to a computer to bypass the body entirely for such chores as guiding vehicles or machines. [40:p. 56]

Alan Gavins, Director of the EEG Systems Laboratory, explains that the model of the brain currently being used is that of a local computer network. He compares this with the model of the steam engine, which was used during the latter half of the nineteenth century; the telephone switchboard model, which was used in the early twentieth century; and the cybernetic guidance and control system model, which has been in use since the late 1940s [40].

The computer industry is also aiding the growth of the new field of molecular electronics, which is of immense importance to neuroscience. Biochemists and biotechnologists are using molecular electronics to work on the production of a bioprocessor, which has far-reaching implications for impact on human brain studies. Kathleen McAuliffe, who describes this phenomenon as the "biochip revolution" explains:

> The bioprocessor will be a molecular latticework that can grow and reproduce. Capable of logic, reason, perhaps even feeling, its three-dimensional organic circuitry will not process data in the rigid linear style of earlier computers, but network-fashion, like the living brain. Small enough to mesh directly with the human nervous system, biochip implants may restore sight to the blind and hearing to the deaf, replace damaged spinal nerves, and give the human brain memory and number-crunching power to rival today's mightiest computers. [31:p. 53]

James McAlear, president of EMV Associates, Inc., of Rockville, Maryland, intends to build a living computer that can design and assemble itself. This computer would use the same genetic coding mechanism as other living things. McAlear's projects in the field of artificial intelligence are reminiscent of science fiction but are being taken very seriously by other researchers. He has recently been awarded a National Science Foundation grant to test the first living interface between the brain and the electrode-studded chip. McAlear comments on artificial intelligence:

> After all, we are looking at conductive velocities about a million times faster than nerve cells, circuit switches one hundred million times faster than neuronal junctions, or synapses, and packing densities of the functional circuit elements a million times greater than are formed in the brain.
> This factor of ten to the twentieth power is truly incomprehensible in terms of any present concept of intelligence. It would be expected that the "being" of an individual so equipped would live in the computer part, not in the central nervous system. It is also possible that when the corpus perishes, its implant would survive and could be transmitted to a fresh host. Well, that pretty much fits the specifications for an immortal soul. And if you have something that has intelligence and the ability to communicate at high speed, it might well become a single consciousness—a superior, an omnipotent being. [31:p. 55]

McAlear and others working in the area of artificial intelligence imply that research and development will allow the eventual disappearance of present distinctions between life and nonlife. The implantation of a biocomputer in the human brain will provoke the evolution of a higher type of intelligence. McAlear, emphasizing the revolutionary impact of the biocomputer, states, "We are so accustomed to thinking of ourselves as the crowning glory of evolution that it is difficult even to consider the possibility that we are merely the beginning of life—a potential for intellectual development that is limitless once we take control of our biological destiny" [31:p. 58].

Neurological researchers at the National Institutes of Health are envisioning the implantation of microcomputers in paralyzed limbs, which, activated by brain waves, can be programmed to control basic motor functions. These investigators are concentrating upon discovering how nerve cells communicate [19].

Candace Pert, who was instrumental in the discovery of the opiate receptor, which led to the discovery by two Scottish scientists, John Hughes and Hans Kosterlitz, of endorphins, the body's natural opiates, is currently working on the connection of neurochemical phenomena with circuit diagrams of the brain. Pert is quoted in an interview:

> I'm tinkering around inside the human computer. People are just very complicated electronic mechanisms, and our emotions of love, hate, anger, and fear are hard-wired in our brains.
>
> There's no doubt in my mind that one day—and I don't think that day is all that far away—we'll be able to make a color-coded map of the brain. A color-coded wiring diagram, with blue for one neurochemical, red for another, and so on—that's the neuroscientist's ambition. We'll be able to describe the brain in mathematical, physical, neurochemical, and electrical terms, with all the rigor of a differential equation. [34:p. 64]

The Building Blocks of Behavior

The association of brain activity and complex behavioral patterns has proven to be an extremely complicated endeavor. Some investigators have tried to address behavior as a separate phenomenon. Attempts have been made to discover the simplest elements or building blocks of complex behavioral patterns. This endeavor was largely initiated through the pioneering efforts of Ivan Petrovich Pavlov (1849–1936), a Russian physiologist.

Pavlov conducted experiments with animals that led to the establishment of a paradigm for learning through conditioning. Pavlov, who won a 1904 Nobel prize for his work on the mechanisms of digestion, noticed that his dogs salivated before their food was placed in front of them. Their salivary glands began working when they heard the sounds of food preparation or saw the person who fed them. He began to wonder why this happened and to become interested in the process surrounding the dogs' responses. He performed the now-famous bell experiment, in which he caused a bell to ring just before the dog got its food. The dog salivated when the bell rang. If no food appeared after the bell for a long enough period of time, the dog no longer salivated at the sound. From these experiments, Pavlov ascertained that the cycle of learning was a conditioning process that included four phases—drive, stimulus, response, reinforcement. Pavlov's method is known as *classical conditioning*, because it was the initial method. Sometimes it is called Pavlovian conditioning, in his honor.

Pavlov became a hero in the USSR because of the premise that followed from his findings with dogs, that perhaps man could also be conditioned. His behavior could be shaped and controlled through the same type of process utilized with the dogs. Pavlov worked in Russia until his death, trying to refine his experiments, which the Russians used to support the Marxist doctrine of environment being more crucial to development than heredity.

Three American psychologists, John B. Watson, Edward L. Thorndike, and B. F. Skinner, became tremendously excited at Pavlov's findings and began intensive work on exploration of the conditioning process in man. Watson viewed human behavior from a strictly mechanistic viewpoint and believed, according to Lee Edson, that, "Man . . . was little more than a stimulus-response machine; such humanistic notions as love and desire . . . are really only manifestations of conditioned glandular or muscular responses in the body" [17:p. 36]. Watson himself is quoted as saying, "Give me a dozen healthy infants, well formed, and my own specified world to bring them up in, and I'll guarantee to take anyone at random and train him to become any type of specialist I might select—doctor, lawyer, artist, merchant-chief, and yes, even beggarman and thief, regardless of his talents, penchants, tendencies, abilities, vocations, and the race of his ancestors" [17:p. 36].

Just as Pavlov is remembered for his experiments with dogs, Watson is remembered for his experiments with a single child named Albert. Through the application of the conditioning paradigm, Watson caused Albert, eleven months old, to scream in terror at the sight of a furry white rat. Watson is controversial because of the methods he used on Albert and because he took such an extreme position in viewing man as a completely mechanical being. However, Watson's experiments with Albert and later with other children gave psychotherapists the idea for deconditioning processes used to rid people of their phobias.

Thorndike, who had been performing experiments on cats ten years before Pavlov made his discoveries, attempted to prove through trial-and-error experiments that learning is mechanistic. He believed that one could be taught new behavior through a "kind of mechanical process of 'stamping in' new connections in the brain" [29:p. 151]. Thorndike eventually came up with what is known as the law of effect, "the principle that the outcome of an activity will determine whether it is learned or repeated" [29:p. 151]. Thorndike also theorized that learning would be inhibited by discomfort and increased by reward.

Skinner is the scientist credited with making a profound alteration in learning theory through introduction of operant, or instrumental conditioning, as opposed to classical conditioning. Skinner had been inspired by both Pavlov and Thorndike and built his theories accordingly. Operant conditioning is described by Lyons and Barrell as "a type of behavior conditioning in which a subject learns to make a particular response in order to secure positive reinforcement or avoid negative reinforcement" [29:p. 152]. Pavlov's techniques revolved around the animals' built-in reflexes; Skinner's techniques involved the teaching of new behaviors through *shaping*, which is defined as "an operant conditioning technique in which a desired response is learned by rewarding all close responses initially and by then decreasing rewards until only the desired response is elicited" [29:p. 152].

The idea of the conditioning of man through the process of shaping is controversial, although its power is generally acknowledged. Conditioning techniques have been used widely and successfully in the field of advertising. Skinner has suggested that man and his culture can be reshaped through conditioning. In his book *Walden Two*, he employs a character named Frazier to present his ideas. Frazier explains that joy and love, productive emotions that strengthen, will be reinforced, but "sorrow and hate—and the high voltage excitements of anger, fear and rage—are out of proportion with the needs of modern life, and they're wasteful and dangerous" [17:p. 53]. Consequently, they (the negative emotions) will be systematically eliminated through the conditioning process.

In both *Walden Two* and its nonfiction version, *Beyond Freedom and Dignity*, Skinner clearly advocates the use of behavior modification techniques to rid the world of those things he considers undesirable—injustice, war, pollution, and other "negative influences" upon the population. He implies that man is a machine, insofar as he can be reprogrammed and reshaped just as one would rebuild a machine to be more efficient or less noisy [21].

That man can be reprogrammed has been much publicized. Brainwashing techniques have been reported at various times in different parts of the world. The Russians were said to have used brainwashing in the 1930s to extract confessions from individuals who had once been leading party members or army officers. Mental torture was the primary mechanism used, and it was in the form of a "deprogramming" of everything the accused men knew, instilling in them a hopeless confusion, making them amenable to any suggestion from their accusers. The same type of conditioning was supposedly employed by the Chinese during the Korean war [21].

Behavior modification programs are also in effect in many penal institutions and mental hospitals. These programs are most often built around a reward system. If punishment is used, it is in the form of a withdrawal of privileges rather than physical pain. Conditioning techniques have been employed to cure alcoholics, other drug users, and smokers of their addictions.

Not all individuals who have been exposed to behavior modification programs have been successful in ridding themselves of their negative behaviors. Some individuals have been able to withstand the extreme conditioning techniques used in brainwashing. However, the belief still exists among some investigators that, if enough is known about brain structure and its relation to "mind," it will be possible to reshape all individuals.

When approaching the brain-mind problem, the reductionists who focused on a mechanistic approach to behavior often maintained a dualistic attitude. They divided the self into two parts, its form and its function, just as they had done to the external world. There was the brain with its centers and organ systems, its function to secrete behavior. If one could know the function of the smallest units, the brain cells or neurons, one could induce the function of the organ it (or they) helped to compose.

With regard to the investigation of human behavior, the reductionists and mechanists have generally divided into two groups—the behaviorists and the structuralists. The behaviorists focus on stimulus-response patterns, with the triggering mechanisms in the external environment. The structuralists lean more toward the form of the internal apparatus as responsible for its functions. The structuralists believe that complex functions, such as language, are due to the unique structure of the brain.

Sociobiologists might be included in the structuralists' camp, at least with regard to microscopic structure. They imply that the DNA building blocks that carry codes for the building of cells and organs also carry codes that determine many patterns of behavior.

Howard Gardner writes:

> The structuralists are distinguished first and foremost by their ardent, powerfully held conviction that there is structure underlying all human behavior and mental functioning, and by their belief that this structure can be discovered through orderly analysis, that it has cohesiveness and meaning, and that struc-

tures have generality (otherwise there would be as many structures as behaviors, and little point in spelling them out). [18:p. 10]

Although Gardner states a personal reservation about the concept "human mind" because of its implications of a mind-body dichotomy he rejects, he gives the following two assumptions that distinguish the structuralist philosophy:

One is the belief that through careful examination of groups which, like children or primitives, differ from the contemporary Western adult, new light can be cast on the whole of human experience; the second is the faith that what is distinctive about human beliefs, development, and institutions is a reflection of the fundamental nature of human thought, and hence, the biological structure of the "human mind." [18:p. 13]

Whether searching for the smallest components of the brain or of behavior, investigators have occasionally been compelled to address the question of "mind." Sherrington was convinced that the part of the picture we call mind may never be known and that, therefore, we should have misgivings about our ability to understand the brain. He wrote:

Mind, for anything perception can compass, goes therefore in our spatial world more ghostly than a ghost. Invisible, intangible, it is a thing not even of outline; it is not a "thing." It remains without sensual confirmation, and remains without it forever. All that counts in life. Desire, zest, truth, love, knowledge, "values", and, seeking metaphor to eke out expression, hell's depth and heaven's utmost height. [39:p. 256]

Eccles calls himself a dualist-interactionist who believes that the brain and the mind are independent entities. He also names Sherrington and Penfield as developing dualist-interactionist theories. Eccles postulates a self-conscious mind that "exercises a superior interpretative and controlling role upon the neuronal events [15:p. 226]. He explains further:

A key component of the hypothesis is that the unity of conscious experience is provided by the self-conscious mind and not by the neuronal machinery of the liaison areas of the cerebral hemisphere. . . .
    The experienced unity comes, not from a neurophysiological synthesis, but from the proposed integrating character of the self-conscious mind. I conjecture that in the first place the *raison d'etre* of the self-conscious mind is to give this unity of the self in all its conscious experiences and actions. [15:pp. 227–228]

The study of the machine that runs the machine continues, however, with the hope on the part of many that science will eventually understand the mechanism in its entirety and settle the question of "mind." Lord Adrian discussed the mind-body problem with the idea that natural science must address the question of mind without defining it and that the physiologist, being a natural scientist, must continue the research. He wrote, "So for the present we can set aside these misgivings and go on trying to find out what sort of physical and chemical changes are taking place in the brain when the mind is at work" [1:p. 232].

Numbers of scientists have, indeed, set aside their misgivings, if they have them, and continued to investigate the structure of the brain. Technological advancements, most notably in the area of computers, are aiding them in their search for an understanding of brain mechanisms. There are those who continue to think that the mind and the brain are synonomous. They assert that mind is "the ghost in the machine" and imply that continued research into the physical brain will solve the mystery of the human mind. Others imply that the physical brain is too much of an enigma to allow comprehension. Gevins, after discussing his analogy of the brain to a local computer network, said, "But I don't want to get trapped in this analogy. The brain is more complicated than our machines. Until the next technology comes along, it's convenient to model it after local computer networks, but the brain is basically a different sort of entity" [40:p. 58].

Pert, after calling people "complicated electronic mechanisms" introduced a new note by saying:

> Consciousness is before the brain, I think. A lot of people believe in life after death, and the brain may not be necessary to consciousness. Consciousness may be projected to different places. It's like trying to describe what happens when three people have an incredible conversation together. It's almost as if there were a fourth or fifth person there; the whole is greater than the sum of its parts. [34:p. 112]

The apex of the mechanistic approach to the human brain behavior problem is apparent in the idea of building a machine that thinks. Pamela McCorduck traces the history of this idea in her book *Machines Who Think* and writes:

> But are humans machines? Even machines that clank softly, meat machines? Is the mind a mechanism? We've said yes, then no. We've wanted to put ourselves inside nature that way, yet stumbled over the means, as the histories of both philosophy and psychology have shown us.
>   Well, then, if the properties of mind can be realized by a physical process, they are mechanisms. Does that ease the resistance we feel to the idea of mind as mechanism? . . . Apparently it isn't enough that those mechanisms all around us, our fellow humans, do thinking: historically, at least, we've preferred to postulate the mind-body split. [32:p. 330]

Marvin Minsky, one of the modern researchers in artificial intelligence, discusses the mind-body problem:

> When a question leads to confused, inconsistent answers, this may be because the question is ultimately meaningless or at least unanswerable, but it may also be because an adequate answer requires a powerful analytical apparatus. [32:p. 340]

He implies that the conceptual tools necessary for understanding or solving the problem of mind may become available as research continues in the area of attempting to make computers behave intelligently.

From one perspective, computer simulation of various functions of mind-brain activity appears reductionistic. We may use a mechanical form to accomplish a biologic function. The human body, including the brain may be a "meat machine." Just as mathematics was used first to reify the word world and later to move concepts toward other frames of reference, the computer at first seems to reify a mechanistic and reductionistic approach to the question of human self, mind, and body. However, as we shall see in the next section, mathematics and the science of information processing has catalyzed new concepts that undermine the rigid mechanical world of Euclid and Newton and raise questions of enormous magnitude.

The age of certainty is beginning to wane even while it is making its most inspiring contributions.

References

1. Adrian, L: A physiological approach to the mind. In Flew, A (Ed): *Body, Mind, and Death.* New York: Macmillan, 1964, pp 231–236
2. Bailey, R: *The Role of the Brain.* New York: Time, Inc., 1975
3. Baumer, F L: *Modern European Thought: Continuity and Change in Ideas, 1600–1950.* New York: Macmillan, 1977
4. Bernstein, P, and Green, R: *History of Civilization,* Volume I: *To 1648.* Totowa, New Jersey: Littlefield, Adams, 1976
5. Bernstein, P, and Green, R: *History of Civilization,* Volume II: *Since 1648.* Totowa, New Jersey: Littlefield, Adams, 1976
6. Bowra, C: *Classical Greece.* New York: Time, Inc., 1965
7. Bronowski, J: *The Ascent of Man.* Boston: Little, Brown, 1973
8. Capra, F: *The Tao of Physics.* Boulder, Colorado: Shambhala, 1975
9. Carson, L: *Ancient Egypt.* New York: Time, Inc., 1965
10. Darwin, C: Autobiography. In Loewenberg, B (Ed): *Charles Darwin: Evolution and Natural Selection: An Anthology of the Writings of Charles Darwin.* Boston: Beacon Press, 1959, pp 161–299
11. Darwin, C: The origin of species. In Loewenberg, B (Ed): *Charles Darwin: Evolution and Natural Selection: An Anthology of the Writings of Charles Darwin.* Boston: Beacon Press, 1959, pp 161–299
12. Delgado, J: Triunism: A transmaterial brain-mind theory. In *Brain and Mind,* Ciba Foundation Symposium (69) (new series), Amsterdam, The Netherlands: Excerpta Medica, 1979
13. Descartes, R: Thought comprises every sort of consciousness. In Flew, A (Ed): *Body, Mind, and Death.* New York: Macmillan, 1964, pp 133–137
14. Durant, W: *The Story of Philosophy: The Lives and Opinions of the Greater Philosophers.* New York: Washington Square Press, 1926
15. Eccles, J C: *The Human Mystery.* New York: Springer International, 1979
16. Eccles, J C, and Gibson, W C: *Sherrington: His Life and Thought.* New York: Springer International, 1979
17. Edson, L: *How We Learn.* New York: Time, Inc., 1975
18. Gardner, H: *The Quest for Mind: Piaget, Levi-Strauss, and the Structuralist Movement.* New York: Vintage Books, 1974
19. Garr, D: The healing brain. *Omni,* September 1981, pp 80–85
20. Gazzaniga, M: The split brain in man. In Ornstein, R (Ed): *The Nature of Human Consciousness: A Book of Readings.* New York: Viking Press, 1973
21. Good, P: *The Individual.* New York: Time, Inc., 1974
22. Gorman, J: The case of the selfish DNA. *Discover,* Volume 2, Number 6, June 1981, pp 32–36
23. Gould, S J: *Ever Since Darwin: Reflections in Natural History.* New York: W. W. Norton, 1977
24. Gould, S J: Evolution as fact and theory. *Discover,* Volume 2, Number 5, May 1981, pp 34–37

25. Grunwald, J (Editor-in-Chief): The year in science. *Discover*, Volume 3, Number 1, January 1982, pp 66–79

26. Gurin, J: In the beginning. *Science 80*, Volume 1, Number 5, July/August 1980, pp 44–51

27. Hale, J: *Renaissance*. New York: Time, Inc., 1965

28. Huxley, T H: On the origin of species. In Loewenberg, B (Ed): *Charles Darwin: Evolution and Natural Selection: An Anthology of the Writings of Charles Darwin*. Boston: Beacon Press, 1959

29. Lyons, J, and Barrell, J J: *People: An Introduction to Psychology*. New York: Harper & Row, 1979

30. Mason, S F: *A History of the Sciences*. New York: Collier Books, 1962

31. McAuliffe, K: Biochip revolution. *Omni*, December 1981, pp 52–58

32. McCorduck, P: *Machines Who Think*. San Francisco: W. H. Freeman, 1979

33. McKean, K: Beaming new light on the brain. *Discover*, Volume 2, Number 12, December 1981, pp 30–33

34. Pert, C: Interview. *Omni*, February 1982, pp 61–65, 110–112

35. Popper, K R, and Eccles, J C: *The Self and Its Brain*. New York: Springer International, 1977

36. Rensberger, B: Tinkering with life. *Science 81*, Volume 2, Number 9, November 1981, pp 44–49

37. Rose, S: *The Conscious Brain*. New York: Vintage Books, 1976

38. Sagan, C: *Cosmos*. New York: Random House, 1980

39. Sherrington, C: *Man on His Nature*. New York: Cambridge University Press, 1963

40. Stein, K: Brainstorms. *Omni*, October 1981, pp 52–58, 140–144

41. Thomas, L J: *The Lives of a Cell: Notes of a Biology Watcher*. New York: Bantam, 1975

42. Whitehead, A N: *Science and the Modern World*. New York: Mentor, 1948

The Mechanical World of Form and Function

Commencement Remarks

It is with some pleasure and some sadness that I address those of you who are graduating today. You are beginning your career—I am near the end of mine. Although I would not trade places with you, for my life has been rich and rewarding, I do feel a pang of jealousy that I cannot be with you in the quest, your search for truth. In your scientific endeavors, I hope that you will always strive to seek out those tiny hidden bits of knowledge that will assist you and others to piece together a clearer picture of reality.

There are pitfalls in your quest, dangerous temptations to extend a fact beyond its boundaries, rely on intuition rather than observation, or guess rather than measurement. A newly discovered fact may be so intoxicating in its radiance that you may be lulled into framing it against a teleologic or tautologic background, and though it glows for awhile, the matrix in which it is embedded will corrupt it and nullify its value to you and to others.

Beware of those whose reliance on metaphysics and mysticism, now so prevalent in our culture, offers premature closure on questions of enormous magnitude. They have the ear of the masses, but in the bright light of objective scrutiny, they are as jellyfish on hot sand! There will be those, not, it is hoped, among you, who will counterfeit science or use it for monetary or political reward. Science is, and must always be, its own reward. Each answer must bring new questions, and each hypothesis, new tests for validity. Often, our measurements and observations may have little meaning to us, but if we are meticulous in our pursuits, others perhaps yet unborn may use our data to further human knowledge—the noblest cause for self-dedication.

Best wishes now and may all your publications be validated.
Thank you.

The Relative World
of
Process

Chapter 7

The Return of Uncertainty

The test of the explanations which science offers is that they shall so connect one event with another that we can coherently predict the results of our actions. By this test, its classical methods had toward the end of the last century had two hundred and fifty years without a failure. But by the same test, at the end of the last century classical science failed. This needs to be said roundly, for many people still speak as if the choice between the old and the new picture of nature were a matter of philosophical taste. It is not: it is a matter of fact. [6:p. 35]

Jacob Bronowski, 1955

A detailed investigation of the sources of our ideas has shown that there is only one type of model or picture which could be intelligible to our restricted minds, namely one in mechanical terms. Yet a review of recent physics has shown that all attempts at mechanical models or pictures have failed and must fail. For a mechanical model or picture must represent things as happening in space and time, while it has recently become clear that the ultimate processes of nature neither occur in, nor admit of representation in, space and time. Thus an understanding of the ultimate processes of nature is for ever beyond our reach; we shall never be able—even in imagination—to open the case of our watch and see how the wheels go round. The true object of scientific study can never be the realities of nature, but only our own observations on nature. [21:pp. 364–365]

Sir James Jeans, 1954

The Relativity Theories

As the twentieth century began, the scientific world was still dominated by Newtonian method and thinking. The work of Newton had allowed a new vision, a new way of understanding the world. Newton and many of his followers were religious men who believed that they were to direct their inquiries toward the discovery of a divinely governed universe that operated according to immutable laws of God. The universe was analogous to a clock that had been wound up by the Creator and was running as He had directed.

Newtonian science had been enormously validated by tremendous advances in technology related to measurement. Instruments were devised that could measure time, space, mass, and energy with extraordinary accuracy. These instruments, coupled with other instruments that assisted man's perception, that is, the telescope and the microscope, allowed measurements of relationships in a world that had previously been beyond man's perception. By 1900, we were capable of entering the worlds of the very large and the very small and measuring these worlds with the utmost precision.

Those scientists who studied matter and energy and the interactions between the two thought that they had carried their investigations to a point beyond which nothing much would be added to the general body of knowledge. James S. Trefil commented:

> By the late 19th century, physics had come to the point where it seemed that its original mission—to explain the physical world—had been fulfilled. Most physicists felt that nothing new was going to turn up in their investigations of the world: that all that was left to do was to find the next decimal place in various physical constants and to work out in even greater detail the consequences of the laws that had already been stated. [33:p. 202]

Around the turn of the twentieth century, however, our conceptual frames concerning space, time, and energy began to show flaws. Mathematics, the instrument by which the world of the very small and the world of the very large were measured, began to alter and take on new form. The world of absolutes, the logical, measurable, cause-and-effect mechanical world, began to show cracks in its foundation. This was not totally unexpected, for as Trefil said, "A few physicists realized that, contained within the structure of classical physics, were the seeds of its own destruction" [33:p. 202].

To speak of the death of certainty may be a bit premature, since the search for absolutes remains a major driving force in science. However, the concepts of certainty in a reductionistic approach to form and function aligned in a mechanistic cause-and-effect sequence suffered severe injury in the beginning years of the twentieth century, an injury that was rather insidious in spite of its abruptness. Most of us are not yet aware of all its ramifications. Like an internal hemorrhage in its effects upon the body, the injury to the world of absolutes began to cause major conceptual frames to stagger without apparent reason to the casual observer.

Three papers appeared in the early 1900s that precipitated an enormous change in the laws and concepts of classical physics. The first was the presentation of the quantum theory by Max Planck, in 1900. The other two were Albert Einstein's papers on special relativity (1905) and general relativity (1916). Although these papers are credited with bringing about the changes that have been termed "a revolution in physics," the men who wrote them reflected the thinking of several individuals who preceded them.

Einstein recognized the importance of the work of the many scientists who helped lay the foundation of the new physics. He is quoted as saying:

> In every true searcher of Nature there is a kind of religious reverence; for he finds it impossible to imagine that he is the first to have thought out the exceedingly delicate threads that connect his perceptions. The aspect of knowledge which has not yet been laid bare gives the investigator a feeling akin to

that experienced by a child who seeks to grasp the masterly way in which elders manipulate things. [15:p. 238]

Although it would be impractical, if not impossible, to trace the threads of thought that lead eventually to the theories of special and general relativity and the quantum theory, a few individuals made significant contributions. Not all these individuals were acknowledged by Einstein to have influenced his thinking directly, but they added important information to the data pool. It is often difficult to explain exactly how one's ideas take form or exactly what triggers a so-called inspiration.

In the eighteenth and early nineteenth centuries, theories of electricity were, according to Bertrand Russell, "wholly dominated by the Newtonian analogy" [28:p. 49]. In 1841, Michael Faraday (1791–1867) discovered the process of electromagnetic induction. He also determined the laws governing the direction in which the current in the wire will flow. His work on induction paved the way for James Clerk Maxwell (1831–1879) to adopt a theory of electromagnetism in which he suggested that light and electricity are the same in their ultimate natures. Maxwell's four laws of nature with regard to electricity and magnetism are today known as Maxwell's equations. The equations were based on the work of Faraday and his predecessors. They were to have a direct influence on the work of Einstein. Carl Sagan wrote, "The corrected Maxwell equations implied the existence of electromagnetic radiation, encompassing gamma rays, X-rays, ultraviolet light, visible light, infrared and radio. They stimulated Einstein to discover Special Relativity" [29:p. 39].

Prior to 1900, most physicists conceptualized space as being filled with a fixed, invisible substance called *ether*. However, in 1887, before Einstein's publication, Albert Abraham Michaelson (1852–1931) and Edward Williams Morley (1838–1923) performed a series of experiments that demolished the theory of a stationary ether. Ernst Mach (1838–1916) read the report of the Michaelson-Morley experiments and concurred with the idea that the concept of a stationary ether was incorrect. Although Einstein claimed that the Michaelson-Morley findings had little effect upon his thinking, he credited Mach with being a great influence. He read Mach's *Science of Mechanics* and applauded his skepticism toward Newtonian absolutes. Mach had referred to absolute space and motion as "pure mental constructs, that cannot be produced in experience" [2:pp. 457–458]. Franklin L. Baumer wrote, "Rejecting the abstraction of isolated bodies rotating in an empty universe, Mach also talked much about relative motions. 'For me only relative motions exist.'" [2:p. 458]. Einstein himself credited Mach with convincing him that absolute motion does not exist. He claimed that Mach shook his dogmatic faith in mechanics. Silvio Bergia went to some length to outline Mach's influence upon Einstein and quoted Philipp Frank, one of Einstein's biographers, as claiming that Mach had "ploughed the ground where Einstein could cast his seed" [3:p. 85].

Hendrik Antoon Lorentz (1853–1928), a Dutch physicist and personal friend of Einstein's, made outstanding contributions to the electron theory of matter and the electromagnetic theory of light. He studied the phenomena of moving bodies and worked out the law "the greater the speed, the greater the contraction," which Einstein proved mathematically. Einstein was able to use the Lorentz transformation in elaborating his special theory of relativity. The Lorentz transformation, according to Russell, "tells us what estimate of distances and periods of time will be made by an observer whose relative motion is known, when we are given those of another observer" [28:pp. 52–53]. Einstein, however, was to give Lorentz' theories a fundamentally different interpretation.

Jules Henri Poincaré (1854–1912), a French mathematician, predicted the development of the special theory of relativity and intuitively understood it, as is evidenced by a remark he made in 1904, at which time he predicted a new mechanics that would demonstrate there can be no velocity that exceeds light. He said that the new mechanics would maintain "the principle of relativity, according to which the laws of physical phenomena should be the same, whether for an observer fixed, or for an observer carried along in such a motion" [16:p. 76].

A few scholars have suggested that Einstein merely set forth Poincaré's theory, but others have suggested notable differences. Martin Gardner postulated that Poincaré's belief in a universal time prevented his creating the theory of special relativity. He also suggested that "Poincaré did not see the essential steps that had to be taken in order to carry out such a program" [16:p. 76]. Bergia stated that "There is an all-important difference of method between Poincaré and Einstein" [3:p. 80]. He also claimed that the predictive value of Einstein's theory made it substantially different from that of Poincaré. He noted, however, that Poincaré's results could be carried over into relativity. Einstein was apparently not aware of the extremely close similarity of his thinking and that of Poincaré and Lorentz when he developed the theory of special relativity but acknowledged their achievements years later.

Several physicists had ventured into what would become the new physics, but it took the genius of Einstein to formalize the theory of special relativity, which heralded the revolution in scientific thinking of the twentieth century [14]. His first paper on relativity appeared in Volume 17 of *Annalen der Physik* in 1905, and its impact on the Newtonian world is still being felt.

In order to understand the immensity of Einstein's work, we should review the basic tenets of Newtonian physics. In the Newtonian system, there was absolute space and absolute time, which contained bits of moving matter. Time and space did not change. Changes could occur in time, but time itself flowed along smoothly and uniformly. The earth moved around the sun in absolute time in a sea of motionless ether. Atoms, which were the basic units of matter, were absolute. The total quantity of atoms or matter in the universe was constant, and the only change was in the distribution.

In the Newtonian view it was possible to have a stationary observer who could measure the absolute velocities of moving objects. Copernicus thought that the sun was the governor or ruler of the universe, the fixed observer. Kepler believed that the sun was the center for the Deity. Newton himself believed that God was the stationary and immutable observer and prime mover. He said that the Deity "endures for ever, and is everywhere present, and by existing always and everywhere, He constitutes duration and space. . . . (He is) a Being incorporeal, loving, intelligent, and omnipresent, who in infinite space, as it were in his sensory, sees the things themselves intimately, and thoroughly perceives them, and comprehends them wholly by their immediate presence to Himself" [24:pp. 541–542].

The Newtonian system was a deterministic system best characterized, perhaps, by Pierre de Laplace. In his *Essay on Probability*, written in 1812, he expressed the theory that a certain universe existed that would be predictable in every aspect, if one could know the positions and speeds of all the particles. The Laplace universe was a cause-and-effect universe with a fixed history or, as Baumer described it, "The whole history of the universe, past, present, and future, was fixed, a chain of irresistible (and equivalent) causes and effects" [2:p. 461].

Einstein, in his 1905 paper on special relativity, presented two postulates that made sense only in a universe in which time and length are not absolute. He said that (1) there is no way to tell whether an object is at rest or in uniform motion relative to a fixed ether, and (2) regardless of the motion of its source, light always moves through empty space with the same constant speed. In essence, Einstein claimed that there was no universal absolute time for everyone, only a local time that applies solely to the instant or "now" the observer occupies. He said that both time and length were relative. Gardner explained:

> Length and time are relative concepts. They have no meaning apart from the relation of an object to an observer. There is no relation of one set of measurements being "true," another set "false." Each is true relative to the observer making the measurements; relative to his frame of reference. [16:pp. 53–54]

The theory of special relativity also showed that mass is relative, that there are relative changes in the amount of matter in an object. Einstein formulated his famous equation $E = mc^2$ to express the relation of mass to energy. Energy can change to mass and mass can change to energy under certain conditions. The old ideas of classical physics of an unchangeable total amount of mass and an unchangeable total amount of energy in the universe were seen as not accurate. Every experiment concerning the fundamental postulates of special relativity has established them as fact, and the theory is considered to be sound in all respects.

The impact of the theory of special relativity was so enormous and its postulates so inconceivable to many classical physicists that it was extremely difficult to visualize. In 1908, Hermann Minkowski (1864–1909), Einstein's mathematics teacher, gave a lecture to the Eightieth Assembly of German Natural Scientists and Physicians, making it possible for his audience to have at least a limited understanding of Einstein's theory. In this lecture, Minkowski postulated a four-dimensional space-time universe. He said that objects exist in both time and place. "Nobody has ever noticed a place except at a given time or a time except at a place" [38:p. 40]. He also made the often quoted, beautiful, and unforgettable statement, "Henceforth space by itself, and time by itself, are doomed to fade away into mere shadows, and only a kind of union of the two will preserve an independent reality" [2:pp. 462–463].

Several scholars have theorized that Einstein may well have developed his ideas from his work with Minkowski, who was aware of many of the concepts of relativity, including time dilation. Minkowski's 1907 paper, *Basic Equations for the Electromagnetic Phenomena in Moving Bodies*, plus his other work, is thought to have enabled Einstein to develop the theory of general relativity, in which he was to reorganize our approach to the problems of gravitation.

The Minkowski four-dimensional universe was to emerge even more clearly in Einstein's momentous 1916 paper on general relativity. According to the special theory of relativity, uniform motion is relative, and classical physicists agreed that this was so. They were content to believe that accelerated motion was absolute. Einstein, however, was not satisfied with this idea, and in the theory of general relativity he expounded the view that *all* motion is relative and that gravity and inertia are one and the same thing. The theory was named the *general theory* because it is an extension of the special theory and includes the special theory. In other words, it is a generalization of the special theory.

Einstein was able to prove that his principle of equivalence allows a more efficient and simpler way of looking at the world despite its mathematical complexity. This principle states that gravity and inertia are the same phenomenon. In 1921 in a lecture at Princeton University, Einstein declared, "The possibility of explaining the numerical equality of inertia and gravitation by the unity of their nature gives to the general theory of relativity, according to my conviction, such a superiority over the conceptions of classical mechanics, that all the difficulties encountered must be considered as small in comparison" [16:p. 83].

According to Gardner, the general theory can be stated in this way:

> All the laws of nature are invariant (the same) with respect to any observer. This means that regardless of how an observer is moving, he can describe all the laws of nature (as he sees them) by the same mathematical equations. He may be a scientist working in a laboratory on the earth, or on the moon, or inside a giant spaceship that is slowly accelerating on its way to a distant star. The general theory of relativity provides him with a set of equations by which he can describe all the natural laws involved in any experiment he can perform. These equations will be exactly the same regardless of whether he is at rest, moving uniformly, or moving with acceleration with respect to any other object. [16:p. 89]

The general theory of relativity, which is considered to be wholly Einstein's work, is thought by mathematicians to be elegant and artistic. Lorentz said, "Every lover of the beautiful must wish it to be true" [16:p. 83]. It set forth a world of becoming rather than a world of being—a world in process. According to Baumer, "The new physics, more abstract than the old, collapsed all four Newtonian absolutes, which now became abstractions in their own turn" [2:p. 461].

Einstein said, "There is no more common-place statement than that the world in which we live is a four-dimensional space-time continuum" [2:p. 461]. But while this may have seemed a commonplace statement to Einstein, the world of classical physics was viewing it as something akin to extraordinary. Einstein had given, in his theory of general relativity, the first genuine theory of gravitation, which A. P. French described as "one of the most marvellous products of speculative but disciplined thinking about the physical world" [15:p. 111].

Although several thinkers previous to 1905 had been close to developing the special theory of relativity, and would no doubt have finally produced it, it was Einstein who made a tremendous leap beyond with the general theory. French said, "And of all Einstein's great scientific achievements, the general theory of relativity is perhaps supreme in its originality and intellectual grandeur" [15:p. 111]. Gardner wrote, "If Einstein had not lived, no doubt other scientists would have given physics the same twist, but a century or more might have slipped by before they did so. Few other great theories in the history of science seem so completely the work of a single man" [16:p. 76]

Einstein's work destroyed completely the Newtonian concept of an absolute framework of time and space. Einstein proved that the world of physics is not composed of events but of observations and that those observations are relative to each observer, to his place and velocity. Newton's world was one that looked the same to every observer, a God's-eye view of the world. Jacob Bronowski called Einstein's world a "man's eye view." He said:

> By contrast [to the God's eye view], Einstein's is a man's eye view, in which what you see and what I see is relative to each of us, that is, to our place and speed. And this relativity cannot be removed. We cannot know what the world is like in itself, we can only compare what it looks like to each of us, by the practical procedure of exchanging messages. I in my tram and you in your chair can share no divine and instant view of events—we can only communicate our own views to one another. [5:p. 249]

The man's-eye view of the world is a complete turnaround from the God's-eye view of a law-abiding universe working according to predetermined mathematical laws, a gigantic machine set in motion by its creator. The implications of the man's-eye view are frightening and unacceptable to those whose security rests upon the clockwork universe. Paul Davies said:

> In the old Newtonian picture, the observer did not seem to play an important part: the clockwork mechanism carried on turning, completely oblivious of whether, or by whom, it was being observed. The relativist's picture is different. Relations between events such as past and future, simultaneity, length and interval, become functions of the person who perceives them, and cherished impressions such as the present and the passage of time fade away from the world "out there" altogether, residing solely in our own consciousness. The division between what is real and what is subjective no longer appears to be precisely drawn, and one begins to have misgivings that the whole idea of a "real world out there" may crumble away completely. [8:p. 49]

Einstein may have seen the postulates of the new physics as "commonplace," but the traditional views are still very much dominant in the thinking of most of us. Even for physics, the consequences of Einstein's work are not easily assimilated. It is easy to acknowledge the results of the theory of relativity without incorporating it into our belief systems. Russell said:

> The problem of allowing for the spectator's point of view, we may be told, is one of which physics has at all times been fully aware; indeed it has dominated astronomy ever since the time of Copernicus. This is true. But principles are

often acknowledged long before their full consequences are drawn. Much of traditional physics is incompatible with the principle, in spite of the fact that it was acknowledged theoretically by all physicists. [28:p. 19]

One of the greatest difficulties for all of us in understanding the new physics is that we are bound to our old ideas by the very words we must use to explain the new concepts. Einstein understood this quite well and expressed it beautifully in *The World as I See It:*

> We have forgotten what features in the world of experience caused us to frame (pre-scientific) concepts, and we have great difficulty in representing the world of experience to ourselves without the spectacles of the old-established conceptual interpretation. There is the further difficulty that our language is compelled to work with words which are inseparably connected with those primitive concepts. These are the obstacles which confront us when we try to describe the essential nature of the pre-scientific concept of space. [5:pp. 255–256]

Bronowski elaborated further on the difficulties our language gives us in a discussion of numbers, or the language of relationships, in March 1966, when he said:

> This is a cardinal point: it is the language that we use in describing nature that imposes (by its arrangement of definitions and axioms) both the form and the limitations of the laws that we find. . . . On present evidence, we must conclude (in my view) that the human mind is constrained to conceive physical laws in arithmetical language: the whole numbers are literally an integral part of its conceptual apparatus. If this is so, then the mind cannot extricate the laws of nature from its own language; our formal logic is not that of nature; and we are not at all, as Leibniz and others have thought, in a preestablished harmony with the language of nature. [6:p. 61]

In spite of the many obstacles our language sets before us, we have come to recognize Einsteinian physics as the most productive way in which to view the universe. Our universe can now be conceptualized as a kaleidoscopic, open system of harmonic interacting force fields. In this interacting relationship of systems, properties emerge that we call mass and energy. The interaction of systems and mass and energy we call process. The simultaneity and sequencing of these interacting processes we call events in space-time. The events of mass and energy interacting in a particular space-time we call our universe.

The enormity of the difference in the Newtonian concept of the universe and the Einsteinian concept of the universe was well appreciated by Sir John Collings Squire, who remarked upon Alexander Pope's *Epitaph on Newton* with two most insightful lines. Pope had written:

> Nature and Nature's laws lay hid in night; God said, "Let Newton be!" and all was light.

Squire answered:

> It did not last: the Devil howling "Ho! Let Einstein be!" restored the status quo. [11:p. 1094]

The Quantum Theory and Quantum Mechanics

Einstein, however, was not the only scientist who developed revolutionary concepts that helped form our new view of the universe. The doors of physics were opened wider still by a group of scientists working on the concept of matter, most notably, Lord Rutherford with his work in 1911 on the structure of the atom, Max Planck with the introduction of the quantum theory in 1900, and Niels Bohr, who, in 1913, put the Rutherford atom and the quantum theory together to give us a new model of the atom. Baumer says, "If anything, the concept of matter was more thoroughly 'bolshevized' than were the concepts of space and time" [2:p. 462]. Sir Arthur Stanley Eddington believed Lord Rutherford to be the individual most responsible for the revolution in classical physics. He said, in the Gifford Lectures of 1927:

> When we compare the universe as it is now supposed to be with the universe as we had ordinarily preconceived it, the most arresting change is not the rearrangement of space and time by Einstein but the dissolution of all that we regard as most solid into tiny specks floating in void. [10:p. 1]

Before we discuss Rutherford's work with the atom, however, let us review some of the discoveries that preceded it. J. J. Thomson, as you may recall from Chapter 5, discovered a particle smaller than the atom, an electron. This discovery, which was made in 1897, was important to the study of the atom. The electron is a particle that carries a negative electric charge. The movement of electrons in a wire is the electric current. Once the electron was identified as the carrier of the negative charge, it was established that it existed inside the atom because electric current could be extracted from neutral atoms. Electrons exist within the atom. Scientists began questioning the structure of the atom.

At the end of the nineteenth century, the "raisin bun" atom was the model that was widely accepted. This depicted the atom as a "large blob of positive matter in which electrons were embedded in much the same way as raisins are embedded in a piece of bakery," explains Trefil [33:p. 251]. Physicists were now concerned with the subatomic world, and their investigations opened up a new era in physics. Questions concerning the atomic world revolved around two broad categories—atomic structure and the interactions of atoms and light. The new physics, called quantum mechanics, which would develop around these questions, would give scientists some of the most complex problems yet presented. The problem of wave-particle duality that would arise from investigation into the microscopic world would be momentous.

Let us look for a moment at the genesis of the wave-particle problem, as it will prove to be of enormous consequence. To the classical physicists, everything had to be either a wave or a particle. The idea of light being composed of particles had already been supported by Newton long before Planck was to hypothesize the quantum theory. Newton did not come upon the idea of the quantum theory because he did not, in his day, have the concept of energy. However, Newton's brilliant thesis concerning light particles was to prompt a debate that would reappear in another form in the twentieth century.

Newton, working on the phenomenon of white light and colors, concluded that white light is a mixture of different kinds of corpuscles belonging
to different colors. He said that the differently colored corpuscles behaved as
unchangeable substances,

> . . . which colours are not new generated, but only made apparent by being
> parted; for if they be again entirely mixt and blended together, they will again
> compose that colour, which they did before separation. And for the same
> reason, transmutations made by the convening of divers colours are not real;
> for when the difform rays are again severed, they will exhibit the very same
> colours which they did before they entered the composition; as you see blue
> and yellow powders, when finely mixed, appear to the naked eye, green, and
> yet the colours of the component corpuscles are not thereby really transmuted,
> but only blended. For when viewed with a good microscope, they still appear
> blue and yellow interspersedly. [12:p. 98]

Christian Huygens (1629–1695), a contemporary of Newton's, introduced
a different theory of light. He said that light is not of substance. It is a
transference of energy, a wave. He wrote:

> If, in addition, light takes time for its passage—which we are now going to
> examine—it will follow that this movement, impressed on the intervening
> matter, is successive; and consequently it spreads, as sound does, by spherical
> surfaces and waves, for I call them waves from their resemblance to those
> which are seen to be formed in water when a stone is thrown into it, and which
> present a successive spreading as in circles, though these arise from another
> cause, and are only in a flat surface. [12:p. 105]

According to Huygens' wave theory of light, different colors have different corresponding wavelengths.

The debate between those who favored the corpuscular theory of light and
those who favored the wave theory of light was intense. Newton was very
persuasive and his theory prevailed, most physicists accepting it as the more
plausible explanation. However, in the middle of the nineteenth century, the
wave theory took over after it was used successfully to explain the bending of
light around very small obstacles, something the corpuscular theory could
not do. This was not to be the end of the corpuscular theory. It would turn
up again and prove even more effective.

As scientists proceeded to work in the microscopic field, they found that
properties of both waves and particles could be found in objects on the
atomic scale. This discovery was translated as a wave-particle problem and
believed to be a logical contradiction. The classical physicists were enormously confused by the pictures they were seeing of the microscopic world,
a world in which things were not behaving as they did in the macroscopic
world.

One of the problems that presented itself was known even in the time of
Clerk Maxwell, but no one had been able to solve it and so it had remained
largely ignored. This problem was so puzzling that it was named "the ultraviolet catastrophe" by Paul Ehrenfest, a friend of Einstein's. Although it is not
necessary here to explain the ultraviolet catastrophe, it is necessary to point
to it as an example of a situation that required the bringing together of two

disparate, fundamental theories—the mechanical theory of matter, in which the state of a system is defined by a finite number of mechanical quantities, and the electromagnetic field theory, in which the state of the field is defined by a set of continuous functions.

With the introduction of the quantum theory by Planck in 1900, the ultraviolet catastrophe was solved and a whole new era began in physics. And, as we shall see, Einstein would be caught up in the new ideas concerning the quantum theory and would spend the rest of his professional life trying to reconcile his own ideas with those of quantum mechanics, which would emerge in the 1920s.

Planck hypothesized that, just as there are quanta of matter and quanta of electricity, there are energy quanta. This immediately cast a shadow over the long-accepted identification of light as a wave.

What is a quantum? It can be defined as an indivisible unit of energy. Translated into more ordinary language, an elementary quantum can be defined as a discrete step. In the United States, the elementary quantum of money is a penny. In England, the farthing is the monetary elementary quantum. Einstein and Leopold Infeld described the quantum in terms of continuous and discontinuous change. They wrote:

> Some quantities can change continuously and others can change only discontinuously, by steps which cannot be further decreased. These indivisible steps are called the *elementary quanta* of the particular quantity to which they refer.
> We can weigh large quantities of sand and regard its mass as continuous even though its granular structure is evident. But if the sand were to become very precious and the scales used very sensitive, we should have to consider the fact that the mass always changes by a multiple number of one grain. The mass of this one grain would be our elementary quantum. From this example we see how the discontinuous character of a quantity, so far regarded as continuous, can be detected by increasing the precision of our instruments.
> If we had to characterize the principal idea of the quantum theory in one sentence, we could say: *it must be assumed that some physical quantities so far regarded as continuous are composed of elementary quanta.* [12: 250–251]

Although Planck had postulated that light might exist in quanta, he thought that the emission of light quanta was related more to the structure of atoms rather than to the nature of light. "What Einstein had done," wrote Trefil, "was to take the hypothesis that Planck had made very seriously" [33:p. 282]. It was Einstein who first recognized that a light theory would be needed that would incorporate both the wave theory and the particle theory. The difficulties presented to physicists are apparent in Einstein's and Infeld's explanation of the wave theory of light and the quantum theory of light:

> The state of affairs can be summarized in the following way: there are phenomena which can be explained by the quantum theory but not by the wave theory. Photo-effect furnishes an example, though other phenomena of this kind are known. There are phenomena which can be explained by the wave theory but not by the quantum theory. The bending of light around obstacles is a typical example. Finally, there are phenomena, such as the rectilinear propagation of light, which can be equally well explained by the quantum and the wave theory of light. [12:p. 262]

Once again Newton's corpuscular theory received attention in the explanation of the phenomenon called the photoelectric effect. The old light corpuscles were replaced by light quanta called photons, and it was demonstrated that radiation energy is built up by light quanta. Newton's old theory was revived and took new form as the quantum theory of light.

It is to both Planck and Einstein that we owe the suggestion that light exhibits the properties of both waves and particles. Einstein's work gave us a better idea of Planck's quantum theory. It was Einstein who was the first to recognize the need for a quantum theory of matter, and it would be his papers that would inspire the creation of the field of quantum mechanics.

While physicists were engaged in questions concerning the nature of light phenomena, the most complex problems coming to their attention concerned the interaction of light and atoms. If you recall, the model of the atom at the turn of the twentieth century was that of a raisin bun. In 1911, Rutherford conducted some experiments that showed that the atom was not like a raisin bun but had a very hard center. He proposed the theory that the atom is not indivisible and consists of a small impenetrable nucleus surrounded by revolving electrons.

The Rutherford atom looked very much like our solar system with the sun at the center (the nucleus) and the planets, or electrons, moving around it in orbit. The electrons carry the negative charge, and the nucleus carries the positive charge. The atom, far from being a bit of dense matter, is empty. Trefil wrote:

> It is very important to get some idea of how empty an atom really is. We are used to thinking of atoms as small, compact, dense clumps of matter. In fact, they are not. For example, if the nucleus of a uranium atom were a bowling ball sitting in front of you, the electrons of the atom would be like 92 ping-pong balls scattered over 100 square miles of area. Everything except the bowling ball and those 92 ping-pong balls would be empty space. [33:pp. 288–289]

The Rutherford atom was revolutionary because it, too, challenged Newtonian concepts. If the classical laws were applied, the Rutherford atom would not be able to exist at all. Once the nucleus was established, the problems began. According to the laws of classical physics, the orbiting electrons would eventually lose energy, spiral into the nucleus, and destroy the atom in a very short time. Researchers began to realize that the basic laws surrounding electromagnetic phenomena would have to be modified at the atomic level. Classical physicists were not sure they could "save" the Rutherford model.

Then, in 1913, Niels Bohr (1885–1962), a Danish physicist, adapted the quantum theory to atomic structure. He took the Rutherford atom and Planck's theory of the quantum, put them together, and postulated that the atom represents a dynamic system of electrons rotating in orbit around a nucleus, from which radiation is emitted only during the passage of an electron from an orbit of higher energy to one of lower energy. This meant that there were stable orbits in which the electrons could move without loss of energy.

Bohr's idea that systems of atoms contain a distinct and separate set of possible stationary states greatly influenced the later work of Einstein. Bohr's application of the quantum theory to the structure of the atom lead to the development of wave, or quantum, mechanics. Bronowski wrote:

> Bohr's paper *On the Constitution of Atoms and Molecules* became a classic at once. The structure of the atom was now as mathematical as Newton's universe. But it contained the additional principle of the quantum. Neils Bohr had built a world inside the atom by going beyond the laws of physics as they had stood for two centuries after Newton. [5:p. 337]

Bohr's work explained a number of puzzling facts, but it also presented a problem in that nobody knew why it worked, only that it did work. Questions began to arise concerning the nature of the electron, which had been thought of as a particle but was seen to exhibit some of the properties of a wave. Trefil said, "It is in the interplay between the particle-like and the wave-like properties of an electron that the explanation of a Bohr atom and, ultimately, the development of the science of quantum mechanics is to be found" [33:p. 295].

It is to Louis de Broglie, a French physicist, that we owe the discovery of the wave character of electrons, which explained the Bohr atom and the stable orbits. In 1925, de Broglie proposed an equation, which is today called the de Broglie relation, that linked together the particle properties of electrons and the wave properties of electrons. His contemporaries called the equation the "Comedie Francaise" and did not consider it seriously. Trefil explained:

> We have discussed particles and we have discussed waves. To the classical physicist, these two different kinds of things had to be distinct and separate. The implications of the particle-like nature of light had never been fully accepted by the physics community up to this point. So when de Broglie wrote down an equation that seemed to link these two properties, wave and particle, in an inexplicable way, it was not well received. [33:p. 296]

Although most of his contemporaries may have thought de Broglie to be less than inspired, Einstein took de Broglie's work quite seriously. He said that de Broglie had "lifted a corner of the great veil" [22:p. 148] and found evidence in his own work to support the de Broglie relation. He also suggested other experiments that might serve to detect de Broglie waves. Einstein's contribution to de Broglie's work is considerable, as he provided the experimental proof for the young researcher's speculations, successfully removing the critics' objection, that de Broglie had no evidence for his theory.

At the same time de Broglie proposed his theory, two German scientists were working separately and independently on the problem of subatomic particles. A new science would develop from the mathematical techniques they employed in their work. Werner Heisenberg (1901–1976) and Erwin Schrödinger (1887–1961) would have their names forever linked with quantum mechanics, which Einstein called "the most successful physical theory of our time" [22:p. 150].

Heisenberg, in 1925, in collaboration with Max Born and Pascual Jordan, developed a quantum mechanics based on matrix algebra. According to Martin J. Klein, Einstein, although impressed, was not convinced that this new approach to quantum theory was the answer to all the problems the quantum theory had introduced. Einstein wrote, in a letter:

> The most interesting theoretical work produced recently is the Heisenberg-Born-Jordan theory of quantum states. It's a real witches' calculus, with infinite determinants (matrices) taking the place of Cartesian coordinates. Most ingenious, and adequately protected by its great complexity against being proved wrong. [22:p. 149]

Later in 1925, he was to remark to Born, "An inner voice tells me that it is still not the true Jacob" [22:p. 149]. Born, who was Heisenberg's teacher, is reported by Klein to have taken this negative opinion as "a hard blow" [22:p. 149].

Einstein was to have a much more favorable reaction to an alternative to the Heisenberg-Born-Jordan theory presented in 1926 by Schrödinger, the wave theory of quantum mechanics. He wrote to Schrödinger, "I am convinced that you have made a decisive advance with your formulation of the quantum condition just as I am equally convinced that the Heisenberg-Born route is off the track" [22:p. 149]. Klein said that Einstein was more impressed with Schrödinger's work because the wave theory was more compatible with de Broglie's work.

The arguments over the different forms of basic atomic physics were centered in Göttingen and attracted scientists from all over the world. Several scholars relate the classic story that arose from the dispute surrounding the electron. Bronowski told it this way:

> The quip among professors was (because of the way university time-tables are laid out) that on Mondays, Wednesdays, and Fridays the electron would behave like a particle; on Tuesdays, Thursdays and Saturdays it would behave like a wave. [5:p. 364]

Most of the prominent physicists of the day were engaged in the search for answers to the questions posed by investigation into the world of subatomic particles. Bronowski remarked, "A new conception was being made, on the train to Berlin and the professorial walks in the woods of Göttingen: that whatever fundamental units the world is put together from, they are more delicate, more fugitive, more startling than we catch in the butterfly net of our senses" [5:p. 364].

Born was to give a statistical interpretation of Schrödinger's wave function that would synthesize the two models and aid in the creation of the new quantum mechanics. The two methods, that of the Heisenberg-Born-Jordan theory, with its emphasis on matrix algebra, and the Schrödinger wave function, were shown to be mathematically equivalent and not so different as they had at first appeared [31]. It is here that we must leave Einstein, for he was never able to completely accept the revelations of the new quantum mechanics. "He would not," stated Klein, "admit it as the basis for theoretical physics" [22:p. 150]. Instead of pursuing the answers to the problems posed by quantum mechanics, Einstein would devote the rest of his professional life to finding a unified field theory. He did so, claimed Klein, because, "it was his hope that a complete field theory would provide the basis for all of physics, giving that complete description he missed in the quantum mechanics he had helped so much to develop" [22:pp. 150–151]. What discoveries had led to Einstein's decision to concentrate on formulating a unified field theory?

In 1927, Heisenberg introduced what he called the principle of uncertainty, which says that the electron is a particle that gives only limited information [19]. In explaining this idea, Bronowski said that the more accurate term for what Heisenberg proposed is the principle of tolerance. He wrote:

> The information that the electron carries is limited in its totality. That is, for instance, its speed and its position fit together in such a way that they are confined by the tolerance of the quantum. This is the profound idea: one of the great scientific ideas, not only of the twentieth century, but in the history of science. [5:p. 365]

Although Heisenberg introduced his principle of uncertainty as a new characterization of the electron, Bronowski carried its implications much further, saying, "The Principle of Uncertainty or, in my phrase, the Principle of Tolerance fixed once for all the realisation that all knowledge is limited" [5:p. 367].

What exactly did Heisenberg say about the electron? In order to accurately determine its location, one would have to introduce an interminable and random disruption in its motion. If the motion is controlled, uncertainty is introduced into the position. Obviously, there is no way to get an accurate determination of both the motion and the position of an electron, the requirements to determine each being mutually incompatible. Therefore, only statistical predictions can be made. "We can always predict the probability of finding a particular particle at a particular point in space," explained Trefil, "but we cannot predict what a single particle will do" [33:p. 321].

We again become aware of radical differences between classical physics and quantum physics. In classical physics, objects are described as existing in space and laws are formulated governing their changes in time. In quantum physics, objects are not described in space and their changes are not described in time. Einstein and Infeld gave a very clear explanation of the difference:

> There is no place in quantum physics for statements such as: "This object is so-and-so, has this-and-this property." Instead we have statements of this kind: "There is such-and-such a probability that the individual object is so-and-so and has this-and-this property." There is no place in quantum physics for laws governing the changes in time of an individual object. Instead, we have laws governing the changes in time of the probability. Only this fundamental change, brought into physics by the quantum theory, made possible an adequate explanation of the apparently discontinuous and statistical character of events in the realm of phenomena in which the elementary quanta of matter and radiation reveal their existence. [12:p. 292]

Perhaps the most important tenets of quantum physics are the replacement of continuity by discontinuity and the replacement of laws governing individuals by probability laws [23]. Understanding the significance of the change from certainty to probability is not so difficult when we consider the emphasis the Newtonian world had placed upon knowing about the individual thing or event. In quantum physics the individual is discarded and replaced by statistics. We may say that one of every ten cars passing a shopping center is going to turn into the center, but we cannot say which particular car. We may say that three of every fifteen families in a particular community will have a major illness in the family sometime within the next year, but we cannot say which family or exactly when the event will occur. Statistical laws cannot be applied to individual members of a group but only to the group itself.

The statistical aspect of quantum mechanics differed from classical mechanics, which assumed that we could observe, measure, and predict the future of any particular particle. In quantum mechanics, no particle can be measured without disturbing it and its individual development cannot be traced. Quantum mechanics can predict only probability distributions and not the precise, deterministic results of classical physics [33].

Many physicists and other scientists are unhappy with the blow quantum mechanics and the uncertainty principle have dealt to the mechanistic world view, even though they are constrained to admit its validity. The implications of the theories governing the world of quantum mechanics are undeniable, but as Trefil said, "You may not approve of this kind of statistical theory, but if you don't you ought at least to have the intellectual honesty never to use a transistor radio or solid-state stereo system, because both of these rely on the use of the statistical theory of quantum mechanics as it is applied to the transistor and other solid-state electronic devices" [33:p. 323].

The uncertainty of the uncertainty principle is altogether different from the uncertainty classical physics has always acknowledged as an important element in its predictions. Louis J. Halle explained this difference:

> A measurable element of uncertainty in prediction has always had an important part in classical mechanics. However, unlike the uncertainty of the Uncertainty Principle associated with quantum mechanics, all that this traditional uncertainty represents is the necessary inadequacy of the information available to us limited human beings as a basis for prediction. . . . Under quantum mechanics, the uncertainty of the Uncertainty Principle is not simply a matter of insurmountable obstacles to the prediction of what, because it is predetermined, is predictable in principle. It arises, rather, from the fact that the future is not predetermined—or not precisely predetermined. . . . The quantum of uncertainty defined by h (Planck's constant) is inherent in being, a fundamental property of the physical world. It represents the ultimate limit of precision in the movements and interactions of objects. It is equivalent to an irreducible looseness or play in the mechanism of a watch. [17:pp. 67–69]

Fritjof Capra also emphasized the difference in probability as we generally understand it and the probability of quantum mechanics:

> It is important to realize that the statistical formulation of the laws of atomic and subatomic physics does not reflect our ignorance of the physical situation, like the use of probabilities by insurance companies or gamblers. In quantum theory, we have come to recognize probability as a fundamental feature of the atomic reality which governs all processes, and even the existence of matter. Subatomic particles do not exist with certainty at definite places, but rather

show "tendencies to exist" and atomic events do not occur with certainty at definite times and in definite ways, but rather show "tendencies to occur." [7:p. 133]

The impact of quantum physics upon our world view is enormous. The clockwork universe of Newtonian mechanics is not a given. We must now acknowledge that the concrete world that once seemed so apparent is actually, by nature, insubstantial. Quantum mechanics, which has stood up under every test, has allowed us to make tremendous technological advances. Because of our knowledge of this new physics, we now have use of many items familiar to all of us. These include hand calculators, transistors, miniaturized computers, and phenomenal inventions like the laser, which has many applications, including the delivery of energy to very small systems. We are realizing that our world is a quantum world. We are beginning to think in terms of randomness and indeterminacy rather than precise location and exactness. The implications are, of course, almost incomprehensible. Davies wrote:

> The apparently concrete world around us is seen to be an illusion when we probe into the microscopic recesses of matter. There we encounter a shifting world of transmutations and fluctuations, in which material particles can lose their identities and even disappear altogether. Far from being a clockwork mechanism, the microcosm dissolves into an evanescent, chaotic sort of place in which the fundamental indeterminacy of observable attributes transcends many of the cherished principles of classical physics. The compulsion to seek an underlying lawfulness beneath this subatomic anarchy is strong but . . . apparently fruitless. We have to face the fact that the world is far less substantial and dependable than envisaged hitherto. [8:pp. 90–91]

Klein claimed that Einstein "refused to give up the idea that there was such a thing as the real state of a physical system, something that objectively exists independently of observation and measurement, and which can, in principle, be described in physical terms" [22:p. 150]. Einstein's decision to search for a unified field theory rather than concentrating his efforts in the area of quantum mechanics can better be understood when we consider what the quantum world has done to our old ideas of science and the scientist. Hans Reichenbach described the situation as this:

> The picture of scientific method drafted by modern philosophy is very different from traditional conceptions. Gone is the ideal of a universe whose course follows strict rules, a predetermined cosmos that unwinds itself like an unwinding clock. Gone is the ideal of the scientist who knows the absolute truth. The happenings of nature are like rolling dice rather than like revolving stars; they are controlled by probability laws, not by causality, and the scientist resembles a gambler more than a prophet. [27:p. 248]

One can only contrast this statement with Einstein's famous remark, "God does not play dice" to realize the enormous impact quantum mechanics must have had upon him. Einstein could not, perhaps, see himself as a gambler and the happenings of nature as rolling dice. Those scientists who did pursue the new pathways opened up by quantum mechanics found themselves delving into an investigation of those influences that would decrease the uncertainty we have now acknowledged is a fundamental part of the physical world. Many of them were to turn their attention to systems and information theories.

Systems or Patterns

It is helpful to describe the development of systems concepts from quantum physics. A *system* can be defined as a set of phenomena relating to and influencing each other [32]. The relationship of phenomena in the formation of various patterns is fundamental in quantum theory. In order to study or analyze the physical world, the quantum theorists first divide it into two systems—an observed system, which is the object, and an observing system, which is defined as those performing the experiment and the apparatus they use. The implication that this is a gambler's world is clear when we realize that any description of the observed systems is in terms of probable relationships among the two systems.

Systems concepts are generally stated in terms of patterns, influences, processes, emergent properties, and information. We will try to describe these various phenomena in that order. Let us first examine the idea of *patterns*. In order to form a pattern, we must have an interconnectedness among the various objects or events that constitute the pattern. In experiments concerning the electron, for example, we are required to examine its properties, not in isolation, but as an interconnection between the process by which it was prepared or created for examination and the subsequent measurement. Actually, it is impossible to view the quantum world in terms of entities. We must always look at interconnections and interactions among particles or networks of particles. Niels Bohr said, "Isolated material particles are abstractions, their properties being definable and observable only through their interaction with other systems" [7:p. 137]. However, we do speak of isolated particles because of the practical value in experimentation. As Henry Stapp explained, "The observed system is required to be isolated in order to be defined, yet interacting in order to be observed" [7:p. 136].

With the advent of quantum physics, we see the world not in terms of physical isolated objects obeying deterministic laws but, as Capra defined it, in terms of "wave-like patterns of probabilities." He also explained that these patterns "do not represent probabilities of things, but rather probabilities of interconnections" [7:p. 68]. Throughout the new physics, we find the descriptions given in terms of patterns, unified wholes, interconnections, and probabilities. Capra wrote:

> Quantum theory thus reveals a basic oneness of the universe. It shows that we cannot decompose the world into independently existing smallest units. As we penetrate into matter, nature does not show us any isolated "basic building blocks", but rather appears as a complicated web of relations between the various parts of the whole. [7:p. 68]

Even those who do not agree with some of the mathematical interpretations of quantum physics, still agree with the cosmic interconnectedness that seems to be one of its fundamental features. David Bohm, who has commented upon one of the basic mathematical interpretations of quantum physics, known as the Copenhagen interpretation, wrote:

> One is led to a new notion of unbroken wholeness which denies the classical idea of analyzability of the world into separately and independently existing parts. . . . We have reversed the usual classical notion that the independent "elementary parts" of the world are the fundamental reality, and that the various systems are merely particular contingent forms and arrangements of these parts. Rather, we say that inseparable quantum interconnectedness of the whole universe is the fundamental reality, and that relatively independently behaving parts are merely particular and contingent forms within this whole. [7:p. 138]

It would seem that the idea of a universal interconnectedness of patterns is not something we can choose to believe or not believe but is there before us as a basic tenet of the new scientific view. To repeat Bronowski, "This needs to be said roundly, for many people still speak as if the choice between the old and the new picture of nature were a matter of philosophical taste. It is not: it is a matter of fact" [6:p. 35]. Capra also emphasized that we have little choice in this matter, using the verb *force* in describing the new view given us by quantum theory. He said, "Quantum theory forces us to see the universe not as a collection of physical objects, but rather as a complicated web of relations between the various parts of a unified whole" [7:p. 138].

Seeing the universe in terms of an interconnectedness of patterns among events rather than a collection of physical objects is a momentous departure from the Newtonian world view, which was based upon the idea that each bit of matter has an individual and independent existence and that it can be described at a certain point and time in space. Alfred North Whitehead explains:

> Newtonian physics is based upon the independent individuality of each bit of matter. Each stone is conceived as fully describable apart from any reference to any other portion of matter. It might be alone in the Universe, the sole occupant of uniform space. But it would still be that stone which it is. Also the stone could be adequately described without any reference of past or future. It is to be conceived fully and adequately as wholly constituted within the present moment. [35:p. 160]

Whitehead called this idea of Newtonian physics the doctrine of simple location. He acknowledged that quantum physics had destroyed the theory of the concrete existence of physical things in time and space. In addressing the demise of the idea of simple location, he also implied the idea of a basic pattern or interconnectedness throughout the universe. He wrote:

> My theory involves the entire abandonment of the notion that simple location is the primary way in which things are involved in space-time. In a certain sense, everything is everywhere at all times. For every location involves an aspect of itself in every other location. Thus every spatio-temporal standpoint mirrors the world. [36:p. 87]

In another statement concerning the abandonment of the idea of simple location, Whitehead introduced the idea of *influence* and replaced the doctrine of simple location with the focal region. He said:

Modern physics has abandoned the doctrine of Simple Location. The physical things which we term stars, planets, lumps of matter, molecules, electrons, protons, quanta of energy, are each to be conceived as modifications of conditions within space-time, extending throughout its whole range. There is a focal region, which in common speech is where the thing is. But its influence streams away from it with finite velocity throughout the utmost recesses of space and time. Of course, it is natural, and for certain purposes entirely proper, to speak of the focal region, thus modified, as the thing itself situated there. But difficulties arise if we press this way of thought too far. For physics, the thing itself is what it does, and what it does is this divergent stream of influence. [35:p. 161]

This statement is even more complicated than it at first appears, for Whitehead is stating clearly that a thing is not a thing as we would traditionally define it. The thing is what it does, and what it does is its influence. The idea of influence among systems is evident when we consider the universe as a pattern, a weaving together of a collection of events. We hear it expressed poetically by Francis Thompson:

All things by immortal power,
Near or far,
Hiddenly,
To each other linked are,
That thou canst not stir a flower,
Without troubling of a star. [8:p. 56]

One of the problems with Newtonian physics was the attempt to isolate systems, to remove the system from the influences of its environment, an impossibility in quantum physics. We cannot free a system from the forces that influence it, and neither can we study identical systems in order to predict accurately, for identical systems do not exist. Davies explained, "There are no identical systems. Because the universe changes from day to day and place to place, the cosmic network of forces can never be completely identical" [8:p. 56].

Here we see introduced the idea of *process*, or change. Not only do we have patterns organized into systems, but these systems are forever changing. Baumer summed up Whitehead's ideas concerning the interconnectedness of changing systems or patterns when he wrote:

Whitehead learned to think in terms of physical "fields" and "events," rather than isolated objects, hence of wholes or patterns, rather than parts. Quantum theory further suggested the rhythmic or periodic, as opposed to enduring, character of atomic entities, hence that the patterns were forever changing. Matter conceived as activity or energy, plus the new significance attached to time, convinced Whitehead, once and for all, that process was at the heart of nature. [2:p. 473]

Baumer also quoted Whitehead on process, changing the text slightly:

The actual world is a process, and the process is the becoming of actual entities. . . . How an actual entity *becomes* constitutes *what* that actual entity *is*. . . . Its "being" is constituted by its "becoming." This is the "principle of process." [2:p. 473]

The old mechanistic concepts of form and function are viewed in terms of process by systems theorists. Ludwig von Bertalanffy was the first to develop the ideas we now term *general systems theory*, which, he hoped, would prove to be the paradigm uniting biology as well as all related physiologic and health systems [32]. In his definition of process he differentiated between slow and quick processes, using an example from a living system:

> What are called structures are slow processes of long duration, functions are quick processes of short duration. If we say that a function such as a contraction of a muscle is performed by a structure, it means that a quick and short process wave is superimposed on a long-lasting and slowly running wave. [4:p. 87]

Quantum theory had established that what we are accustomed to think of as particles are actually probability centers of influence as suggested by Schrödinger. The probability centers are defined in terms of their influence, or what they do, as suggested by Whitehead. This is process. Capra wrote:

> Quantum theory has shown that particles are not isolated grains of matter, but are probability patterns, interconnections in an inseparable cosmic web. Relativity theory, so to speak, has made these patterns come alive by revealing their intrinsically dynamic character. It has shown that the activity of matter is the very essence of its being. The particles of the subatomic world are not only active in the sense of moving around very fast; they themselves are processes! The existence of matter and its activity cannot be separated. [7:p. 203]

James G. Miller, one of our foremost authorities in the study of living systems, emphasized process in our conceptualization of the four-dimensional world of the new physics:

> Structure is the static arrangement of a system's parts at a moment in three-dimensional space. Process is dynamic change in the matter-energy or information of that system over time. . . . All change over time of matter-energy or information in a system is process. [26:pp. 83–87]

We may say that the interactions of slow and fast processes mediated through patterns of probability centers of influence compose interconnected patterns or systems. The patterns of process resulting from the interaction of the probability centers of influence are arbitrarily delineated into open systems. It is virtually impossible to study a closed system. As Heisenberg stated, "in atomic physics even approximately isolated systems cannot be observed" [9:p. 1053].

Various properties arise from the interaction of open systems or patterns, which are called *emergent properties*. They may be defined as those properties evolving from interacting systems that are not discernible in the component systems. The properties of the relationship are different or, as some might say, more than the sum of the properties of the interacting systems. Bertalanffy wrote:

> The meaning of the somewhat mystical expression, "the whole is more than the sum of its parts" is simply that constitutive characteristics are not explainable from the characteristics of isolated parts. The characteristics of the complex,

therefore, compared to those of the elements, appear as "new" or "emergent."
[4:p. 55]

The term *emergent* was defined by the zoologist, Lloyd Morgan, in his
book, *Emergent Evolution*, in 1923, as something different from a mere resultant of something lower. An emergent is something novel and qualitatively
new. According to Baumer, "It was this, 'the something more' in Morgan's
phrase, which distinguished the doctrine of emergence from mechanistic
doctrine" [2:p. 472].

An example of emergent properties is a crystal of salt, which is composed
of sodium and chloride atoms. The crystalline property of a grain of salt is
not that of the sodium and chloride atoms but that of their relationship. The
same atoms have different properties if they are not combined. Sodium is a
solid quite different from table salt, and chloride is a yellowish gas. The
crystalline properties that are the emergent properties are not present if the
relationship of sodium and chloride ions is placed in a solution of water [32].
Bronowski commented, "Salt is a compound of two elements: sodium and
chlorine. That is remarkable enough, that a white fizzy metal like sodium,
and a yellowish poisonous gas like chlorine, should finish up by making a
stable structure, common salt" [5:p. 321].

We see, then, that interacting open systems produce emergents that cannot be ascertained by studying the properties of the subsystems that are
interacting to form the given system. In other words, patterns of influence
interacting with other patterns of influence may result in properties not
discernible in any of the component patterns.

We have examined briefly the phenomena of patterns or systems, influences, processes, and emergent properties. We have left the concept of information until last. If you recall, we suggested that many scientists would try
to decrease the uncertainty introduced by the world of the new physics by
turning their attention to systems and information theories. We have seen the
complexity of systems. We have also introduced the term *information* in
Miller's statement, "All change of matter-energy or information in a system
is process" [26:p. 83]. We have yet to define what we mean by information or
how we link it with matter-energy. And how do we conceptualize information as a reduction of uncertainty?

Reducing the Uncertainty

Information may be defined as any influence that decreases the uncertainty in
a system. Some influences may be visualized as particles, in which case we
may say that the information has matter for a carrier. Other influences may
be seen as waves, in which case we may state that the information has an
energy carrier. We know that mass and energy are properties of patterns of
influence, so we may postulate that mass and energy are information. Carl
Friedrich von Weizsacker stated this clearly in *The Unity of Nature*:

> Mass is information. . . . Energy is information. The relativistic equivalence
> of mass and energy enables us to transfer to energy all we have said about mass.
> [34:pp. 291–292]

We do not, however, say the reverse, that information is mass and energy, even though it may be carried by either of these patterns of influence. Norbert Wiener emphasized this point, "Information is information, not matter or energy. No materialism which does not admit this can survive at the present day" [37:p. 132].

Kenneth Sayre defined information as reduced uncertainty:

Although "information" may signify such different matters as notification, knowledge, or simply data, in any case the imparting of information is the reduction of uncertainty. "Information" thus signifies the positive difference between two uncertainty levels. [30:p. 23]

We may define information, therefore, as any influence that decreases the uncertainty of a system. We must realize that no influence completely eliminates uncertainty, and so our definition must be relative. There are influences that inhibit activity, and there are influences that increase the activity of systems. If either type of influence increases the statistical probability of this increased or decreased activity, it may be termed information. Sayre explained, "In this more specific terminology, we may define information simply as increased probability" [30:p. 23].

Miller seemed to agree with the notion that information is reduced uncertainty. He wrote:

Information is the opposite of uncertainty. It is not accidental that the word *form* appears in *information*, since information is the amount of formal patterning or complexity in any system. [26:p. 57]

In differentiating between information and meaning, Miller said:

Meaning is the significance of information to a system which processes it; it constitutes a change in that system's processes elicited by the information, often resulting from associations made to it on previous experience with it. *Information* is a simpler concept: the degree of freedom that exists in a given situation to choose among signals, symbols, messages, or patterns to be transmitted. [26:p. 57]

Concepts of information have their antecedents in the work of some of the physicists we mentioned earlier, especially those who studied thermodynamics, such as Helmholtz, Boltzmann, Maxwell, and Planck. In order to understand these concepts, we must have some comprehension of the terms *entropy* and *negentropy* as they relate to information.

According to the second law of thermodynamics, or the law of the degradation of energy, thermodynamics degradation cannot be revoked or retracted over time. A building that has been burned cannot be unburned. As Miller explained it,

Even though there is an equivalence between a certain amount of work and a certain amount of heat, yet in any cyclic process, where a system is restored to its original state, there can never be a net conversion of heat into work, but the reverse is always possible. [26:p. 60]

The changes that take place in a system when we convert an amount of work into its equivalent amount of heat, when expressed in statistics, show that the system has gone from an ordered state to a state of chaos or disorder. *Entropy* is the name given to this disordered, disorganized, random state. Sayre wrote:

> According to the Second Law of Thermodynamics, the entropy of a closed system tends generally to increase, and the system accordingly tends to diminish in structure. [30:p. 61]

The term *negentropy* was introduced by Schrödinger to indicate increased structure, or order, the opposite of entropy, which is loss of structure, or disorder.

Claude Shannon, who was one of the founders of communications theory, and Wiener, who was instrumental in developing the science of cybernetics, noted that Schrödinger's concept of negentropy, or the negative of entropy, has the same statistical measure as that for information. It is not necessary to have a complete understanding of thermodynamics or the statistical measures involved. We have introduced these data to help explain the derivation of the terms entropy and negentropy as related to information. Entropy signifies lack of order or randomness, and negentropy signifies an increase in order. If entropy progresses, information, or negentropy, decreases. Miller gave a clear and simple example of this concept:

> One evening in Puerto Rico I observed a concrete illustration of how information decreases as entropy progresses. Epiphany was being celebrated according to Spanish custom. On the buffet table of a large hotel stood a marvelous carving of the three kings with their camels, all done in clear ice. As the warm evening went on, they gradually melted, losing their precise patterning or information as entropy increased. By the end of the evening, the camels' humps were nearly gone and the wise men were almost beardless. [26:p. 61]

Whereas the idea of force was a central focus in Newtonian mechanics, information is a key concept in the quantum world of open systems. Shannon was led to his theory of information by noting that open systems could be altered by other impinging influences in a statistically probable way that decreased the uncertainty in any given system. Defining information as any influence that alters a system in a statistically probable manner, and keeping in mind the idea that emergent properties of systems become information to other systems, we reach the next step of conceptual complexity, called cybernetics. By the process termed *cybernetics*, a system, via its emergent properties, may influence another system, thereby altering the second system's emergent properties. These altered properties now become new information to the original system. In this arrangement we have a feedback loop in which emergent properties of a system serve as information to the second system, which alters its emergent properties, resulting in new information being fed back to the original system.

The close relationship between cybernetics and information theory was emphasized by Anatol Rapoport, who also linked it to the idea of reduction of uncertainty:

> Cybernetics is the science of communication and control. As such, it does not examine transformations of energy. It examines patterns of signals by means of which information is transmitted within a system and from one system to

another. Transmission of information is essential in control, and the capacity of a system to exercise control depends on how much information it can process and store. In fact, the concept "quantity of information" is central in cybernetics. In this context, "quantity of information" is unrelated to the meaning of the information, its significance, or its truth. Quantity of information is related simply to the number of "decisions" which must be made in order to reduce the range of possible answers to the questions one asks; to put it in another way, to reduce uncertainty. [18:p. 107]

Wiener's work in cybernetics led us to appreciate how information might be reciprocally exchanged among two or more systems in a feedback loop so that as one system influences another, the subsequent influence on the second system produces new information back to the first, or original, system. By combining systems and information theories with the science of cybernetics, we may postulate that all systems within the universe are involved in a cybernetic exchange of influences. When these influences decrease the uncertainty in a system, the influence is termed *information*.

To rephrase this rather complex concept, the emergent influences of a system may affect a second system, altering its emergent influences, which affect the original system, resulting in a servoemergent relationship, or feedback loop, consisting of alteration and realteration in an infinite recursion. By *servo* we imply a feedback phenomenon; by *emergent* we mean properties that cannot be observed in any of the isolated components of a given system. This recursive readjustment process among systems and their emergent influences may lead to a harmonic oscillation, or synchronized resonance pattern of long duration, so that we speak of these dynamic relationships as though they are entities.

Since we have already stated that alterations that decrease the uncertainty in systems may be called information, we may now state that information is a pattern of recursive influence among systems. Therefore, the continuous recursive readjustment among a given set of systems in response to information, whether the information emanates from within the relationships of these systems or from without, causes a constant adjustment and readjustment of all systems involved, resulting in decreased uncertainty.

At our present state of conceptual organization, we must consider all systems as open, that is, susceptible to influence. This is another way of stating that all systems may be informed. Regardless of where we arbitrarily bound a system—atomic, cellular, organic, individual, or social—we may speculate that the given system is composed of subsystems and is in itself a subsystem of a larger system or suprasystem. As our delineated open system reciprocally adjusts and readjusts to influences from other similar systems, subsystems, and suprasystems, we have a continuous recursion with a simultaneously associated infinite regression of adjustments and readjustments in subsystems of the given system and an infinite progression of adjustments and readjustments in all suprasystems.

This interdependency of subsystems, systems, and suprasystems is difficult to conceptualize, especially when the continuous flow of information among systems makes the relationships dynamic rather than static. Perhaps we might glimpse this complexity even in a two-dimensional model if we keep in mind that we have distorted process by making our model static and

Figure 1

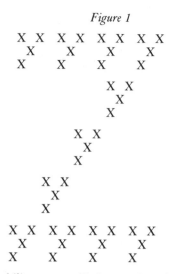

1. Subsystem X is a probability center of influence. Its influence radiates throughout the diagram.
2. System Y has emergent properties that are different from the four X's. One could not deduct from studying X that four X's would compose Y.
3. Suprasystem Z has emergent properties different from subsystem X or system Y.
4. The properties of subsystem X, system Y, and suprasystem Z reciprocally influence each other.

(Even this overly simplified model indicates the complexity of servoemergent properties and recursive readjustment. An alteration in any subsystem, system, or the suprasystem would affect the emergent properties of these interacting patterns resulting in a recursive or reciprocal exchange of information.)

have no way of representing the space-time element. Suppose we start with a subsystem we may term *X*, which is continually varying. When several *X*s interrelate to form a system, we have the emergent property *Y*. Similarly, when a group of *Y*s are organized into a suprasystem, we have an emergent property *Z*. We could not observe property *Y* from studying *X* alone or emergent property *Z* from studying *X* and/or *Y* (see Figure 1).

Using this conceptual frame, we may speculate that a quantum shift in a very small system, such as a hydrogen atom, would influence all the systems in the universe. Of course, these influences would be extremely subtle. We must emphasize that any alteration of a system affects the chain of influences, and vice versa, whether the influences are associated with change, equilibration, or stability. If we arbitrarily select a system in this oscillating chain of reciprocal and recursive interactions, we may state that the system involved has received and processed information.

It seems appropriate to end this subsection with another illustration from the world of relativity and quantum physics and probability theory. Geoffrey Chew has originated a theory or philosophy of nature known as the "bootstrap hypothesis," which he has used, according to Capra, "to construct specific models of particles formulated in S-matrix language" [7:p. 286]. The bootstrap philosophy is the final rejection of the Newtonian mechanistic world view, and it expresses the oscillating chain of reciprocal and recursive interactions that make up the world of systems and information. Capra explained:

> In the new world view, the universe is seen as a dynamic web of interrelated events. None of the properties of any part of this web is fundamental; they all follow from the properties of the other parts, and the overall consistency of their mutual interrelations determines the structure of the entire web. Thus, the bootstrap philosophy represents the culmination of a view of nature that arose in quantum theory with the realization of an essential and universal interrelationship, acquired its dynamic content in relativity theory, and was formulated in terms of reaction probabilities in S-matrix theory. [7:p. 286]

Practical Considerations

The "purists" who work in developing systems theories, information theories, and theories of cybernetics would argue that they should not be completely identified with each other. Information theory, for example, was originally designed to study the transmission of information in systems of electronic communication. That it has been used in work with electronic communications systems does not mean that it can be equally applied to general systems theory, which is concerned with living systems. The same might be said of cybernetics. Bertalanffy discussed the problem of confusing and intermixing cybernetics and systems theories:

> *Cybernetics* is a theory of control systems based on communication (transfer of information) between system and environment and within the system, and control (feedback) of the system's function in regard to environment. As mentioned and to be discussed further, the model is of wide application but should not be identified with "systems theory" in general. [4:p. 21]

There are some who argue otherwise, however, and believe that the theories do have widespread application. Stafford Beer wrote:

> Cybernetics is the science of communication and control. The applied aspects of this science relate to whatever field of study one cares to name: engineering, or biology, or physics, or sociology. . . . The formal aspects of the science seek a general theory of control, abstracted from the applied fields, and appropriate to them all. [18:p. 106]

Ralph Parkman commented:

> Cybernetics may be described as the study of brainlike processes or equilibrium-seeking processes and in these kinds of terms it is subject to very broad and often disparate interpretations. It overlaps such fields as general systems theory, theory of automata, semantics, information theory, logic and invades important areas of the physical, natural and social sciences. [18:p. 106]

Most scholars would agree that we are becoming more accustomed to thinking in terms of systems. Bertalanffy wrote:

If someone were to analyze current notions and fashionable catchwords, he would find "systems" high on the list. The concept has pervaded all fields of science and penetrated into popular thinking, jargon and mass media. Systems thinking plays a dominant role in a wide range of fields from industrial enterprise and armaments to esoteric topics of pure science. [4:p. 3]

We are also experiencing another revolution in technology, which is emanating from the relationship or interconnectedness of the new physics, systems theories, and information theories. With all the advances made in the field of electromagnetism, we have entered and are well into what Marshall McLuhan referred to as "the new electric age" which he equated with the "age of information." This is clearly an era of systems, electricity, and information. McLuhan wrote, in 1964, in *Understanding Media: The Extensions of Man:*

Today it is the instant speed of electric information that, for the first time, permits easy recognition of the patterns and the formal contours of change and development. The entire world, past and present, now reveals itself to us like a growing plant in an enormously accelerated movie. Electric speed is synonomous with light and with the understanding of causes. So, with the use of electricity in previously mechanized situations, men easily discover connections and patterns that were quite unobservable at the slower rates of mechanical change. [25:p. 305]

It is interesting to note that, along with his early acknowledgment of the enormous explosion in information processing made possible by the technological advances in the use of electricity, McLuhan hinted at the search for causes in our accelerated recognition of patterns and systems. It implied an investment in the cause-and-effect ideas of the Newtonian world. And yet, McLuhan definitely understood the impact of electronics automation upon the mechanical world. He wrote that "the lineal and sequential aspect of mechanical analysis . . . has been erased by the electric speed-up and exact synchronizing of information that is automation" [25:p. 303].

The computer is the principal technological invention that has accelerated the processing and storing of electrical information. Although computers had their origins much before the birth of the relativity and quantum theories, their ability to process and store vast quantities of information was greatly enhanced by the development of the transistor, which was a result of the application of quantum mechanics. The computer, which handles and stores information, is having an impact upon our lives that we are scarcely able to conceive. According to Frank Herbert and Max Barnard, "We say flatly that computers will have more influence on what people do than all of the effects laid at the door of both fire and the wheel" [20:p. 15].

We must keep in mind that information is defined as an influence that decreases uncertainty within a system. The meaning we assign to information is relative to the observer and the other systems involved. This point is important in understanding information processing machines, or computers. With these technological tools we have learned to process, code, and store information more rapidly than ever before and we have assigned meaning to this information.

We had developed numbers as a means of quantitating relationships. In one sense, computers are mechanized operations for quantitating relationships. Often, we translate computer activity into mathematical symbols. Essentially, however, the computer is an option chooser. It selects options by following a preset program and by selecting those options in a stepwise fashion, decreasing uncertainty in the symbolic system, or problem, with each step. It generates and organizes information by rapidly decreasing uncertainty. It does so by continually choosing one of two possible choices in a series of choices.

The functions of the computer are to process and scan information, to store information, and to make decisions based on the information it has processed and stored. A calculator handles numbers, but the computer handles information, which may be defined as anything that can be expressed by an electromagnetic signal and quantified. Such information can come in many forms, including verbal, graphic, or numeric.

Rapidity is a key concept in understanding the effects of computers on the age of information. Herbert and Barnard illustrated this phenomenon by saying, "To give you some idea of that pace, at four million cycles a second (a common pulse rate), a computer could handle four million bytes a second. That's four million actions every second" [20]. (A bit, or binary digit, is the smallest unit of information, and a byte is a string of eight bits.)

Philip A. Abelson has pointed out that minicomputers can process 10^7 bits per second and said, "During the past 15 years there has been an exponential increase in the volume of communications and in the bit rate that can be achieved" [1:p. 752]. He also notes that the earth stations operated by Satellite Business Systems have terminals that have "a throughput capability of 12 million bits per second [1:p. 752].

The computer is faster than the human brain. Herbert and Barnard illustrated the rapidity of the computer by comparing how long it would take a computer to solve a problem with how long it would take a person to solve the same problem. They called the computer a "time cruncher" and wrote:

> Perhaps now you can begin to understand what we mean when we call the computer "a time cruncher." Pause for a moment and consider that. If a computer had your time sense, it would be as though it accepted your problem, followed your instructions to produce an answer, and then had to wait seven or eight years for you to pick up the answer and get on the next instruction. If you took a few minutes to read a "printout" while composing the next steps in your head, the computer would be counting off a wait of centuries. And that's for computers with millionth-of-a-second responses. Computers are now in the works with trillionth-of-a-second responses. [20:p. 36]

With the advent of the computer age, many comparisons would be noted between the human central nervous system and various computer models. Some brain researchers would use computer models to describe brain functions. We will address computer-brain comparisons in the next chapter on living systems. We will note here, however, the two major types of computers generally used for comparison purposes.

The two major formats of information processing used by computer technology are (1) the analog format, in which the information is arranged as a continuous but varying flow, and (2) the digital format, in which information is arranged in discrete, or discontinuous, quantitized units. Ralph W. Gerard discussed the differences between the two formats:

> An analogical system is one in which one of two variables is continuous on the other, while in a digital system the variable is discontinuous and quantitized. The prototype of the analogue is the slide rule, where a number is represented as a distance and there is continuity between greater distance and greater number. The digital system varies number by integers, as in moving from three to four, and the change, however small, is discontinuous. The prototype is the abacus, where the bead on one half of the wire is not counted at all, while that on the other half is counted as a full unit. The rheostat that dims or brightens a light continuously is analogical; the wall switch that snaps it on or off, digital. In the analogical system there are continuity relations; in the digital, discontinuity relations. [13:p. 13]

The feedback concept is extremely important in understanding the information explosion. Computers utilize information loops or circuits rather than a one-way mechanical sequence. McLuhan wrote:

> Feedback is the end of the lineality that came into the Western world with the alphabet and the continuous forms of Euclidean space. . . . The programming can now include endless changes of program. It is the electric feedback, or dialogue pattern, of the automatic and computer-programmed "machine" that marks it off from the older mechanical principle of one-way movement. [25:pp. 307–309]

The automation of the computer world and the mechanization of the industrial world are not the same. The electric age has presented us with a network of information that encompasses the entire globe. To borrow some of McLuhan's terminology, electric information is processed at the rate of electric instant speed. We are beginning to characterize our world as flowing information. McLuhan wrote:

> In the case of electricity, it is not corporeal substance that is stored or moved, but perception and information. As for technological acceleration, it now approaches the speed of light. . . . It is strange, then, that electricity should confer on all previous human organization a completely new character? [25:p. 305]

According to Herbert and Barnard, "It is inevitable that computers will permeate almost every aspect of our lives. The positive rewards make this a certainty. They will kick in a dramatic speedup to the changes and evolution of our world" [20:p. 75].

Where are we in this rapidly evolving universe of information? The work of scholars and scientists during the twentieth century has necessitated a complete reorganization of our conceptual frame. We must shift our manner of organizing information to conceive entities as fluid harmonic patterns. Particles seem to be transient emergent properties of wave periodicity. Probability has replaced certainty, the interaction of influences has replaced simple location, and form and function are merged into processes of varying duration. We can no longer confidently differentiate mass and energy or waves and particles. These "things" are all relative to the way we organize information. As our concept of our world alters, we are forced to adjust our ideas of ourselves, our minds, and our bodies. We will now examine the concept of living systems as process.

References

1. Abelson, P A: The revolution in computers and electronics. *Science*, Volume 215, Number 4534, February 12, 1982, pp 751–753
2. Baumer, F L: *Modern European Thought: Continuity and Change in Ideas, 1600–1950*. New York: Macmillan, 1977
3. Bergia, S: Einstein and the birth of special relativity. In French, A (Ed): *Einstein: A Centenary Volume*. Cambridge, Massachusetts: Harvard University Press, 1979
4. Bertalanffy, L von: *General Systems Theory: Foundations, Development, Applications*. New York: George Braziller, 1968
5. Bronowski, J: *The Ascent of Man*. Boston: Little, Brown, 1973
6. Bronowski, J: *A Sense of the Future*. Cambridge, Massachusetts: MIT Press, 1977
7. Capra, F: *The Tao of Physics*. Boulder, Colorado: Shambhala, 1975
8. Davies P: *Other Worlds: A Portrait of Nature in Rebellion, Space, Superspace and the Quantum Universe*. New York: Simon and Schuster, 1980
9. Eddington, A S: The constants of nature. In Newman, J (Ed): *The World of Mathematics*, Volume Two. New York: Simon and Schuster, 1956, pp 1074–1093
10. Eddington, A S: *The Nature of the Physical World*. New York: Macmillan, 1928
11. Eddington, A S: The new law of gravitation and the old law. In Newman, J (Ed): *The World of Mathematics*, Volume Two. New York: Simon and Schuster, 1956, pp 1094–1104
12. Einstein, A, and Infeld, L: *The Evolution of Physics from Early Concepts to Relativity and Quanta*. New York: Simon and Schuster, 1938
13. Foerster, H von: *Cybernetics: Circular Causal and Feedback Mechanisms in Biological and Social Systems*. New York: John Macy, Jr., Foundation, 1951
14. Forsee, A: *Albert Einstein: Theoretical Physicist*. New York: Macmillan, 1963
15. French, A (Ed): *Einstein: A Centenary Volume*. Cambridge, Massachusetts: Harvard University Press, 1979
16. Gardner, M: *The Relativity Explosion*. New York: Vintage Books, 1976
17. Halle, L J: *Out of Chaos*. Boston: Houghton Mifflin, 1977
18. Handy, R, and Harwood, E: *A Current Appraisal of the Behavioral Sciences*. Great Barrington, Massachusetts: Behavioral Research Council, 1973
19. Heisenberg, W: The uncertainty principle. In Newman, J (Ed): *The World of Mathematics*, Volume Two. New York: Simon and Schuster, 1956, pp 1051–1055
20. Herbert, F, and Barnard, M: *Without Me You're Nothing: The Essential Guide to Home Computers*. New York: Pocket Books, 1980
21. Jeans, J: Some problems of philosophy. In Commins, S, and Linscott, R (Eds): *Man and the Universe: The Philosophers of Science*. New York: Washington Square Press, 1954
22. Klein, M J: Einstein and the development of quantum physics. In French, A (Ed): *Einstein: A Centenary Volume*. Cambridge, Massachusetts: Harvard University Press, 1979
23. Laplace, P: Concerning probability. In Newman, J (Ed): *The World of Mathematics*, Volume Two. New York: Simon and Schuster, 1956, pp 1325–1333
24. Mason, S F: *A History of the Sciences*. New York: Collier Books, 1962
25. McLuhan, M: *Understanding Media: The Extensions of Man*. New York: Signet Books, 1964
26. Miller, J G: Living systems: Basic concepts. In Gray, W, Duhl, F, and Rizzo, N (Eds): *General Systems Theory and Psychiatry*. Boston: Little, Brown, 1969, pp 51–133

27. Reichenbach, H: *The Rise of Scientific Philosophy*. Berkeley, California: University of California Press, 1973
28. Russell, B: *The A B C of relativity*. New York: Mentor, 1959
29. Sagan, C: *Broca's Brain*. New York: Ballatine, 1980
30. Sayre, K: *Cybernetics and the Philosophy of Mind*. Atlantic Highlands, New Jersey: Humanities Press, 1976
31. Schrödinger, E: Causality and wave mechanics. In Newman, J (Ed): *The World of Mathematics*, Volume Two. New York: Simon and Schuster, 1956, pp 1056–1068
32. Spradlin, W W, and Porterfield, P B: *Human Biosociology: From Cell to Culture*. New York: Springer-Verlag, 1979
33. Trefil, J S: *Physics as a Liberal Art*. New York: Pergamon Press, 1978
34. von Weizsacker, F: *The Unity of Nature*. New York: Farrar, Straus, Giroux, 1980
35. Whitehead, A N: *Adventures of Ideas*. New York: Mentor, 1955
36. Whitehead, A N: *Science and the Modern World*. New York: Mentor, 1948
37. Wiener, N: *Cybernetics*. New York: John Wiley and Sons, 1961
38. Wolf, F: The man behind Einstein. *Science Digest*, Volume 90, Number 2, February 1982, p 40

Chapter 8

The Emergence of I

It is the same elements that go to compose my mind and the world. This situation is the same for every mind and its world, in spite of the unfathomable abundance of "cross-references" between them. The world is given to me only once, not one existing and one perceived. Subject and object are only one. The barrier between them cannot be said to have broken down as a result of recent experience in the physical sciences, for this barrier does not exist. [32:p. 137]

Erwin Schrödinger, 1956

Even without going beyond them (the bounds of scientific inquiry) one can say that, just as the Greek temple is more than an aggregation of stones, so each of us human beings is more than an aggregation of molecules. This is no less true of the eagle that rides the wind, the fish that darts through the pondweed, the butterfly that waves its patterned wings, or the crocus that spreads its petals to the sun. Matter, as it builds up from less to more, acquires form, and form represents the order that arises out of the original chaos. [20:p. 109]

Louis J. Halle, 1977

Life as Process

What are the implications of the recent advances in physics and systems and information theories for our concepts concerning life? They are, as we shall see, enormous. Although the implications are clear, however, the final impact upon biology is still to be felt, for the biological sciences are just now beginning to apply the theories emanating from the momentous changes that have occurred in related fields. While physicists have become increasingly concerned with the role of the human mind in defining all physical events in a relative world of process, biologists have until recently tended to be even more involved in the reductionistic approach to life and have concentrated on determining our place in the mechanical world of form and function. During the twentieth century, physicists have focused on relationships within systems and among systems, defining the human mind as an integral aspect of those relationships. "It is," says Harold J. Morowitz, "as if the two disciplines were on fast-moving trains, going in opposite directions and not noticing what is happening across the tracks" [27:p. 34].

Although Morowitz sees the split as still being definitive, there are others who believe that the gap is beginning to close. "The meeting of biology and physics," claims Jacob Needleman, "seems just around the corner" [28:p. 59]. As we look at biology today, however, we can still perceive the desire to pursue the old reductionistic goal of finding the basic building blocks of life. Even so, there has been tremendous advance in our thought concerning living systems. Until the seventeenth century, with the invention of the microscope and the subsequent discovery of the cell, our definition of life remained intertwined with our definition of soul, the spirit that gave each of us individual and meaningful existence. After the discovery of the cell, we would become more sophisticated in our arbitrary differentiation between life and nonlife. We would assign the designation of life to both plants and animals, claiming that they are alive because they are composed of cells that are themselves composed of living matter. We had begun to define life in terms of functions, and living matter manifested itself through its functions, that is, metabolism, growth, response to stimulation, and reproduction.

One of the biggest hurdles we have had to overcome in applying scientific theories to ourselves is our perennial desire to differentiate between ourselves and the rest of the kingdom of living things. This is no less true today than it was when Darwin's theories concerning evolution threw the conventional thinkers into confusion. "It is strange but true," wrote Sir Charles Sherrington, "that one among the animals should have been led to fancy itself so different from the rest as actually to forget that it was an animal" [33:p. 121]. Sherrington believed the discovery of microscopic life to be "a revelation comparable with the expansion of the nine Ptolemaic spheres to the immensities of the Galileo-Newton universe" [33:p. 64].

Although we gradually learned to accept the idea of cellular life, we were still reluctant to recognize ourselves as a part of the animal kingdom without insisting upon a uniqueness that allowed but little admission of significant similarities. Lewis J. Thomas refers to our obsession with setting ourselves apart from the rest of life as our "most consistent intellectual exertion down the millennia" [35:p. 1]. It takes little imagination, then, to anticipate the resistance that has occurred in applying the theories of relativity, systems, and information to living systems, that is, ourselves.

Another hurdle we have had to overcome concerns disagreement about what constitutes life. "To ask the definition of life," said Sherrington, "is to ask a something on which proverbially no satisfactory agreement obtains" [33:p. 63]. We have already said that the distinction between life and nonlife is arbitrary. Our ideas about the differentiation between life and nonlife have developed very slowly. [18,19] "Just as there is no particular moment in an infant's or an embryo's life," wrote J. Arthur Thomson, "when we can say, 'Mind has awakened,' so in the world of life as a whole we cannot say. 'Lo, here,' or 'Lo, there' " [20:p. 106]. Louis J. Halle elaborated upon this thought:

> I would speculate that the property of matter we call life began to manifest itself some 3,500 million years ago simply as a continuing intensification of a tendency somehow inherent in being as a whole. There is a continuous devel-

opment between the pre-life that the snow crystal represents and the life that the reader represents. The crystal does not know in itself a drive to survive and to perpetuate what it represents, but the reader does know such a drive in himself. The difference can be defined in terms of a spectrum of intensity without drawing a categorical distinction at any point. (No one can say, "Lo, here," or "Lo, there.") [20:pp. 120–121]

What we are discussing is the dividing line between the animate and the inanimate, if, indeed, there is one. What do we actually see when we progress from the inanimate to the animate? If we look at the chemistry and the construction of the ultimate parts of the inanimate and the animate, we see that they are fundamentally alike. We can systematize and notice that the animate is part of a series with the inanimate, just as Halle suggested. "The animate," wrote Sherrington, "then becomes merely a special case within the more general" [33:p. 122].

Perhaps it would be more advantageous to talk in terms of increasing complexity in proceeding from the inanimate to the animate and to the more elaborate forms of cellular life. Halle described this process:

> Elementary particles combine to make atoms, atoms to make molecules, molecules to make primitive organic cells, primitive organic cells to make developed organic cells, and developed organic cells—to make ever more highly organized forms of life—until in our own time, going from small to large, we come to human beings, and blue whales. [20:p. 130]

What is essential for what we call living matter is a combination of the ingredients, their exact proportions, and a very definite and precise geometrical arrangement [7]. What we are looking for are particular relationships, and these relationships themselves are constantly changing in various patterns or systems. The materials that constitute living matter must be assembled into packets of just the right kind, and these packets must be able to exchange information with the environment in order to maintain life. Erwin Schrödinger, in addressing the question of what characterizes life, wrote:

> When is a piece of matter said to be alive? When it goes on "doing something," moving, exchanging material with its environment, and so forth, and that for a much longer period than we would expect an inanimate piece of matter to "keep going" under similar circumstances. [32:p. 74]

Schrödinger's definition of life is almost identical to Alfred North Whitehead's explanation of physical things as defined in terms of what they do and what they do is influence. Although we quoted Whitehead at length on this in the preceding chapter, we shall repeat a portion. "For physics," explained Whitehead, "the thing itself is what it does, and what it does is this divergent stream of influence" [36:p. 161]. The thing that living creatures do that assures them of life is import negentropy, or, as Schrödinger declared, "It (life) feeds on negative entropy" [32:p. 75]. This fits neatly with the idea of increasing complexity in living systems, for the more complex the organism the more it moves toward the decrease of entropy. "When an organism grows from the germs in the egg-cell to become, at last, an elephant," wrote Halle, "the process . . . is in the direction of decreasing entropy" [20:p. 82].

The living world evolves toward increased order and organization, or negentropy. Most natural events tend toward the state of disorder, the final event seeming to be the destruction of order. This is not true of life. Ludwig von Bertalanffy wrote:

> In open systems, however, we have not only production of entropy due to irreversible processes, but also import of entropy which may well be negative. This is the case in the living organism which imports complex molecules high in free energy. Thus, living systems, maintaining themselves in a steady state, can avoid the increase of entropy, and may even develop towards states of increased order and organization. [1:p. 41]

In our study of open systems we are often tempted to consider individual plants and animals as closed systems. The new physics has made us aware that even the carbon atom, that extraordinary system of influence seen throughout the chain of living tissue, is an open system. The same carbon atom may participate successively in the patterned relationship of a blade of grass, the muscle of a cow, and the brain of a human. In each relationship it participates in the emergence of different properties and, by a feedback loop we have previously termed servoemergence, is itself altered. As we realize that all those probability centers called atoms are continuously changing even if their patterns continue to be statistically probable, we appreciate the dynamic quality of molecules, cells, and living tissues.

As cells and tissues evolve into more complex patterns via importation of negative entropy, we may state that these tissues have enhanced their ability to code, move, and store information. Life may be viewed as a process of coding and storing dynamic information in molecular arrangements. DNA is an enormous library of data. Even the cell, previously delineated as the basic building block of life, is a colony or conglomerate of living things [25,30]. All the different constituents that make up the system known as the complex cell are exchanging information to promote the realization of the whole [22]. Halle referred to the cell as a "community operating on the basis of a division of labor among its variously specialized members" [20:p. 126]. "The developed cell," he speculated, "may well be a community of primitive cells that, with the passage of time, became integrated into one another to form the complex unit we know today" [20:p. 126]. The cell is a colony, or conglomerate, of living things, including mitochondria, centrioles, and basal bodies. Thomas says that cells are "ecosystems more complex than Jamaica Bay" [35:p. 2].

We must now admit that the cell itself is a conglomerate of living systems, and we are also faced with other molecules that bridge the gap between living and nonliving things. We might also say that viruses are alive. The virus is a submicroscopic agent that consists of a nucleic acid core surrounded by a protein coat. It has the ability to reproduce inside a living cell. Researchers at the University of California at San Francisco have now isolated a mysterious organism much smaller than a virus that can proliferate and infect although it has no genetic material of its own. They have labeled this organism a prion and are suggesting that it may constitute a new form of life [16].

Whitehead, in emphasizing process, cautioned against the delineation of specific boundaries between living and nonliving systems, preferring to define life in terms of what it does. The encoded information is what determines the definition. There are electrons, for example, both within and without living systems. "Thus an electron within a living body is different," explained Whitehead, "from an electron outside it, by reason of the plan of the body. The electron blindly runs either within or without the body; but it runs within the body in accordance with its character within the body; that is to say, in accordance with the general plan of the body" [37:p. 76]. If an electron is inside a cell, it is considered part of the coded information that constitutes the cell and is, therefore, in one sense, alive.

All living things are patterns of influence that are continually in the process of harmonic interaction. The processes of interaction may be divided into fast processes, for example, energy, and slow processes, for example, matter. All these patterns or systems of interaction also have emergent properties. The emergent properties of the slow processes are usually defined as *form* and those of the processes of shorter duration as *function*. Within the human body, a process of longer duration may be called a muscle and a process of shorter duration a muscle contraction. Or, to use another example, we may call the body a process of long duration and a thought a process of short duration [34].

Those emergent properties of slow processes, because they are perceptible to our sensory organs, have a tendency to seem more real than those emergent properties of fast processes. We must remind ourselves that organized patterns of influence respond differently to other patterns of influence, some reflecting light, some not reflecting light, some resisting impingement of other patterns so that they appear solid and have the ability to register touch sensation, others not giving the appearance of solidity. We cannot say that one is more "real" than the other. We might be able to perceive a stone both by its resistance to our palpation and by its reflection of light. We might not be able to perceive electromagnetic activity radiating from a radar screen. The stone is no more real than the electromagnetic activity emanating from the radar screen. If we step in front of a giant radar screen, our existence is immediately threatened and our tissues will disorganize into a nonliving pattern of organization quite rapidly, even though those influences involved in this reorganization can neither be seen, felt, nor heard.

To primitive thinking the rock is very real since it can be perceived by the sense organs; the force fields emanating from a radar screen are quite magical. Even those of us who consider ourselves more sophisticated in our thinking and armed with our present theories may find it difficult to comprehend that the influences in the stone and those in the radar screen represent only different patterns of organization. Our concepts of the stone and the forces emanating from the radar screen are in themselves patterns of organized influence derived either from direct tactile and sight experience or from the observation of effects.

When the dynamic interactions of the patterns of influence become disrupted or unstable so that the total emergents of all systems are not within the boundaries that we call life, we say that death occurs. Schrödinger defined death as a state of maximum entropy. When the living organism ceases to draw negentropy from its environment, it will die. To define death in systems terms we say that it is a dissolution of systems, or patterns of interacting processes, with the processes of short duration dissipating more quickly than those of long duration.

Since muscle contractions and other short-duration processes, including thought and movement, dissipate more rapidly, we have what appears to be a residue of long-duration processes, namely, the body. Although the short-duration processes may appear to dissipate more rapidly, we must keep in mind that the time element, whether we call it rapid or slow, is completely relative to our point of observation. If we were to move our time frame to a more rapid sequencing of events, we could observe the slow processes evolving and dissipating quite quickly. As an analogy, we may speculate that a snow crystal is a harmonic pattern of influences resulting in those properties we call crystalline. At room temperature we may see some of the processes dissipate so that we have the residue, or drop of water, which represents the processes of long duration. We may choose to poetically consider the drop of water a dead snowflake.

As those processes of even longer duration, namely, hydrogen and oxygen in chemical union, dissipate into widely dispersed water molecules, we say that the water has evaporated or that the body of the dead snowflake has disintegrated. In a process of extremely long duration, the water molecules themselves may break up into their components of hydrogen and oxygen, and under extreme duress, these systems of influence, namely, the atoms of hydrogen and oxygen, may in themselves dissipate into patterns of influence that we call energy. The latter, of course, requires a nuclear reaction to be observable in a given human's lifetime.

In the analogy of the snowflake, we are aware that all the different organized patterns of influence have emergent properties, depending on the dynamics of the interacting subsystems of influence. The individual human unit is also comprised of multiple systems and patterns of organized influence with fast and slow processes that we have arbitrarily divided into mind and body. These fast and slow processes are not clearly delineated but are a continuum, so that anything that affects a process of short duration inadvertently affects all systems, even those of longer duration. Conversely, anything that affects processes of longer duration affects the resonance patterns of those interactions of shorter duration.

Whereas all open systems, living and nonliving, radiate influences and are influenced by other systems, living systems actively absorb or import influences. We may say that all systems process information. Living systems actively acquire information [34]. Some of the emergent properties of those relationships we term life have been characterized as metabolism, reproduction, and irritability.

A nonliving system, such as a stone, may passively absorb heat and light from the sun. Its relationships are temporarily altered by the addition of these fast processes to the slow processes of its molecular arrangement. When the sun sets and the stone cools, its internal pattern of relationships returns to its previous state. A living system, such as a plant, absorbs the fast processes, light and heat, and utilizes them by means of a series of changes and actions called photosynthesis to arrange and rearrange its molecular patterns into a slow process that remains after the sun has set. The plant has organized and stored the information via metabolism into new patterns. The plant has grown. The cell and all the living things that make up the cell have the ability to catch and store energy in this process termed *metabolism*. Plants can convert energy, which is a fast process, into matter, which is a slow process. Animals are able to do the reverse and take the matter of the plant and transform it into energy. Both plants and animals are patterns of influence continually in the process of harmonic interaction.

The statement that the study of life is the study of the movement of coded information incorporates the processes of metabolism and reproduction. Metabolism is the interchanging or interaction of fast and slow processes to result in function and form. In reproduction, coded information is moved from one generation to another in the genetic blueprint, or molecular codes, of DNA.

One of the most peculiar emergent properties of protoplasm is its response to stimuli, called *irritability*. By this process protoplasm codes, organizes, and alters its arrangement in response to changes in its external or internal environment. Irritability is based on stimulation or a difference in environment. In its less complex form, irritability appears to be a type of metabolism, and indeed, the two processes are inseparable. However, as the complexity of tissue arrangement increased, cells and tissues have specialized (emphasis on different) emergent properties. As cells developed into colonies, specialization became more evident, with various groups of cells concentrating on nutrition and metabolism, others on reproduction, and still others on adjusting rapidly to changes in the environment. We will be concentrating in this discussion on the properties of those cells and tissues that specialized in response to environmental change, again emphasizing that this response is a type of metabolism.

In the early stages of evolution cells that specialized in irritability were involved in sensory and motor activity. Later, sensation and locomotion were again subspecialized. By having cells that were labile to environmental alterations the colonies of cells could better adjust to their environment and hence increase their chances of survival.

How do the individual cells, arising from a single egg, know how to specialize? At our present level of knowledge this question must go unanswered and remains one of the great mysteries of living systems. We can speculate that the information necessary for specialization is somehow processed by signals transmitted among the membrane, the nucleus, the cytoplasm, and the external environment. We do know that, as tissues in living organisms became more specialized, complex groups of cells with similar functions consolidated into organs, those groups of cells we designate in mammals skin, muscle, bone, gut, genitalia, and central nervous system.

The tissues most specialized in irritability are the nervous system, which includes the perceptive organs, nerves, and brain. This subsystem is responsible for organizing and responding to influences in the environment of the individual.

Living Systems and Information Processing

In a sense, we may say that the nervous system has specialized in coding, moving, and storing information usually arising from processes of short duration, that is, light waves in sight, sound waves in hearing, pressure gradients in touch and position, and molecular arrangements in taste and smell. All these stimuli initiate patterns or waves of electrochemical activity in cells and nerve tissue. In these waves of activity, information is coded, moved, and organized or stored. How these experienced waves are processed is one of the most complex and fascinating problems we have addressed.

As we have just emphasized, we separated slow and fast processes into form and function. Since nerve cells are processes of longer duration than those processes of short duration we call stimuli, we called the cells the brain and the body since they had form, and the function of information processing we called mind. We immediately encounter difficulty if we attempt to use a reductionistic approach to the study of the central nervous system. The processes of mind and brain are not reducible to the study of the individual atoms composing the specialized tissues involved [21]. We cannot determine which atoms and cells are responsible for the information processing activity involved in any single decision of the brain. Sir Arthur Stanley Eddington explained:

> But it is physically improbable that each atom has its duty in the brain so precisely allotted that the control of its behaviour would prevail over all possible irregularities of the other atoms. If I have at all rightly understood the processes of my own mind, there is no finicking with the individual atoms. I do not think that our decisions are precisely balanced on the conduct of certain key-atoms. Could we pick up one atom in Einstein's brain and say that if it had made the wrong quantum jump there would have been a corresponding flaw in the theory of relativity? [10:p. 445]

We may reduce the slow processes, the brain, to its component parts, cells. But we soon find out that a cell is not a tiny brain. It still may maintain its information processing capabilities, but these activities are different from brain activity. We are reminded of systems theory, which emphasizes that the whole is different from the sum of its parts [34]. The patterned relationship of cells results in emergent properties not evident in an individual cell.

We may, by studying individual cells, discover analogies that will help us conceptualize brain activity as mind. A nerve cell does respond to stimuli it receives, and it does code information. Often the information is of continuous flow so that the cell continually stores information until a sufficient level is reached, at which time it will send a signal to another cell. These signals are periodic, coming in interrupted bursts as packets of information. If we study the neuron's information processing patterns, we may divide these patterns into the continuous and the interrupted. The continuous describes the organization of incoming data, and the interrupted may be defined as the discharge of discrete unitized signals.

One is reminded of the wave and particle theories of light. When we consider light a continuous flow we conceive it as a wave. When we quantitize light into packets we consider it a particle. Once again we encounter difficulty when we attempt to utilize a reductionistic approach, and we are met with the necessity of looking at the whole, which is, as we have emphasized again and again, different from the sum of its parts. Sir James Jeans discussed this phenomenon with poetic intensity:

In the particle-picture, which depicts the phenomenal world, each particle and each photon is a distinct individual going its own way. When we pass one stage further towards reality we come to the wave-picture. Photons are no longer independent individuals, but members of a single organization or whole—a beam of light—in which their separate individualities are merged, not merely in the superficial sense in which an individual is lost in a crowd, but rather as a raindrop is lost in the sea. The same is true of electrons; in the wave-picture these lose their separate individualities and become simply fractions of a continuous current of electricity. In each case, space and time are inhabited by distinct individuals, but when we pass beyond space and time, from the world of phenomena towards reality, individuality is replaced by community. [24:p. 395]

We first addressed information processing as continuous and interrupted in the last chapter when we spoke of computer activity as being analog, or continuous, and interrupted, or digital. We may use an analogy here in an individual neuron, which also might be said to use an analog and digital format. The continuous, or analog, flow of information waves is unitized, or digitalized, into packets of condensed information. "The nervous system," said Walter Pitts of the Massachusetts Institute of Technology, "treats the continuous by averaging many of the discretes" [17: p. 51]. Ralph W. Gerard of the University of Chicago, in referring to the analogic and digital mechanisms in the brain, has stated plainly that "both types of operation are involved in the brain" [17:p. 12].

Perhaps the brain does process information in dynamic interacting chemicoelectric wave patterns that would be similar to an analog format. Gerard emphasized the analogic functioning of the brain:

In the first place, everyone agrees that chemical factors (metabolic, hormonal, and related) which influence the functioning of the brain are analogical, not digital. . . . Second, much of the electrical action of the nervous system is analogical. The brain waves themselves, the spontaneous electrical rhythmic beats of individual neurons, particularly the well known alpha rhythm, are analogical. [17:pp. 12–13]

The brain may simultaneously differentiate these experienced sets into units or blocks of information, which would be similar to a digital format.

The analog and digital systems form a continuum and are overlapping in many areas. The process of evolving biologic systems is replete with many examples of different types that overlap in function. The respiratory systems of some amphibia have gills, a phylogenetically older system operating simultaneously with the lung. In the central nervous system of mammals there are several overlapping systems of motor control, for example, the extrapyramidal and pyramidal systems, the former phylogenetically older but integrated with the more recently evolved cortical structures.

With respect to the analog-digital system, we may state that the analog is phylogenetically older, consisting of innate molecular programs, such as respiration, progressing through those systems, such as mother–child relationships, which are semi-innate but require imprinting on to the more recent substrate for data processing, language. The process of language is a striking example of the digital system, although all data processing can be unitized and is, therefore, to some degree digital. These two processes, analog and digital, are intimately interrelated and are considered parallel only for conceptual purposes.

The extent that the continuous and interrupted systems are interrelated depends on the processing of data from the internal and external milieu in a smooth fashion. The analog system allows less flexibility in one sense, in that it is genetically programmed and thereby affords less predictability of contingent variations. It is more flexible in another sense, in that it is a continuous operation and not distorted into arbitrary digital units.

Digital data processing accentuates differences; analog data processing seems to focus more on simultaneity. The analog is more efficient in familiar situations, whereas the digital paradigm allows a more efficient processing of new situations. Both work from data bits, or units of information. The digital system quantitates or unitizes its output as opposed to the analog, which translates data into pictures or feeling states. The rules of linear logic apply only to the digital operation. The analog paradigm may combine feelings or emotional states and perceptions relating to these emotions into large complex patterns, or gestalts [34].

Using the terms digital and analog to describe the two ways by which the human central nervous system processes information is a relatively recent addition to the list of words and phrases to describe this phenomenon. They are popular at the present time because of the ease with which they allow comparison of the two modes of thought with the perhaps easier to understand functions of modern computers [23].

The analog and digital differentiation allows us to form working concepts. Although the terms analog and digital are adapted from the computer field, their use in a discussion of brain functions is not synonomous with their use in descriptions of the computer system of data processing. By *analog* we are implying a gradient or proportional response to stimuli or data. By *digital* we are implying the unitization of data.

Brain researchers have, for many years, realized that there is a significant difference in the way in which the two sides of the human brain process information [14,15]. The evidence is growing that we think in two different ways. As early as 1864, Hughlings Jackson was speculating about the possibility of expression and perception residing in the two different hemispheres, expression in the left and perception in the right. He was able to support his speculation by observation of a patient with a tumor in the right hemisphere who had lost the power of perception. She was not able to recognize objects, persons, or places. Jackson called this defect "imperception" and regarded it in the same light as aphasia, which is loss of the power of expression or speech.

Although Jackson was extremely interested in the possibilities presented by investigation of the separate functions of the two hemispheres, most researchers chose to concentrate their efforts on studying the functions of the left, or dominant, hemisphere, and it was not until many years later that any real effort was put into looking at the special capacities of the right, or nondominant, hemisphere. The preoccupation of neurologists with the left hemisphere was so emphatic that the general impression given was that there was relatively little reason to attend to the right hemisphere.

The impetus for increasing interest in the functions of the right hemisphere came with split-brain research, which allowed investigators to examine both sides of the brain. With the advent of split-brain surgery, researchers were able to delineate clearly the two major types of consciousness each human being seems to possess. These modes of consciousness are described as analytic and synthetic, rational and intuitive, symbolic and perceptual, interrupted and continuous, differential and existential, and analog and digital.

Clinical neurological research into these two major modes of information processing has been done most extensively by Roger Sperry of the California Institute of Technology and his associates, Michael Gazzaniga and Joseph Bogen. Sperry had begun his research on animals, severing the corpus callosum, which joins the two cerebral hemispheres anatomically. The split-brain operation is called a commissurotomy. It was first performed upon humans to treat severe epilepsy. These procedures upon humans, which first occurred in the 1960s, revealed that definite and separate cognitive capabilities are related to each hemisphere.

By restricting the information going to the independent hemispheres, investigators were able to ascertain what functions each hemisphere was capable of performing. The old models of brain function based upon the so-called dominance of the left hemisphere quickly gave way before the evidence that each hemisphere could perform cognitive tasks independently of the other and without the awareness of the other. Although the right hemisphere is mute, it is able to comprehend some spoken language at the level of a very small child, perhaps at the age of two or three. It can also express itself verbally through what is described as "automatic speech"—emotional outbursts, swearwords, or such simple and much used expressions as "yes" and "no" and "I don't know." The most outstanding characteristic of the right hemisphere is its superiority in handling nonverbal tasks and in visuospatial thinking.

Split-brain research has clearly demonstrated that each person possesses two different and separate modes of data processing that operate simultaneously. The left hemisphere is the domain of analytical, verbal, and logical thinking. It specializes in logic, mathematics, speech, and abstract conceptualizations. The left hemisphere promotes the linear sequencing of information in a digital or interrupted format using one symbol at a time. The right hemisphere is the domain of the pictorial, or visuospatial mode of processing information, in which perceived relationships occur simultaneously in a continuous, or analog, format.

There is also evidence that the two hemispheres are different in their physiological organization. Josephine Semmes and her associates at the National Institute of Mental Health are performing experiments on the relation of language to handedness, which suggest that there is a specific brain organization in each hemisphere related to specialization. Semmes has hypothesized that the right hemisphere is more diffusely organized than the left. The left hemisphere is more focally organized than the right. There are short distances between the nerve cells in focal organization. Semmes found that left hemisphere damage resulted in a localized disturbance of function as contrasted to the less focal results of right hemisphere damage.

There is also ample research evidence to suggest plasticity and overlap of the two separate modes of information processing. Sperry, for example, was convinced in his early split-brain studies that calculation was confined to the left hemisphere. His more recent studies, however, support the idea that the right hemisphere does possess the ability to calculate. Stuart J. Dimond and J. Graham Beaumont have also performed experiments that demonstrate the calculating ability of the right hemisphere.

Essentially, split-brain studies have shown that we do indeed possess what has been termed by many scientists a fundamental duality of consciousness. The clear demarcation in the reasoning processes in split-brain patients has dramatically illustrated the propensity of the human brain to differentiate between analytic, or digital, and synthetic, or analog, and to perform these processes simultaneously. This phenomenon is certainly reminiscent of the wave-particle theories in modern physics. A fundamental question for physicists has been whether the smallest unit of our universe is a wave or a particle. Is it a field of force or a packet of mass? Perhaps the questions facing modern physics more accurately reflect our inside world, namely, our way of organizing information that we perceive or receive through our sense organs.

Lateral specialization of the human brain into two different modes of information processing is thought to be related to the evolution of language. Language is the tool by which we organize our world in a sequential manner, and it is evident that the left hemisphere has specialized in a serial processing of information employing elements or units that change over time. The right hemisphere has specialized in analogic codification or the nonverbal pictorial maplike configuration of the world. This duality of consciousness is unquestionably there and is recognized throughout the literary and scientific worlds.

Each person utilizes a mode of information processing that is predominantly digital or analog, depending on his or her particular physiological and psychological bias. Artists and musicians are thought to be more analogic in their thinking, and mathematicians and linguists might presumably be more digital. That these modes of information processing often conflict within the human individual is also a widely accepted proposition. Literature is replete with examples of characters who suffered great anguish because of their conflict between the forces of reason and those of emotion.

Although it is generally acknowledged that each person possesses and utilizes both the analog and digital modes of information processing, Western thinking is largely biased toward the digital as the more desirable. Comparisons are often made between concrete and abstract thinking or rational and emotional thinking with the implication being that the discursive or digital is the more acceptable. Bogen related this preference in our culture to language. "More likely this evaluation is not cultural in origin, but arises from the fact that the hemisphere which does the propositioning is also the one having a near monopoly on the capacity for naming" [2:p. 121].

Individuals differ enormously in the way in which they view the world. Each person processes information according to the bias of his or her particular mental constructions. Our sense organs are involved in the gathering of information, which our brains then sort, code, store, and modify. The organization of the information processing system may be seen as a filtering or transferring process so that stimuli are patterned in a prearranged format. The filtering process is evident throughout the information processing operation. It filters out all but a small amount of the information in our external environment. Aldous Huxley has suggested that while "each one of us is potentially Mind at Large" [29:p. 19], our individual brains must, in order to allow us to survive, reduce sensory input to that "measly trickle of the kinds of consciousness which will help us to stay alive on the surface of this particular planet" [29:p. 19].

Electromagnetic waves have to be within a certain frequency to chemically alter the retina and evoke a potential in the brain. Sound wave frequencies have to be within a certain range and of sufficient magnitude to register in the brain. The brain has to be at a certain state of arousal for the information to come to our attention. We have become accustomed to conceptualizing our world as having only those properties that are acceptable to the filters of our information processing system.

We are restricted by our evolution to experiencing the world only in ways permitted by our sensory organs. Research psychologist Robert E. Ornstein wrote:

> If we do not possess a "sense" for a given energy-form, we do not experience its existence. It is almost impossible for us to imagine an energy-form or an object outside our normal receptive range. What would infrared radiation or an X-ray "look" like? What is the "sound" of a one-cycle note? Or, as in Zen, what would be the sound of one hand clapping? [29:p. 21]

The human being has evolved to appreciate only certain aspects of the physical world related to seeing, hearing, smelling, tasting, and touching. We are, because of these limitations, inclined to believe that what we are experiencing is the whole of the known universe, that our mode of processing information is the true reality. We take this position even further and assume that what we term *I* or *me* is the only entity "seeing" the true picture of reality. Ornstein related the following story:

> A father said to his double-seeing son, "Son, you see two instead of one."
> "How can that be?" the boy replied. "If I were, there would seem to be four moons up there in place of two." [29:p. 15]

What we call ordinary consciousness is thought to be the personal or private construction of each individual. Whitehead said:

> Thus nature gets credit which should in truth be reserved for ourselves; the rose for its scent: the nightingale for his song: and the sun for his radiance. The poets are entirely mistaken. They should address their lyrics to themselves, and should turn them into odes of self-congratulation on the excellency of the human mind. Nature is a dull affair, soundless, scentless, colorless; merely the hurrying of material, endlessly, meaninglessly. [37:p. 55]

In some strange way, we have done exactly what Whitehead proposed but we have not always been aware of it. For, if we consider the basic tenets of quantum mechanics and the world of the new physics, we are describing a subjective environment while labeling our observations with objective terms. In atomic physics the investigator is describing his interactions with the objects he is studying and not any properties inherent in the object itself. As Werner Heisenberg explained, "What we observe is not nature itself, but nature exposed to our method of questioning" [5:p. 140].

Scientists who work in atomic physics do not view themselves as objective observers detached from the phenomena they are studying but are directly involved in the observed phenomena to the extent that they influence the properties of the objects they are describing. Renowned physicist John Wheeler calls our universe a "participatory universe," which cannot be removed from its observers. He does not recommend the word *observer* because of the connotation of an objectivity that does not exist. Wheeler wrote:

> Nothing is more important about the quantum principle than this, that it destroys the concept of the world as "sitting out there", with the observer safely separated from it by a 20 centimeter slab of plate glass. Even to observe so miniscule an object as an electron, he must shatter the glass. He must reach in. . . . To describe what has happened, one has to cross out that old word "observer" and put in its place the new word "participator". In some strange sense the universe is a participatory universe. [5:p. 141]

Nowhere, of course, is our participation more evident in our discourse on nature than in our studies pertaining to that particular function termed the human mind. What is the mind on whose excellency Whitehead remarked?

The Nature of Mind

Mind is a phenomenon beyond our instruments of perception. Therefore, when we study the mind, we adjust our conceptual analogies and scrutinize similarities and differences in analogous models, remembering that these conceptual frames are rough, simulated models or distorted metaphors. We engage in the same type of endeavor in studying the human mind as that which occupies physicists when they study subatomic phenomena. Neils Bohr emphasized the situation when he wrote, "Isolated material particles are abstractions, their properties being definable and observable only through their interaction with other systems" [5:p. 137]. We try to create images of the mind that give us some idea of that we are attempting to describe. As we do so, we are also constrained by the limitations of the language we must use. In this context, Bohr wrote, "When it comes to atoms, language can be used only as in poetry. The poet, too, is not nearly so concerned with describing facts as with creating images" [3:p. 340].

Even in our attempts to create images, frequently we become lost in semantics. Questions concerning mind and thinking machines or artificial intelligence, for example, hinge to a large degree on definitions of such global terms as mind, think, and intelligence. The term mind is used with relative ease by anyone who speaks the English language, and yet it is exceedingly difficult to define. Equivalent terms in German, for example, translate as intent, spirit, soul, memory, intellect, reason, and opinion, but there is no one word that embodies all the meanings we assign to mind. The *American Heritage Dictionary* defines mind as "the consciousness that originates in the brain and directs mental and physical behavior" [8:p. 449].

Words have long been our most effective tool, and we have spent long and arduous moments compiling books of word definitions, which are supposed to clarify these tools so that they may be maximally utilized. Often we get the impression that we are the servants of this word system. Although such words as mind may enlighten us to some degree, at other times they cloud the fragile data processing operation we call logic. When we say, "I have a mind," what is the I and what is the mind? We are implying that the I is separated from the abstraction mind.

The implication from the dictionary definition is that mind is synonomous with consciousness. Consciousness, in itself, is a most interesting word. It wasn't until the 1600s that we used the word *conscious* to refer to a personal or individual state of awareness. The Latin word had originally meant "to share knowledge with one another" or "to know with." The word took on a new connotation in the seventeenth century, when it began to refer to inward awareness. We now see it used synonomously with that all-encompassing word *mind* in referring to the individual's state of awareness or state of arousal.

In relating conscious activity to the brain and to the two hemispheres, we recall that recent brain research emphasizes that the left hemisphere is digitalizing, analyzing, and articulating and the right hemisphere is analogizing, synthesizing, and engaging in visuospatial information processing [9]. Most daily activity requires the shifting from one mode to the other with simultaneous integration. However, during periods of hyper- or hypoarousal, the shift is definitely from the major, or logical discursive, hemisphere to the visuospatial, or continuous minor, hemisphere [12]. States of arousal, then, are contingent on sensory-to-motor ratio, and vice versa. Roland Fischer described this phenomenon:

> While a hemisphere-specific task is solved by the appropriate hemisphere, the activity of the other is repressed or inhibited. Moreover, Aristotelean logic and language may be interhemispherically integrated with Platonic imagery. But when levels of subcortical arousal are raised (as during creative, hyperphrenic, catatonic and ecstatic states) or become lowered (as in the hypo-aroused meditative states), there is a gradual shift of information processing from the Aristotelean to the Platonic (cortical) hemisphere. [11:pp. 29–30]

Each cell has its analog and digital computation, digital input, analog programming and processing, and digital output. This occurs in cell interaction, not only in neuron-to-neuron activity but also in neuron-to-organ interchange. Analog and digital data processing of sensory input is continuous with motor activity. When the digital operation is included with self-referencing components, we say we are conscious of the movement, or will the movement. When the analog coding system of muscle and data processing go on without digital coding, we describe the movement as automatic, unconscious, or involuntary.

The synchronization of sensory and motor activity is related to the state of arousal but may have a cross-referencing cybernetic effect on the sensory input as to the analog and digital ratio. The digital system, when tied to motor activity, may increase the state of arousal, shifting the resultant sensory feedback more toward the digital coding system even though the analog is continually involved. Once the given motor activity becomes standardized via repetition, the sensory-motor relationship may become almost totally analog, as in shifting gears in a car without the self-referencing awareness of the digital operation.

May we say, then, that human consciousness, or mind, is self-awareness and orientation to our surroundings, contingent on the analog-to-digital ratio of data processing. Mind, then, would vary in cybernetic relationship with our state of arousal. For example, when our state of arousal decreases, as in sleep, the data processing system shifts toward the analog side of the ratio. We are alive and breathing, but during dreamless sleep we are not conscious of ourselves or our environment. However, if the state of arousal is altered by data input, that is, stimuli, we become more alert and awake and orient ourselves to the situation. Similarly, in hyperaroused states and emergency or life-threatening situations, we may perform complex acts using our analog set without being completely conscious of how we did what we did.

It is obvious that we are once again utilizing a mechanical approach to define a process. We are trying to use a combination of words that denote form and function so that we may get some image of the abstraction, mind. Not only does the dictionary definition give mind form and function through its association with consciousness, it also gives its location—the brain. We think of the brain as the seat of the mind, but we have also separated the mind from the brain. Yet, that separation cannot be complete, for the human self is definitely viewed as a function of the brain [13]. We consider with relative ease the idea of a kidney or heart transplant. If, however, someone were to suggest a brain transplant we would react in horror, for we see the brain as the self, the repository of mind, that which makes us unique.

The assertions of the newer theories relating to physics, systems, and information processing imply that the process we term mind is the emergent property of those simultaneous and interwoven patterns of information processing we have just described at length as analog and digital, or continuous and interrupted.

In order to avoid resuming a form and function dichotomy we must reiterate that the information coded, stored, and moved by the neuronal system is an integral part of the system, since neurons are themselves processes regulated by information. So, we have patterns of influence, neurons, responding to other patterns of influence, stimuli, with the entire process termed mind. Some might object to this concept of mind as so general that it could be applied to all living and even nonliving systems. There are those who have defined mind as an all-pervasive process. However, each pattern responding to influence is quite unique and we may define human mind as a special set of these processes. Even with this delineation we would emphasize that no two human minds are alike and that within a given individual the mind process is extremely fluid and never the same from one moment to the next. Patterns of organized process are, of course, statistically similar within a given species and within a given individual, so that we recognize these patterns even though they are continually varying.

Those processes we have termed human mind have been arbitrarily subdivided into thoughts, concepts, perceptions, and symbol production. Information reflective in nature, that is, information about the patterns of information processing within the individual, may be abstractly symbolized as the "self" or the "I" or the individual.

Our ideas about some kind of "magic within" that has led us to separate mind from other processes have resulted in conflicting conceptual formats and increased difficulty in organizing information concerning human behavior and emotional phenomena. Human thought has been one of the great mysteries, and the human self or I has been difficult to study with our present concepts. That process we term mind is nearly impossible to define because it is a process and therefore not easily amenable to a digital description that divides it into segments. We have wanted to separate it from everything else as we differentiate ourselves from the rest of nature. We cannot divide mind and process, just as we cannot divide nature and process. Whitehead wrote:

> Thus nature is a structure of evolving processes. The reality is the process. It is nonsense to ask if the colour red is ingredient in the process of realisation. The realities of nature are the prehensions in nature, that is to say, the events of nature. [37:p. 70]

How, then, are we to study the process we have labeled mind?

Perhaps our most productive efforts to investigate the phenomena of mind, I, and self have been those that have utilized analogies between central nervous system activity and information processing equipment, which has evolved through our advancing technology. Often technology is the development of instruments to extend or elaborate human functions. We can speculate that a hammer is an extension of our hand. The telescope and microscope are extensions of our eye. It does not seem too far-fetched to consider our information processing equipment extensions of our central nervous system. A television camera records visual phenomena, stores it in electrically coded memory banks, and can play it back. An audio tape recorder may record sounds. If we play it back, we hear words. A computer calculates using analog and digital models. It may monitor, set up goal-seeking programs, or anticipate, reflectively monitoring like the self. We are reluctant to see this system of information processing as mind, and yet it has many similarities to the processes in the central nervous system we call mind.

Comparing brain activity to technologic instruments used in information processing seems to have merit, since we build our instruments to organize information in a manner that has meaning to our internal information processing systems. We must be careful to remember that these comparisons and analogies are extremely crude and often spurious. A silicon-based chip is not a carbon-based neuron, and the hard-wired electrical circuits of computers are very dissimilar to the dynamic activities of a living system. However, the continuous and interrupted modes of processing information are, as we have previously illustrated, a characterization of both computers and the human brain. This seems to be a major point in surveying our concepts of ourselves and our world, our mind and our brain.

One of the most recent uses of technology to explain the human mind has been the comparison of mind with the hologram [6]. If you recall from the last chapter, Erwin Schrödinger implied that all matter and energy could be conceptualized as wave patterns of influence. Particles of matter and quanta of energy might be thought of as synchronous and dissynchronous waves in fields of influence. The hologram is a static representation of wave interferences. The information coded on film freezes the kaleidoscopic, dynamically interacting patterns of influences. We may say that the holographic plate captures some of the properties of these interrelated systems of influence at a point in space-time. In a sense, the hologram records those influences that affect the systems involved in a statistically probable way. This is another way of saying that the hologram stores information. At one level this information is a record, a memory of wave phases, some waves being in harmony and others out of phase. The hologram is a code of wave phase and wave interference patterns.

Paul Pietsch, the author of *Shufflebrain: The Quest for the Hologramic Mind*, is convinced that his hologramic theory "relates mind to the principle involved in the hologram" [31:p. 1] and that his research supports his theory. The basic assertion postulated by hologramic theory is "that the brain stores the mind as codes of wave phase" [31:p. 2].

The first researcher to propose a connection between the human brain and the hologram was Karl Pribram, who, in the 1960s, speculated that the model of the hologram could explain many questions concerning memory. Pribram's ideas were not open to clinical investigation, however, until it became possible to record brain activity not just as waves but as a power-spectrum processing images in the same way as the hologram.

The hologram is a simple analogy of the emergent properties of interacting patterns of influences. Some scientists have suggested that the entire world is a hologram. This idea is reminiscent of Huxley's phrase "mind at large," which might be used as a description of all that is. If we stretch our imaginations a little further, we may conceive of ourselves and our universe as emergent properties of interacting fields of influence. From the tiniest probability center of influence, whether it is called neutrino or quark, to the largest galaxy, the cosmos resonates in harmonic patterns of influence. Any emergent property of these interactions may be termed *information*. The manner in which those patterns of influence we call human code and store information is our concept of all that is.

We may go further and state that the process of recording, integrating, and storing data is itself a pattern of waves of influence that are synchronous and dissynchronous and exhibit dynamic harmonic patterns of interference. We may speculate that the periodicity and the duration of these interactions predicate the classification of the experiences into perceptions of form and function, or mass and energy. Those periodic patterns of long duration that affect our internal system we call form and those patterns of short duration we call function. The mind-body dichotomy is an illusion based on differentiating the continuum of process into long and short duration. We cannot deny that those processes, or interacting fields of influence, that we call body are more stable and of longer duration and that those we call mind are more fluid and of shorter duration. Our point is that these processes form a continuum, and in living systems we cannot have one without the other.

We cannot separate out one emergent property of a system without completely altering the system, even for purposes of illustration. We might study the body after the mind is no longer present, but then we are performing an autopsy and not studying a living system. Perhaps our major problem is as usual a problem of word definition. We often limit a definition of mind to those emergent properties of short duration that are found only in the human brain. We must remember that these properties are the emergents of the fast and slow processes of millions of smaller systems we call cells, molecules, atoms, and subatomic particles. We can, if we wish, speak of the mind and body of a cell, but this conceptual frame is probably as nonproductive as separating the mind and body of the suprasystem we call a human being.

We cannot accurately differentiate between processes of long duration, called the body, and processes of short duration, called the mind. Nor can we interrupt the interacting systems into internal and external environment by using the skin as a boundary. The social system of influences is completely intertwined with those organized patterns of influence we call the individual. Relativity, information, and systems theories imply that the human individual, like the atom, might be defined as a probability center of influence radiating to infinity and being influenced by all the other influences in the Universe. Rather than a delimited object, the individual person is a fluid pattern of processes, an open system within an open system. Those influences that have a statistically probable effect on these systems we term information. Organized patterns of this information comprise the abstractions we catagorize by our digital, or interrupted data processing, system as our selves, our bodies, our minds, and our world.

In the commerce of social interchange it seems imperative that we act as if this information processing scenario were reality. When we accept this point of view as a certainty we are like Plato's prisoners in a cave—we abandon our concepts to the world of illusions. The greatest of the illusions is our certainty about any of the dynamic servoemergent properties of process. And, the illusion that haunts us all is the illusion of self, that process of interacting relationships we each consider unique and separate from all other selves. Yet, one of the most productive ways of studying the human self is by studying it in the context of society.

If you recall, the Latin word for conscious meant to know with or to share knowledge with one another. The individual mind is, in this sense, a collective mind. The germ plasm of the human species continually generates new individuals upon whom are imprinted cultural patterns that have evolved by continuous and rhythmical process. Humanity is the continuous rhythm of culture whose cadence is kept by the life spans of individuals.

Mind in Society

Individual mind or consciousness cannot be separated from social mind or consciousness. We emphasize that we are looking at processes and not entities. How, therefore, can we separate the process of the individual self from all those other centers of influence with which it interacts? Social systems, like the individual self system, are always open systems, continually exchanging information with the environment. Each shift in data processing within a culture influences all other information processing functions of the cultural system, including each individual. The process we call the individual self is an emergent of all the dynamic biosocial processes that interact in the system of relationships we call society, or the social mind or self. The study of the human being in the context of society is a relatively recent phenomenon. There is still a tendency to want to idealize the individual self system, to remove it from the rest of nature and to give it an exalted position. No one, perhaps, has seen our struggle to remain isolated entities more clearly than Trigant Burrow, who wrote:

> Although . . . the scientific world in general has turned more and more to the study of functioning wholes, the accustomed approach to man's behavior in relation to his fellows is still essentially atomistic. It is true that we speak much today of the organism as a whole and of the interrelatedness of behavioral process. But even where there is the recognition of a unifying principle underlying man's behavior, it is still largely on a verbal or theoretical plane. It has not yet been incorporated into the vital motivational processes that shape and determine our behavior. In our feeling-life we are all isolationists. We are discrete and often conflicting entities, prejudiced in favor of the self and what we conceive to be its unilateral advantage. [4:p. 63]

It is obvious in reviewing Burrow's writings and life work that he took exception to the atomistic viewpoint, which he defined as that "which exalted the fragment, part or element to a position of major importance" [4:p. 62]. He was optimistic that our focus was changing and said:

> Today this atomistic tendency has receded into the background, and investigators recognize with increasing surety that the whole is something more than the sum of its parts; that they must study the intricate modes of interfunctioning among the parts and the emergent properties of the whole if phenomena are to be rightly understood and basic principles formulated. [4:p. 62]

Sociologists were concerned with the question of self in society even before Burrow stated his position. Emile Durkheim is most famous for his concept of anomie, which may be defined as a state of confusion or normlessness brought about when social adjustment is disrupted and experienced by the individual as psychic pain. Durkheim argued that human thought, which we have stated is an arbitrary subdivision of the process of mind, depends on language, which depends on society. Durkheim also believed that the origins of our concepts of time, space, and causality are found in the rhythms of group existence.

It seems apparent upon scrutiny that all the parameters by which we measure ourselves are in the context of a group, but we seldom consider this phenomenon when we think of our self systems. There would be no need to measure time or space or to think in cause-and-effect terms unless this were an exercise performed in relation to other individuals. In addition, all the roles the individual assumes are societal roles. The child learns to be an adult by assuming the various roles that constitute the adult system or identity. We see children playing at being teachers, mothers, firemen, or soldiers. They are in the process of organizing their responses as they deem required by those others who are playing the game with them.

George H. Mead, another leading sociologist, began to influence American sociologists around the turn of this century with his theories concerning the individual personality, in which he claimed that there is no individual consciousness outside social experience. He believed that unity of self was given to the individual by the social group or community. He called this self "the generalized other." One of his most important contributions to sociological thought was his idea that the individual is a reflection of group behavior that manifests itself in social behavioral patterns involving all other members of the society.

Mead's theories are also reflected in the work of Charles H. Cooley, whose "looking-glass theory" had a profound influence upon contemporary sociology. The concept of the looking-glass self is stated in his two-line verse:

> Each to each a looking-glass
> Reflects the other that doth pass.

The looking-glass self is similar to William James' social self. The social self is a reflective self that comes about as a response to, or reaction to, the opinions of others. Most of us go through three stages in reaction to another person, although we don't stop and label them. First, we imagine what we look like to the other person; second, we imagine what his judgment of our appearance is; and third, we get some kind of feeling about ourselves as a result of our first two thought processes. We are either proud, embarrassed, indifferent, or anxious. If we turn that process around somewhat, we can see that the personality, or consciousness, if you will, of any other person is only a group of ideas or system of thoughts we associate with symbols that stand for that individual. The effect upon our self systems of the imagined thinking of others and our effect upon them is profound. If we were confined to a mechanical reflection, it might be less impactive, but we are concerned with our opinions of the other's opinion.

Cooley believed society to be a mental phenomenon consisting of relationships among personal ideas. He wrote:

> The imaginations people have of one another are the solid facts of society. Society exists in my mind as the contact and reciprocal influence of certain ideas named "I," Thomas, Henry, Susan, Bridget, and so on. It exists in your mind as a similar group, and so in every mind. [26:p. 344]

The individual self is certainly a relationship phenomenon. We can illustrate this even further with simple examples, such as that of a hermit or a miser. There could be no hermit if there were not a society that recognized that individual as set apart and alone. There would be no defined miser if others did not notice his stinginess.

Another area of thought that emerged from contemporary sociology concerns the hypothesis that the individual self is an emergent of the many roles it must play in the context of society. The self does not exist prior to the roles it plays but only as an emergent property of those social interactions that give it identity. This is a thesis opposed by many theologians, for it suggests that the soul does not exist in the beginning but is an emergent. The soul creates itself or evolves from many beginnings throughout the course of a lifetime.

Florian Znaniecki interpreted the concept of roles in terms of functions and was the first sociologist to do so. His concept is that a person is an organic psychological self, which may be defined as a system incorporated in a more comprehensive system, the social circle. The individual self system exists within a social system or circle that is part of a cultural system, and it has certain functions to perform in order to meet the requirements of its individual roles.

The culture of which we are all members is a fluid process, not a concrete entity. This fluidity is perhaps more apparent at present than in previous times due to the rapid flow of information. Every cultural shift in any designated group of humans directly or indirectly affects all other cultural patterns over time. The management of information in a culture finds expression in social mores and laws.

We have elected to differentiate. The realization of one's individuality and one's selfhood implies the use of differentiating instruments. This includes the use of language symbols that have common meaning. Self is like a word. The printed word is information coded on ink and paper. The spoken word is information coded in a series of air vibrations. The word in an individual's brain is information coded in chemical and electrical interactions among many cells. Yet, we cannot say a word does not exist. The self might be seen as a word used as a reference point for other words. It is information about the information coding process and the association of information stored and presently impinging upon our data processing systems. The amount of information flowing through our self systems is enormous and is coded in interrupted bursts as units or packets of data. This concept is reflected by Percy Bysshe Shelley in his poem, "Mont Blanc":

The everlasting universe of Things
Flows through the Mind, and rolls its rapid waves,
Now dark—now glittering—now reflecting gloom—
Now lending splendour, where from secret springs
The source of human thought its tribute brings
Of waters,—with a sound but half its own,
Such as a feeble brook will oft assume
In the wild woods, among the Mountains lone,
Where waterfalls around it leap for ever,
Where woods and winds contend, and a vast river
Over its rocks ceaselessly bursts and raves.
[37:p. 82]

Among the universe of things that flow through the mind are our social perceptions and conceptions of other persons, particularly those involved in our childhoods. Through our perceptive organs we knew what people looked like, the sound of their voices, their smells, and their touches. Is it any wonder that our idea of this process called individual mind is anthropomorphic and atomistic? Since our concepts are relative to the data we wish to organize, if we rely only on unaided perceptions and the words of perceivers for developing these concepts, we may expect an anthropomorphic format for organizing this information.

The impact of sociological thought combined with systems, relativity, and information theories upon our ideas of self is yet to be fully realized. The self system becomes a patterned relationship of interacting probability centers of influence. These patterns can never be absolute but only statistically probable. In this format, we may adopt any conceptual frame we like concerning the individual, whether it is souls, fairies, or multiple personalities, as long as we recognize that these data arrangements are "as-if" paradigms. The number of these as-if paradigms is infinite in the expanding field of nebulous interacting influences, all relative and all uncertain.

One of the paradoxes that occurs, then, when we divide our world into units, resides in the question, "Is the world a continuous process or is it a sequence of discrete units?" An analogous question is, of course, "Is light a wave or a particle?" Jeans wrote:

> It seems at least conceivable that what is true of perceived objects may also be true of perceived minds; just as there are wave-pictures for light and electricity, so there may be a corresponding picture for consciousness. When we view ourselves in space and time, our consciousnesses are obviously the separate individuals of a particle-picture, but when we pass beyond space and time, they may perhaps form ingredients of a single continuous stream of life. As it is with light and electricity, so it may be with life; the phenomena may be individuals carrying on separate existences in space and time, while in the deeper reality beyond space and time we may all be members of one body. [24:p. 395]

Our answer to the question, "Is the world a continuous process, or is it a sequence of discrete units?" is, "It is both." Our choice between these modes of information processing is relative to the situation. We can say that self is a continuous fluid process and that self is a discrete unitized phenomenon. The choice depends on the information processing paradigm we are using. If we are forced to choose one as the truth and exclude the other, we have a distortion.

For most social interactions we choose to use a differentiating format of me and not-me, and in this format, the self is a discrete entity in opposition to the not-me. Perhaps the arbitrary nature of this choice may be illustrated in the following anthropomorphic vignette.

A wave and a particle happened to be transversing the same space-time parameter, and since they were on the same beam, the particle, being more self-contained, attempted to synchronize or converse with the attractive wave that was accompanying him. The particle admired the wave's form, although she was, for the most part, informal, and the wave in her own way had noticed the self-contained assuredness of the particle. She was at first somewhat reluctant to interchange because of his apparent formality. However, since neither seemed to be accelerating, a brief synchronization seemed like a way to pass time-space.

As a means of opening the interchange, the particle stated that he noticed that the wave had been glancing at harmonic scales and suggested that he, too, was interested in this type of phenomenon, particularly in the sense that it lent itself well to mathematical operations and could be digitalized oftentimes into whole numbers. "Whole numbers," the wave said with a slight shudder, "I was not aware that numbers still existed." "Oh yes," the particle said, encouraged by the naiveté of his curvaceous partner, "In any digital operation whole numbers become the backbone of modulating influences. One of the chief goals in information processing is an analog-to-digital conversion in which we can obtain a whole number representation of all events and entities." His enthusiasm seemed quite friendly, and even though a bit arrogant, he seemed to be an intelligent fellow, so the wave decided to synchronize more freely. "You think, then," she said, "A to D conversion moving from the continuous to the interrupted has a great deal of advantage over harmonic continuums?" "Indeed," said the particle, "if you will note, harmonic continuums do have nodal points of harmony which indicate probability centers of influence, or psi entities, as they are called by those adroit in digital operations, and even though we must keep within the tolerance factors predicated by the uncertainty principle, using statistical operations, we can say with a fair degree of certainty that the cosmos contains entities." Seeing that his listener was not overly disturbed by his rather brash statement, he pulled himself together in a tighter sphere of influence and continued. "Although I certainly hope not to give affront to such a lovely phenomenon as yourself, waveforms themselves can be digitalized and in many practical situations be considered particles."

The wave, who was listening very tolerantly, smiled gently with her rippling contour and after a brief time-space lapse, questioned, "Is it possible to go the other way?" "I am not sure what you mean," said the particle, checking his boundaries. "Could particles then becomes waves, if one elected not to use whole numbers in the operation?" "Of course, that would be possible," said the particle, looking a bit uncomfortable, "but that eliminates boundaries. Without boundaries, we could not logically sequence influences into information.

"I am not good at logic," the wave said rather demurely, "could you elaborate?" "Well," said the particle looking a little embarrassed, "if one used the continuous mode of addressing a phenomenon, we have the problem that you seem to be having at the present time. Without boundaries, without at least as-if boundaries, everything merges together so that there are no discrete entities and no way of really conversing about things, no cause-and-effect sequencing, and indeed, no way of communicating." "Is communication really that essential?" said the wave. "If one wants to be someone," said the particle. "What if one wishes only to flow?" asked the wave. "In that case, everything would be everything," said the particle "and there would be little to talk about." He obviously was becoming somewhat indignant and turned to give his best lecture about reality versus nonreality, when he realized his mild companion had fused into his own boundaries, causing him frantically to rearrange his periphery lest he too fade imperceptibly into a continuum.

The particle shuddered a bit as he observed another particle in front of him lapse into waveform. "One must be careful," he said to himself, "it is so easy to lose boundaries." He was still quite restless when a particle emerged near him. He seemed friendly enough, well boundaried, and of good form, so to speak. "It's nice to have a differentiated companion," he thought to himself. "Waves are so seductive and illusive, it's impossible to predict where these processes start and stop." "How are you today?" he said to his new companion. "I'm fine," the new particle replied, "could we discuss your views on whole numbers some more?"

In reviewing the mind-body dichotomy often attributed to Descartes, we find the form and function dilemma dissolving into a continuous process. The I, rather than being the motivating force of information processing, becomes an emergent property. The I does not do the thinking. The I and the thinking emerge from the same processes. Of course, we may attempt to isolate a part of this servoemergent process and call it I, self, or ego for reference points in relating patterns of activity, but the I then represents a pattern of influences and is not the originator of these influences. To say, "I think; therefore, I am" would be better phrased "When thinking, I am." Or, more abstractly, "When external and internal information processing systems interact in a certain statistically probable harmonic pattern, I emerge."

The emergence of the I phenomenon may, in a crude way, be analogous to the emergence of the note C when a violin is fingered and bowed in a certain manner. The C note is different each time it is played on the same instrument and different for each violin, but there is enough resemblance in this emergent sound pattern that we recognize it each time it is played.

Our emergent I is even more fluid, varying continuously with the patterned processes from which it emerges and certainly different in different individuals, or human probability centers.

We may question, "Is this process unique to man?" The answer is "yes" if we boundary our definition to contain only human characteristics, and furthermore, it is unique to a given individual and unique to a given set of influences. If we become more general, the I is everywhere. If we become more specific, it is nowhere. We may view the I arbitrarily as a delineated entity, a particle, so to speak, or more abstractly as a wave. It again depends on the information processing paradigm we use.

The open-ended conceptual frame presented by the newer theories has led to a recrudescence of ancient Eastern philosophy as a way of addressing our present dilemma, a philosophy apparently appreciated by sages many thousands of years ago. We will discuss some of these ideas in the concluding chapter. In this philosophy all is one and nothing is everything. Those who know can't say, and those who say can't know. This awakening of Eastern thought in the Western world has led some scholars to postulate that East has met West in our search for meaning, as though the differentiating and integrating circles had come full round.

References

1. Bertalanffy, L von: *General Systems Theory: Foundations, Development, Applications.* New York: George Braziller, 1968
2. Bogen, J: The other side of the brain: An oppositional mind. In Ornstein, R (Ed): *The Nature of Human Consciousness.* New York: Viking Press, 1974, pp 101–125
3. Bronowski, J: *The Ascent of Man.* Boston: Little, Brown, 1973

4. Burrow, T: *Science and Man's Behavior*. New York: Philosophical Library, 1953
5. Capra, F: *The Tao of Physics*. Boulder, Colorado: Shambhala, 1975
6. Comfort, A: *I and That: Notes on the Biology of Religion*. New York: Crown, 1979
7. Crick, F: Francis Crick: The seeds of life. *Discover*, Volume 2, Number 10, October 1981, pp 62–67
8. Davis, P (Ed): *The American Heritage Dictionary of the English Language*. New York: Dell, 1970
9. Dimond, S, and Beaumont, J: Experimental studies of hemisphere function in the human brain. In Dimond, S, and Beaumont, J (Eds): *Hemisphere Function in the Human Brain*. New York: John Wiley and Sons, 1974, pp 48–88
10. Eddington, A S: Reality, causation, science, and mysticism. In Commins, S, and Linscott, R (Eds): *Man and The Universe: The Philosophers of Science*. New York: Washington Square Press, 1954, pp 411–470
11. Fischer, R: Hallucinations can reveal creative imagination. *Fields Within Fields*, Number 11, Spring 1974, pp 29–33
12. Fischer, R: The perception–hallucination continuum. *Diseases of the Nervous System*, Volume 30, March 1969, pp 161–171
13. Furst, C: *Origins of the Mind: Mind-Brain Connections*. Englewood Cliffs, New Jersey: Prentice-Hall, 1979
14. Gazzaniga, M: Cerebral dominance viewed as a decision system. In Dimond, S, and Beaumont, J (Eds): *Hemisphere Functions in the Human Brain*. New York: John Wiley and Sons, 1974, pp 367–382
15. Gazzaniga, M: The split brain in man. In Ornstein, R (Ed): *The Nature of Human Consciousness*. New York: Viking Press, 1974, pp 87–100
16. Geneless wonder. *Discover*, Volume 3, Number 4, April 1982, p 15
17. Gerard, R W: Some of the problems concerning digital notions in the central nervous system. In von Foerster, H (Ed): *Cybernetics: Circular Causal and Feedback Mechanisms in Biological and Social Systems*. New York: John Macy, Jr. Foundation, 1951, pp 11–57
18. Gould, S J: *Ever Since Darwin: Reflections in Natural History*. New York: W. W. Norton, 1977
19. Gurin, J: In the beginning. *Science 80*, Volume 1, Number 5, July/August 1980, pp 44–51
20. Halle, L J: *Out of Chaos*. Boston: Houghton Mifflin, 1977
21. Harth, E: *Windows on the Mind: Reflections on the Physical Basis of Consciousness*. New York: William Morrow, 1982
22. Hockett, C: *Man's Place in Nature*. New York: McGraw-Hill, 1973
23. Jaki, S: *Brain, Mind and Computers*. New York: Herder and Herder, 1969
24. Jeans, J: Some problems of philosophy. In Commins, S, and Linscott, R (Eds): *Man and the Universe: The Philosophers of Science*. New York: Washington Square Press, 1954, pp 361–410
25. Life's start: A chance duet. *Science Digest*, Volume 90, Number 3, March 1982, p 20
26. Martindale, D: *The Nature and Types of Sociological Theory*. Boston: Houghton Mifflin, 1960
27. Morowitz, H J: Rediscovering the mind. In Hofstadter, D, and Dennett, D (Eds): *The Mind's I: Fantasies and Reflections on Self and Soul*. New York: Basic Books, 1981, pp 34–42
28. Needleman, J: An awkward question. *Science 81*, Volume 2, Number 5, June 1981, pp 58–59
29. Ornstein, R E: *The Psychology of Consciousness*. New York: Viking Press, 1972
30. Patrusky, B: How do cells know what to become? *Science 81*, Volume 2, Number 4, May 1981, p 104

31. Pietsch, P: *Shufflebrain: The Quest for the Hologramic Mind.* Boston: Houghton Mifflin, 1981

32. Schrödinger, E: *What Is Life? Mind and Matter.* New York: Cambridge University Press, 1967

33. Sherrington, C: *Man on His Nature.* New York: Cambridge University Press, 1963

34. Spradlin, W W, and Porterfield, P B: *Human Biosociology: From Cell to Culture.* New York: Springer-Verlag, 1979

35. Thomas, L J: *The Lives of a Cell: Notes of a Biology Watcher.* New York: Bantam, 1975

36. Whitehead, A N: *Adventures of Ideas.* New York: Mentor, 1955

37. Whitehead, A N: *Science and the Modern World.* New York: Mentor, 1948

The Relative World of Process

Seminar Conclusion

In our discussions we have considered cosmic evolution. In addressing the cosmos, which includes ourselves, we often conceptualize large bodies swirling around in space. We postulate that everything emanated from a "Big Bang." Perhaps by use of analogy we may change our perspectives. Let us attempt to perceive the continuing event as a cosmic symphony.

The symphony begins with the crashing, explosive bang of all percussion instruments and, after a brief pause, as echoes reverberate throughout the dark void, a soft, almost plaintive melody of flutelike quality emerges, growing softly in volume and pitch. One after another the voices of other instruments join in, and their entrance is so imperceptible that, even as they gain full voice, it is as though they were always there. Their harmony swells, until at last the cosmos is filled with a resonating cadence, rising and falling and shifting in tone and volume.

Out of the periodicity of reverberating harmony, we know time; out of the tone, we know energy; and from the volume, we know mass. Amid the shifts in melody, we know space. Since we are part of the cosmic symphony, we do not hear it. We are its waves, but we sense its echo in the sunlight, in a snowflake, and in a rose. Of course, we are speaking in metaphors as we must in addressing interacting probability centers of influence, whether we bound them large or small.

At present, we speak of influences as waves analogous to sound waves because this format best fits our words and mathematical symbols. We must keep in mind that in our metaphors we are incorporating the patterns by which we organize information equally with those influences we term information. Thus, space, time, mass and energy, and particles and waves represent our patterns of organizing information, which we attribute to all those influences of which we are an integrated continuum. When we speak of ourselves as isolated objective observers, we are perpetuating a myth.

Myths often seem comforting.

Conclusion

Chapter 9

The Death of Certainty

When Western physics was born in Greece in the fifth century B.C., science, philosophy and religion were not considered separate fields; they were united in a search for the fundamental nature of all things, an ultimate essence they called *physis*, the root of our word *physics*. [4:p. 42]

Mary Long, 1981

What is the meaning of a pelican, a sunflower, a sea-urchin, a mottled stone, or a galaxy? Or of $a + b = b + a$? They are all patterns, dancing patterns of light and sound, water and fire, rhythm and vibration, electricity and spacetime, going like
  Thrummular, thrummular thrilp,
  Hum lipsible, lipsible lilp;
    Dim thricken mithrummy,
    Lumgumptulous hummy,
Stormgurgle umbumdular bilp. [9:p. 118]

Alan Watts, 1966

Increasing Uncertainty—An Overview

In the previous chapters we have attempted to illustrate the progress of a conceptual evolution, a search for certainty. This search began with a rather nebulous, poorly differentiated animistic or anthropomorphic way of viewing our world, through progressive differentiation via linguistic tools and other cultural instruments, to a religious conceptual frame in which man and his gods were differentiated from the world. With religion came ritual, dogma, and increased certainty. From the misty continuum of the beginning we became convinced of a standardized reality. Our certainty was bolstered by revelation and reified by a specialized social segment dominated by priests and shamen whose power rested heavily on words.

Naming and, finally, measuring by the new language of numbers, our confidence grew until we began to place more and more faith in our powers of reason and logic. In the West, the Greek culture and later the Western cultures of Europe entered a period of thought in which most intellectuals were convinced of the absolute power of differentiation and reductionism and a mechanistic world of form and function that could be known beyond doubt. By reason and objective observation we could know all.

The reign of certainty was mildly disturbed by the petulant protests of the Rational Empiricists, Locke, Berkeley, and Hume and shuddered under a smashing blow from Kant and his *Critique of Pure Reason*. But Copernicus, Galileo, and Newton had built a strong fortress. Rapidly advancing technology erected on the power of differentiation all but precluded doubt in a rational mechanistic frame of reference for all concepts.

Then, in the late nineteenth and early twentieth centuries, our instruments of differentiation, whose pointer readings were the bulwark of our differentiated world, began to oscillate nervously. Tremors began to radiate through our island of certainty. These tremors escalated and were followed by a tidal wave of unique concepts generated by Einstein, Heisenberg, Schrödinger, and others. When this wave subsided, our world of certainty lay in ruins.

The new concepts hinging on theories of relativity and information processing, which began to spring up quickly, were exhilarating but confusing. Everything was seen as relative. Mass, energy, space, and time, all the building blocks of past centuries, became fluid processes. Let us quickly review what happened to our conceptual world that caused it to collapse.

Many of the new concepts responsible for our growing uncertainty were initiated in the fields of mathematics and nuclear physics. For most of us who were not trained in these areas, the new ideas seemed somewhat bizarre and removed from everyday life. For example, when we thought of an atom, which is beyond our capability of immediate perception, we generally thought of a tiny ball with other smaller balls revolving around it—a miniature solar system. We conceptualized the difference in elements as depending on the size of the central ball and the number of smaller balls that revolved around it. We learned in chemistry that the properties of basic elements depended on the configuration of the atoms that make up these elements. Since we could not see the atoms, this taxed our imagination somewhat but did not in any great degree conflict with the older word-world concepts, in which larger elements can be made from smaller elements.

We accepted the fact that houses can be made of bricks and that cakes and pies can be made from mixing various ingredients. We rarely questioned that the structures that emerged from either simple building blocks or mixing elements differed from the original units that were placed or mixed together. That a house does not resemble bricks or that a cake does not taste like eggs, flour, and sugar seemed to be a given. We were, therefore, not surprised to learn that when various atoms join together, the emergent properties of these interacting building blocks might be different from the blocks themselves.

We were told that sodium and chloride when separate have totally different properties than the crystalline properties that result when they are mixed together. This did not in any way seem magical. The problems arose when we asked the questions, "Where do the extra properties come from? What happens to the salt crystal when it is dissolved in water?" Our attention was now drawn to properties of relationships that began to strain our older concepts, which were derived from differentiation and describing phenomena as discrete entities.

The study of relationships that result in properties different from the elements that interact in the relationship was our first glimmer of insight into systems theory. We still felt fairly safe knowing that the atoms were the basic building blocks. Even though, when mixed together in various arrangements, the properties of relationships might vary, the atoms could now, as before, be thought of as discrete little entities very similar to the bricks we used in building.

Around the turn of this century, however, our neat building block model began to dissolve. The nuclear physicists, in proving the structure of the atom, indicated that the neat little packages or building blocks, were not stabilized units but were in themselves systems. To say that an atom is a system sounded rather simple until we asked, "a system of what?" We attempted to rely on our older concepts by defining it as a system of tiny pieces of matter. This explanation sufficed temporarily, but we began to divide the pieces of matter into smaller and smaller pieces. We now began to realize that each subatomic piece of matter was in itself a system, so that we regress to smaller and smaller systems until matter disappears.

What happened to this basic building block of the world around us? We felt a little panicky to realize that matter itself is an emergent property of systems and that matter disappears as we continue to divide the system. Nuclear physics had now carried us beyond matter by illustrating beyond any doubt that matter and energy are interchangeable. Einstein's famous theory of special relativity, $E = mc^2$, had been graphically demonstrated in atomic explosions. Until the atomic bomb most of us were content to let these mathematical abstractions about mass and energy remain as the toys of physicists and mathematicians. Nagasaki and Hiroshima brought the world of relativity into public awareness as a horrifying reality. Shifting mass to energy was no longer a bland abstraction or a philosophic exercise.

Although we might wish to return to the old concepts of considering matter as a basic building block and forgetting systems and relativity, international events precluded a return to naiveté. Lay persons began to question the phenomenon that resulted in catastrophic destruction.

What was this tiny atom that, when molested, could exhibit such enormous influence? Unfortunately, the answer from the physicists and mathematicians was not comforting. Atoms were described no longer as tiny solar systems of interacting chunks of mass but as resonating force fields that could not be adequately described using our old coordinates of mass and energy and time and space. Mass and energy were said to be interchangeable, and time and space were said to be on a continuum. When those small systems of resonating force fields we call atoms were measured they gave continually varying results. We were made aware that those properties we call mass and energy depended on fluctuations within the interacting systems of force. This is another way of saying that whenever we decide that an electron, that is, one of the force fields surrounding the atom, has a given mass and energy, we have distorted the system and the space-time continuum.

The picture was further complicated when the physicists informed us that there was no way of predicting the behavior of any given atom at any given time. The best we could do in this nebulous situation was to rely on probabilities and calculated uncertainties. Heisenberg's formulation of this uncertainty into the uncertainty principle further removed the possibility of returning to a more comfortable cause-and-effect way of viewing our world.

We were now becoming aware that no definite entities exist and that our world is composed of resonating force fields interacting in various patterns. These patterns or systems of interaction are processes of long and short duration that result in various emergent properties.

When describing the atom, Schrödinger spoke of it as a "psi entity," implying a probability center of influence with influences radiating from this center in all directions to infinity. We were reminded that even the center is probable and not a definite point. We were told that the influences that radiate from any probability center influence other probability centers throughout the universe, so that our entire cosmos became a kaleidoscopic pattern of force fields influencing and being influenced.

At first brush, this theoretical frame engendered a feeling of hopeless ineptitude in developing any conceptual frame about ourselves and our world. Many believed that it would be easier to dismiss all the information coming from mathematics and nuclear physics as metaphysical and mystical and return to our familiar world as though waking from a bad dream. After all, we have to live as if something were real and tangible, because all our perceptive organs continually reinforce our "knowing" that things do exist and that we ourselves exist. This, indeed, might be a solution if we were willing to take Rousseau's advice and return to the level of noble savage by burning all information and destroying all records. However, most of us would like to continue with our present comforts of life, including those technologies and creature comforts to which we have become accustomed. We would still want to maintain electrical appliances and communication devices, including the telephone and television and the computer technology that makes it possible for us to live in a very populous society. If we are to continue our technologically assisted life-styles, we must somehow reconcile our conceptual frames with those of physics and mathematics, which have been instrumental in developing this technology.

There are those who now question whether technology runs our lives or whether we run the technology. This, of course, is a spurious question, in that here again we are looking at the emergent properties of a system. This system is the human information processing system, and those phenomena that we label technology are the emergent properties of the interaction of the systems we call human and the systems we call nature.

If we elect to accept these new conceptual frames as inescapable, perhaps we may apply some of the theoretical concepts to systems larger than the atom. If we were to take a cell at the tip of one of our fingers, which we might identify under a microscope, we could apply concepts from nuclear physics and mathematics to this phenomenon and appreciate that this is a fairly large system of atomic interaction. This is another way of saying that each cell contains millions and millions of atoms, which in themselves are a resonating force field. Even though each set of force fields that we have termed an atom is somewhat unpredictable, the summation of an enormous number of these atoms gives a somewhat predictable pattern of activity, a certain probability of what patterns of interaction we can expect and what properties we can expect from these interacting patterns.

One of the problems in conceptualizing a cell as a patterned relationship of atoms is our continued difficulty in comprehending the size of an atom. It has been speculated that if one glass of water were poured into the oceans of the world and all the oceans mixed equally well, the hydrogen and oxygen atoms within the glass of water are sufficient in number that, when they are mixed through all the ocean, if we were to take glass of water from any ocean, some of the atoms in our second glass were in our original glass of water before mixing. This would mean that every day we probably drink a hydrogen atom that Caesar or Cleopatra drank or one that was used by Attila the Hun or Kublai Khan. We must be careful in delineating the size of atoms not to forget that these probability entities are centers of radiating influence and that each center of influence influences every other center of influence in the cosmos.

So, within the cell in our fingertip are centers of influence that are so small that they defy our imagination and so influential that they influence all the force fields in the cosmos. This baffling arrangement of force fields is interacting transiently in a pattern of relationship from which emerge those properties we recognize as a human cell.

If we are not already overwhelmed by the magnitude of these complexities within the cell, we may be when we realize that this patterned arrangement of force fields, which Schrödinger called psi entities, contain within the patterned relationships all the coded information necessary not only to reduplicate a cell but to reduplicate the relationships that we call our body. If we can overcome the impact of this new theoretical way of conceptualizing systems of relationships, we can appreciate that our body is composed of millions of these tiny libraries of information that we call cells.

Again, we may apply Schrödinger's concept of psi entities in that the interaction of these cells and their specialized relationships results in a larger system of interacting relationships that we call ourselves. These relationships are not stable entities but exhibit dynamic fluctuations, so that the properties at any given moment of all the interacting relationships are only probable. We may then assume that the entire set of interacting systems that we call the human individual resembles Schrödinger's psi entity, that is, a probability center of interacting force fields.

A New Concept of Mind and Body

We are now ready for the greatest leap of all—the application of these conceptual frames to those properties of the human individual that we call mind and body. If we continue to extend our concepts, what we have termed body, mind, self, or psyche is the interaction of influences among external and internal systems, those systems we call our environment and those systems we have delineated as ourselves. We are now speaking of an astronomical number of systems, both within and without.

The radiating spheres of influence of this enormous number of systems make it impossible to predict what influence any given system will have on the total pattern of activity. For example, if a hydrogen atom in the cell at the tip of our finger were to be activated by a quantum of energy, it would influence every system within our body. Of course, we realize that our body is composed of billions and billions of atoms. They are continually fluctuating, each fluctuation influencing every atom within our body. We are also aware that our environment consists of billions of these tiny force fields, which are also fluctuating. We are now back to Schrödinger's original concept of probability centers of influence.

When we summate all these multiple influences, we may utilize the psi concept and state that the summation of these patterns of influence will result in a probable pattern of relationships. Some of the properties of this probable pattern will be those we are able to perceive through our perceptive organs.

Using Schrödinger's concept, we may utilize all the vectors that make up the pattern we call a person interacting in his environment as a psi entity, one that is not absolutely predictable, but one that exhibits probable properties at a given time. By addressing the human entity as a psi entity, we become aware of the relativity of those relationships and systems that have been consolidated into the self each one of us takes for granted.

In this new world of fields and systems of fields, I or the self is a latecomer, a transient pattern in the shifting patterns of interaction, where any unit of interaction is relative, depending on the system in which it is arbitrarily included and the sum of the influences cybernetically impinging on the given system from the incorporating system called the cosmos.

This new concept of self has been one of our major sources of unrest, for in the dominant world of words, *I* was and is king. Among the oldest of our abstractions, the cornerstone of cause-and-effect sequencing, I is served by all—I live, I feel, I think, and I die.

Why was the concept I so late in visiting the world of relativity? It has been largely a language problem, for the I is linked to word information, which is our principal medium of social exchange. Words and meanings are of no value in themselves, but the I concept lives on in words in sequence, units of absolutes and retained meanings it has formulated. As molecular biologist Gunther S. Stent wrote:

> The obstacle in the way of giving a satisfactory account of the semantic component appears to reside in defining explicitly the problem that is to be solved. That is to say, for man the concept of "meaning" can be fathomed only in relation to the self, which is both ultimate source and ultimate destination of semantic signals. [7:p. 1057]

When we cross the threshold of the world of relativity, we become mute. Words do not fit and must be left outside as we leave outside some of our animal pets. In the world of relativity, I fades into oblivion. It is not that we are thrown out if we use words, but that the world of relativity vanishes before these crude semantic instruments. It is as if we pruned a rose with a bulldozer or dissected a cell with an axe. Without words the self fades away from lack of support. Living and nonliving systems merge, so that life and death have no meaning even if we could conceive of the information in these human concepts or systems without words. In the world of relativity the only language available is advanced mathematics, and even that seems primitive, especially whole numbers.

We, who began as other animals in the preword world many millions of years ago and who developed through the word world what we call civilization have, in the twentieth century, entered the transword world of relativity. From the time we differentiated ourselves via our digital operation, our world was essentially a study of mass and energy plotted against a grid of time and space. During our generation the format has shifted to considering information plotted on a lattice of relativity and probability. We study patterns and relationships rather than actions of entities. Form and function merge into a continuum of process, slow and fast. We no longer observe objects, we study the interrelationship of systems and subsystems of which we are a process. Those properties we attributed to entities are now viewed as information emerging from relationships. The soul or psyche translated into self has shifted from an image of God to a fluid pattern of information organized by biologic and experiential processes.

Prior to this century we were convinced that human language was the most effective mode of information exchange. Now we know that our central nervous system is involved in processing coded information using templates thousands of years old. Our systems are influencing and being influenced by stars millions of light-years away. That these complex instruments can also negotiate in the very imprecise medium of human language is perhaps their least impressive accomplishment but the one we continue to value most because it is the property that differentiates us as human. The language processing of information is our source of technology, science, myth, and religion. It allows anticipation of pain and death and hope for better worlds.

The human word language we prize so highly still reflects the word world of differentiated entities of mind and body, mass and energy, and space and time. In contrast, the new world of information theory has given us the language of influences and relationships that necessitates appreciation of relativity and probability against a background of continuously interacting systems of influence. We have developed information patterns that may be roughly translated into relational and probability codes of mathematics, but these are difficult to translate into the social medium of words. Our linguistic patterns are insufficient. As Neils Bohr recognized,

> The goal of science is to augment and order our experience, every analysis of the conditions of human knowledge must rest on considerations of the character and scope of our means of communication. Our basis (of communication) is, of course, the language developed for orientation in our surroundings and for the organization of human communities. However, the increase of experience has repeatedly raised questions as to the sufficiency of concepts and ideas incorporated in daily language. [7:p. 1054]

Considering the implications of recent discoveries in the world of relativity, almost any pronouncement that we make concerning the events of the twentieth century that have catapulted us into the state of increased uncertainty will be an understatement. Obviously, the theories of relativity and quantum mechanics and information and systems theories have made it difficult to organize our concepts along reductionistic and mechanistic lines. For example, if we make the materialistic statement that all our behavior emanates from a chemical substrate we would, of course, be correct. But the statement is rather superficial. It is true that our behaviors and our observations about our world and ourselves are the emergent properties of chemical reactions. But lest we become too confident in this materialistic approach, we must examine the concept of chemistry.

Chemicals are themselves emergent properties of probability centers of influence. What is that influence? We may call it strong and weak forces, electromagnetic forces, or whatever, but we must inevitably return to harmonic and dissynchronous waves of influence radiating to infinity. Our materialistic particles are wave interference patterns and harmonic wave patterns of influence. We are then left with our observations being emergent patterns of influence interacting in a servoemergent pattern with other similar patterns in an infinite progression and regression. We are left with the picture presented by Alan Watts in the quotation at the beginning of this chapter and reified by Sir Arthur Stanley Eddington in his description of the nature of electrons:

> We see the atoms with their girdles of circulating electrons darting hither and thither, colliding and rebounding. Free electrons torn from the girdles hurry away a hundred times faster, curving sharply round the atoms with sideslips and hairbreadth escapes. . . . The spectacle is so fascinating that we have perhaps forgotten that there was a time when we wanted to be told what an electron is. The question was never answered. . . . *Something unknown is doing we don't know what*—that is what our theory amounts to. It does not sound a particularly illuminating theory. I have read something like it elsewhere:
> The slithy toves
> Did gyre and gimble in the wabe.
> There is the same suggestion of activity. There is the same indefiniteness as to the nature of the activity and of what it is that is acting. [9:pp. 118–119]

Does this mean that we should abdicate our search for knowledge? Unfortunately, or fortunately, we do not seem to have that choice. We are gatherers of negentropy. As living systems humans must continue to influence and be influenced and to organize those influences into patterns of information.

Two Modes of Organizing Information

How do we attempt to bring some order to our thinking now that we appreciate the relativity of all our concepts? Perhaps we may start with the pragmatic assumption that the study of ourselves and our world is the study of the movement, coding, and storage of information in systems. As we have emphasized repeatedly, information processing may be arbitrarily divided into two main formats, the continuous, or analog, and the interrupted, or digital.

We may appreciate ourselves and our world as modes of organized information. If we use an interrupted, or digital, mode we have the world of things and events. If we use the continuous mode, we have a flowing process without definite boundaries. Which is correct? Is it a wave or a particle? It is both. The differentiation is in our process of organizing information. Using the continuous format, all information has a wavelike quality without definitive boundaries. Using the interrupted format, information has a particlelike quality with circumscribed boundaries.

Since our central nervous system seems to use both formats simultaneously, we may appreciate the difficulty that occurs when we focus on one format to the exclusion of the other. Yet, this is what we attempt to do, for most of us are uncomfortable with the concept of "both" and want an "either-or" paradigm. However, we have always used both formats, as illustrated by our appreciation of pictures and words, pictures being a continuous, or analog format of coding data and words being an interrupted format.

A picture of a horse has a much more fluid continuum of data than the simple word *horse*. It would take many words to describe a picture in enough detail so that we could convert these digital units to the exact likeness of the horse we can see in the picture.

In studying the digital and analogic modes of organizing information from a historical perspective, we are impressed that they are so distinct in Eastern and Western cultures. Certain Eastern cultures have emphasized the continuous, or analog, format in a philosophic orientation that views us and our world as a flowing process. In Western culture, heavy emphasis has been placed on the digital, or interrupted, with the eventual evolution of word and number systems and instruments for differentiating, which we call technology.

Western culture had every opportunity to develop the philosophy of a "thingless universe," for Eastern thinking was influential among many of the early Greeks. Some scholars feel that Pythagoras is responsible for moving the West in the direction of the digital mode when he espoused the belief that mathematics, or the language of numbers, is inherent in nature and not just a method for measuring. By coupling religion and mathematics, Pythagoras introduced the Western world to a type of discursive or logical philosophy that was to dominate our thinking [1]. Bertrand Russell believed this to be a significant step in deciding the direction in which the Western world would go in determining its interest in reasoning over intuition:

> The combination of mathematics and theology, which began with Pythagoras, characterized religious philosophy in Greece, in the Middle Ages, and in modern times down to Kant. . . . In Plato, St. Augustine, Thomas Aquinas, Descartes, Spinoza and Leibniz there is an intimate blending of religion and reasoning, of moral aspiration with logical admiration of what is timeless, which comes from Pythagoras, and distinguishes the intellectualized theology of Europe from the more straightforward mysticism of Asia. [6:p. 37]

The Western world, with its increasing interest in scientific proof as opposed to mystical intuition, turned in the direction of the digital mode that then permeated every aspect of Western life and thinking. If the early mathematicians had espoused the view that mathematics is no more a part of reality than any of our other concepts, civilization would, no doubt, have taken a much different turn [2]. The Greeks were suspicious of the unfamiliar or exotic quality of Eastern philosophy, with its emphasis upon the illusory nature of our conceptual world, and embraced the more familiar and practical or "provable" digital mode of thinking. This was a fortuitous route for the West to take as far as science is concerned. According to Alex Comfort:

> It was a signal dispensation of Providence, so far as science was concerned, that the Greek sense of practicality, which separated charismatic aspects of philoso-

phy from brass-tack applications such as mathematics, the Greek zest for life, which was highly inimical to "detachment," Buddhist-style, and the Greek distrust of Oriental exoticism generally, made the illusory character of experience an unpopular philosophical postulate. [2:p. 50]

As the Greek and Roman worlds became involved in Christianity the inclination was toward a belief system that incorporated ideas of good and evil and right and wrong and that connoted the idea of a real world of ethics rather than an illusory world free of ethics. If we examine the Greek world closely, we find that Greek philosophy was always intertwined with ethics and ideas concerning the duties of citizens [2]. The Gnostics, who used a more analogic format of thinking, were not a part of the digitalized religion, which became an integral part of the Western world. However, as Comfort remarked, "A Gnostic church might have produced yogis, but never science or technology" [2:p. 50].

There are similarities in the philosophic systems of East and West. No one can deny, for example, that intuitive thinking is as important to the scientist as to the mystic. Neither can we state that Eastern philosophy denies a practical or scientific side, but it is significant that the description of the two cultures leaves us with a mystical analogic Orient and a mechanistic digital West. It has not been until the twentieth century that the Western world has shown any great appreciation of the analog format as evidenced in Eastern philosophy. This awakened interest is due to the discoveries that have been made by those scientists working in the areas of relativity theories and quantum mechanics.

The similarities in the modern world of physics and the ancient world of Eastern philosophy are startling. The "participatory universe" of modern physics, to give one example, is analogous to the Hindu universe in which one can achieve states of mind that can alter ordinary perceptions in such a way that they are seen as probable rather than inevitable. The Hindu mystic has long understood that the observed cannot be separated from the observer, a premise now accepted by all the modern scientific world and formulated in the Heisenberg uncertainty principle.

The link between modern physics and Eastern philosophy has been described at length by Capra in *The Tao of Physics:*

> Modern physics has confirmed most dramatically one of the basic ideas of Eastern mysticism; that all the concepts we use to describe nature are limited, that they are not features of reality, as we tend to believe, but creations of the mind; parts of the map, not of the territory. Whenever we expand the realm of our experience, the limitations of our rational mind become apparent and we have to modify, or even abandon, some of our concepts. [1:p. 161]

If you recall from Chapter 5, the Greeks believed all the heavens were of perfect geometrical design and that, as Plato said, "God is a geometer." The world of classical physics embraced the idea that space and time are absolutes and that geometry or mathematics is of divine origin. Only with the theory of relativity was the Western world to entertain the notion that mathematics might be a construct of the intellect. In the Eastern world the concepts of space and time have long been viewed as emanating from the mind. Capra quotes a Hindu text:

> It was taught by the Buddha, oh Monks, that . . . the past, the future, physical space, . . . and individuals are nothing but names, forms of thought, words of common usage, merely superficial realities. [1:p. 163]

The belief that our word system is also part of the superficial reality has made it extremely difficult to translate the "thingless universe" of the Eastern mystics into our digital paradigm. Lao-tzu, the legendary Chinese philosopher, encompassed this difficulty in his pronouncement of over 2000 years ago:

> He who knows does not speak,
> He who speaks does not know.

The Taoist philosophy, which is so similar to the new philosophies of physics, presents us first and foremost with the barrier of language, the idea that one cannot express in words that which is inexpressible. As Al Chung-Liang Huang wrote:

> We do not hear nature boasting about being nature, nor water holding a conference on the technique of flowing. So much rhetoric would be wasted on those who have no use for it. The man of Tao lives in the Tao, like a fish in water. If we try to teach the fish that water is physically compounded of two parts hydrogen and one part oxygen, the fish will laugh its head off. [10:p. xiii]

Watts also pointed out, "This is where problems of language relate to Taoist philosophy, for the *Lao-tzu* book begins by saying that the Tao which can be spoken is not the eternal (or regular) Tao" [10:p. 7].

The Taoists believe there is a different way of understanding the universe other than describing it in words. They do not believe that the universe is a linear phenomenon but that it, or nature, is a simultaneous interaction of an infinite number of variables, a universe of patterns of relationships. This leaves those of us who have been attuned to the Western world of words strangely frustrated, for we must find other ways to communicate that transcend our ordinary realm of language. We enter, as we stated earlier, a transword world, or what the Taoists call the world of the unthinkable, *acintya*.

Heisenberg's uncertainty principle also presents us with the idea of complementarity, which is basically, in physics, that any description of reality must be presented by both the particle picture and the wave picture, each one in itself being only partly accurate. The idea of complementarity has been an essential component of Chinese philosophy for thousands of years, as is evident in their principles of yin and yang, the polar opposites. The great physicist, Niels Bohr, was so impressed by the similarities between the new physics and Eastern philosophy that he adopted the Chinese yin and yang symbol of t'ai-chi as his coat of arms [1].

The Taoist views the polar opposites as not in conflict but in harmony, as representing the necessary sides of a unified whole. They are inseparable, for one cannot have the one without the other. Lao-tzu wrote:

> When everyone knows beauty as beautiful, there
> is already ugliness;

When everyone knows good as goodness, there
is already evil.
"To be" and "not to be" arise mutually;
Difficult and easy are mutually realized;
Long and short are mutually contrasted;
High and low are mutually posited; . . .
Before and after are in mutual sequence.
[10:pp. 22–23]

The unified whole, which is a basic tenet of Taoist philosophy and which
is expressed through the yin-yang principle, is not a dualistic philosophy as
we in the Western world might formulate it. Nature is a process, and we are
part of that process. Nature as process expresses itself in opposites, each
necessary for the existence of the other. Is it a wave or a particle? It is both.

Although the new discoveries of physics have awakened an interest in
Eastern philosophy and although their similarities are striking, the difficulties in combining these two disparate ways of thinking, the Eastern analogic
and the Western digital, are not to be underestimated. The whole idea of
Western discursive thinking and of Western religion is to define the universe
in terms of words and numbers and laws and ethics. The Tao of Eastern
philosophy, which is sometimes defined as merely "that which happens," is
not amenable to description or translation into words and numbers and is not
attuned to laws and rules. The Western world, however, seems to be faced
with the paradoxical situation of having to attune itself to an analogic-digital
combination that, although apparently manifest in brain physiology, is almost unthinkable in Western terms.

We know from studying Taoist philosophy that one of the basic beliefs of
the Taoist is that the world as expressed in things and events can be what it is
only in relationship to everything that is. "The Taoists are saying, then,"
explains Watts, "that seen as a whole the universe is a harmony or symbiosis
of patterns which cannot exist without each other" [10:p. 51]. How can we
escape the comparison between this viewpoint and the world of quantum
theory, which, as Capra says, "forces us to see the universe not as a collection
of physical objects, but rather as a complicated web of relations between the
various parts of a unified whole" [1:p. 138].

The idea of an interdependent and interconnected cosmic web in which
the observer cannot be separated from the observed is not entirely alien to
Western philosophers or even to Western theology. The Gnostics, for exam-
ple, were attuned to a more abstract or Eastern analogic way of interpreting
Christianity, but their lack of interest in rules and church dogma made them
enemies of the organized Church and they were gradually forced out. The
Gnostics did not translate the sayings of Jesus literally. In the case of the
Kingdom of God they scorned a literal translation, believing the Kingdom of
God to be a state of self-discovery. In the Gospel of Thomas, Jesus is quoted:

Rather, the Kindgom is inside of you, and it is outside of you. When you come
to know yourselves, then you will be known, and you will realize that you are
the sons of the living Father. But if you will not know yourselves, then you
dwell in poverty, and it is you who *are* that poverty. [5:p. 128]

One cannot separate individual consciousness from the web of things and
events. The Kindgom is both within and without. The individual is manifest

only in relation to the cosmic interconnectedness of all diversities. The Buddhists elaborate continuously upon the theme that everything is a creation of the mind, the same mind that incorporates the Gnostic Kingdom of God. According to the Buddhist Yogacara school:

> Out of mind spring innumerable things, conditioned by discrimination. . . . These things people accept as an external world. . . . What appears to be external does not exist in reality; it is indeed mind that is seen as multiplicity; the body, property, and above—all these, I say, are nothing but mind. [1:p. 277]

The participatory universe in which human consciousness is an integral part of the cosmic whole is as much a framework for modern physics as it is for ancient Eastern philosophy. As physicists experience their inability to reduce the universe to a fundamental particle they encounter Eastern mysticism, which has long held that there is no fundamental particle and that everything is linked to everything else. The properties that identify or characterize each differentiated part are servoemergent, determined by their interaction with all other parts.

The particle and wave pictures of the universe are not confined to mystics and physicists. The duality of our perceptions and our thinking is evident in all aspects of our lives. We are accustomed or, one might more accurately say, programmed to think in both verbal and nonverbal, or digital and analogic modes. The simultaneity of these processes disguise or cloud their interaction so that we take them for granted. Neither the particle nor the wave picture is accurate in itself. Neither the digital nor the analogic is the "true" picture of reality. We cannot have one without the other. The Eastern mind has been trained to think analogically, the unity of the whole being the fundamental picture with the "ten thousand things" springing from that unity, the wave picture of the universe. The Western mind is more inclined to differentiation, a reduction of the unity into parts, the particle picture of the universe.

Capra hypothesizes that science and mysticism are merely "two complementary manifestations of the human mind; of its rational and intuitive faculties" [1:p. 306]. The mystic, whether Eastern or Western, starts from the inside with an analog conceptual paradigm of the unified whole. The scientist begins from the outside and, using a digital paradigm, studies the parts that comprise the whole, the mechanistic approach that has given us our advanced technology.

Perhaps relativity and quantum theories and the uncertainty principle help us appreciate the continuous quality of the universe. This shared concept between mysticism and science may have isomorphic qualities or elements, but they are not identical. Both nuclear physics and ancient mysticism utilize a continuous, or analogic, format, in which differentiation and isolation are viewed as distortion, but there is a marked difference in the antecedent derivation of the conceptual frames. Science utilizes a digitalized form of reductionism, and Eastern philosophy utilizes a continuous format. When science unitizes the continuum, the result is empirical systems that are continually subject to validation and relative to the observer. When mysticism attempts to interrupt the continuum in any cause-and-effect sequence, it is left with magic.

When we carry the two modes of processing information to the extreme, we begin to appreciate the distortion. When mathematics and measuring are pushed beyond their limits, we begin to appreciate the continuous or relative nature of process. When all differentiation is abdicated, we resemble other primates, with no technology and deteriorating culture. The interaction of these two modes and the hybridization of Eastern and Western philosophic thought we are witnessing in the twentieth century may produce some profound changes in our thinking, especially in our theories concerning ourselves.

The Self—A Wave or a Particle?

What happens to our concepts concerning self and its place in the universe when examined through the analogic and digital formats? Many of us conceptualize our bodies as particles, since they are composed of processes of long duration. We rely on the digital, or interrupted, format, since our perceptive organs give us indication of boundaries for our bodies. Paradoxically, we conceptualize the mind more as a wave phenomenon, since it is composed of processes of short duration that are not readily accessible to our senses. This means that we use the digital when speaking of the body and the analog when speaking of the mind, even though we realize that both are continuing, interrelated series of processes.

To make matters more confusing, we abstractly term the information that we process about the information processed in the mind-body continuum as *self*. The self is considered at times as an entity, a particle or thing, and at other times as a wave or a continuum. This abstraction, or metainformation system, is the source of continuing difficulty. Is the self a reality or an illusion? Is it a wave or a particle?

The self system is a fluid conglomerate that fluctuates and pulsates with every set of information that impinges on the central nervous system. The self is used as a digital unit even though it is more like an analog function. As an analogy, we might consider the self a constant mediating the relationship between perceiving organs and that which is perceived. It is like pi in determining a relationship between a center and the periphery of a circle. Inadvertently we assume the self to be the center and not the relationship. The self is open-ended, as is pi, and varies continually with the relationship between points of center and periphery. The self is, then, the area of a pulsating circle and not the center point. It is a composite of all the shifting information, past and present, between the external and internal environment. Like pi, it is never completely whole and, like pi, it has no meaning without reference points in a relationship. There is no self without relationship.

Using the analog format, I am the star I see, the thought I think, the ground beneath my feet. I am the world. Using the digital format, I am different from all other things. I stand alone. I have a beginning and an end. I am a unique, delineated entity.

Western thinking, as we have discussed, leans very heavily toward the idea of a delineated self system. The situation of deteriorating absolutes, which has resulted from relativity theory, quantum mechanics, and systems and information theories, is forcing us to shift our concept of self from that of a delineated entity to that of a fluid system. The self has changed from a rock to a river. Form has moved more and more into function and subsequently into a fluid process of varying duration leading to phrases like "the formlessness of becoming." The fluidity of data processing has resulted in speculation concerning the infinite plasticity of being and the emergence of a relativistic philosophic set concerning the self. That process we term self or ego can be conceptualized as the nebulous interface of two large information processing systems, the biologic and the social. The I is a linguistic constant in our social and symbolic operation. All systems, including the biologic, social, and self systems, are relative probability centers of radiating influence and not entities. The theologic argument of immanence versus transcendence loses its meaning in a fluid amalgamation in which both abstractions are integrated into a continuum.

There has been and will continue to be a considerable resistance to the liquidation of entities or absolutes. Primitive religious groups, for example, will continue to insist upon a return to absolutes in which the soul is embroiled in a binary system of ethics—right and wrong, good and bad, and saved and unsaved. Some psychotherapy paradigms will continue to be organized around an ego or self system, which is seen as an absolute to be realized by the individual after enough hours in narcissistic speculation. These two types of activity are dependent upon the existence of a concrete boundaried self system, or they lose their meaning and their impact.

That an objective, or concrete, self or I is an illusion has been postulated by us for many centuries, but not until the twentieth century has science joined the mystics by approaching from the same theoretical stance; that is, the I is a process rather than an entity. We might speculate that Einstein catalyzed our appreciation of the analog format and a consequent emergence of bridging concepts between cultural and religious philosophies concerning our place in the universe and the definition of self.

We might even speculate that the joining of the Eastern analog and the Western digital paradigms concerning the self system represents a maturational process. During our early years, we are influenced by reproductive functions, which later stabilize and diminish in intensity. In early life there is a tendency to self-reification, increased differentiation, and projection of self. In later years, there is a tendency to integrate patterns of information, a move toward synthesis. There is also a growing sense of relativity. Time is measured against many years rather than a few. Time therefore becomes shorter and less differentiated. Previous travels and memories make new events and places less unique and less stimulating. The earlier stages of life signify the emergence of the digital operation. In later phases, decreasing central nervous system ability and repeated experience lead to more emphasis of the analog functions.

As children we may wonder if other people really feel themselves to be people or are they just things in our imagination, like trees painted as a backdrop for a play. In early adulthood we realize the autistic character of this type of thinking, especially when comparing notes with others who may admit similar childhood fantasies. As age approaches, we begin to appreciate the wisdom of childhood. We only occasionally sense the personal "meness" of children and spend most of our hours as a backdrop—a perceptive illusion existing only in the minds of those young enough and perhaps naive enough to value the concept of an individual self. Self-disillusionment, which is the fear of the adolescent, becomes the balm of the aged. The being and the nonbeing slowly merge into the painless twilight of undifferentiated existence, and we realize that our deaths will exist only for those still young enough to rigorously maintain the illusion of differentiation.

Our ultimate anxiety is the fear of death. Death is not a thing but the absence of things. The more things are utilized in the data processing function called self, the greater anxiety over losses or threatened losses of things. The Chinese Tao or Christian Kingdom is the appreciation of the relativity of self and the relationship of self to things. The self is accepted as not a thing (nothing). However, it is not until our declining years that we seem able to accept the relativity of self and the concept of the continuum of being where the boundaries between life and death are dissolved. Watts once remarked:

> Especially as one grows older, it becomes ever more obvious that things are without substance, for time seems to go by more rapidly so that one becomes aware of the liquidity of solids; people and things become like lights and ripples on the surface of water. . . . The faster the tempo, the more it would appear that we were watching, not so much a succession of things, as the movement and transformations of one thing—as we see waves on the ocean or the movements of a dancer. [10:p. 94]

To some degree, the twentieth century relativistic approach to the concept of self resembles the mystical conceptual frames of early Gnostic Christianity in which Christ represented the merger of God and man. With the dissolution of absolutes, we may speculate that old concepts like man and God died in each other or dissolved into each other to form a unified continuum. From this point of view, the merger of God and man is a conquest of death, which moved from a definitive event or entity to a fluid process in which life and death are relative organizational patterns.

Our Western emphasis upon the digital, or reified, self in a world of things makes it extremely difficult to conceptualize a unity, a continuum in which self boundaries are eliminated. The Chinese philosopher, Chuang-tzu, wrote:

> The knowledge of the ancients was perfect. How perfect? At first, they did not know that there were things. This is the most perfect knowledge; nothing can be added. Next, they knew that there were things, but did not yet make distinctions between them. Next, they made distinctions between them, but they did not yet pass judgments upon them. When judgments were passed, Tao was destroyed. [10:pp. 54–55]

Although our digital format may have "destroyed" the Tao or at least turned our attention away from the unified whole or wave picture toward the particle picture of self, we are now beginning to entertain the premise that the boundary between the external and internal environments is very arbitrary and often spurious. Those emergent properties we call the self and mind are fluid information processed by neural and cultural systems that are interdependent. Far from being reductionistic, the new theories open the door to the most complex view we have ever envisioned of self, mind, and body. All are integrated in the systems of the world and unified in a fluid process without the definitive boundaries of time or space. These concepts are the most exciting and perhaps the most awe inspiring in our history of concepts. For most of us, they are overwhelming.

One of the most gratifying parameters or conditions of the new theories concerning our place in the universe is its extreme tolerance and flexibility. As long as we appreciate that the manner in which we organize information is relative and more or less arbitrary, we may use any "as-if" paradigm we wish. We may utilize an anthropomorphic, a mechanistic, or even a relativistic model. We cannot, at present, state that any particular way of organizing information is the true and only way. We may never be able to do this. Each paradigm we utilize may lead us only into more questions. We can be assured that no one model will give us the complete world picture for which we have searched through the centuries. Have our gods died? Have our souls dissolved into infinity? It is not a matter of "yes" or "no". It *is* a matter of which concepts we find most productive and comforting.

God as process rather than a discrete entity can only be appreciated as a frame of reverence if we adjust our concept of the human self to that of a process rather than entity. If we go the particle route and differentiate ourselves from the rest of being, we must utilize forms or entities for relating to functions, that is, self to object. The differentiating format incorporates data effectively and, at times, appears more validatable, as when we "see" the sun coming up in the east and going down in the west. It is functional to talk about the movement of the sun, especially in the realm of poetry and common parlance. When we try to integrate information from astronomy, we must utilize the data in another format in which the earth rotates rather than the sun.

Perhaps just as we presently need both the wave and particle theories concerning light in order to integrate our information about this form of electromagnetic energy, we will continue to need theories to differentiate self and God into entities as well as those that integrate self and God into fluid processes. This lack of closure will continue to emphasize the relativity of all our information and the human conceptual frames we use to organize this information. The differentiated and integrated formats are complementary, and we must use both to continue our journey called civilization. Focusing entirely on one or the other format has proven and will continue to prove less productive. The analog format leads to stagnation. The digital format leads to alienation.

That we will continue to differentiate and describe is undeniable. Without interrupting the continuum there would be no books about concepts concerning self, mind, and body, no search for the fundamental unit of the universe, and no technological innovations. It will be difficult to remind ourselves that we are part of the process, that it is a participatory universe. Watts gave an excellent description of our situation:

> For the game of Western philosophy and science is to trap the universe in the networks of words and numbers so that there is always the temptation to

confuse the rules, or laws, of grammar and mathematics with the actual operations of nature. We must not, however, overlook the fact that human calculation is *also* an operation of nature, but just as trees do not represent or symbolize rocks, our thoughts—even if intended to do so—do not necessarily represent trees and rocks. . . . Although thought is in nature, we must not confuse the game-rules of thought with the patterns of nature. [10:p. 42]

What is a self, that nebulous phenomenon called the I or the me, that intangible ruler that controls my mind and body and perhaps even my soul? I is the master craftsman that carves fate's rigid surface into my destiny. A being of such omnipotent powers with such vast domains of influence must be one of the most evident forces in all of creation. We have paid homage to this tyrant for centuries and yet, when we search for this seat of power, we always seem to lose our way.

As we have recently begun to question our cause-and-effect sequencing of information, we are beginning to reorganize our search for the self. Although it seems blasphemous to our Western minds, there are those who are beginning to murmur that the self is an effect and not a cause. Rather than saying, "I cause my thoughts," they suggest that "My thoughts cause my I." "I" don't allow myself to see, hear, or touch. My perceptions allow "me" to exist. I am a reflection of the interaction of internal and external environment, especially those biologic and social elements that allow the processes of differentiation and speech. The I is being altered from an absolute to an abstraction, from a potentate to a process. The regal emperor has become a relative emergence.

If I weep for my dissolving self, then my I is sad. If I laugh at my self-centeredness, then my I is happy. I am beginning to suspect that my wonderful self is an echo or a mirror reflecting all those information processing activities of long and short duration that have been arbitrarily delineated by my social system as an individual human and given a name said to be mine. "The whole dear notion of one's own Self," writes Lewis Thomas, "marvelous old free-willed, free-enterprising, autonomous, independent, isolated island of Self—is a myth" [8:p. 142].

I, then, am a social shadow, a reflection of evolving culture. I grow more or less distinct, depending on social interaction. I may maintain myself temporarily by the stored light of social memories. Every shift in the biosocial processes is reflected in my shadow self. If the fires of those processes that fashion this crucial information burn less brightly, I fade into the shadowless glow of the universe. Without my shadow to maintain my uniqueness, I merge into the undifferentiated all. Is it better to be all or a part of the all? Only my shadow seems to care.

Just as Sir Isaac Newton described himself as a lonely child on the beach, we may see ourselves as lonely children by the sea. To one side are the continuous waves of our beginning and on the other the granular world of differentiation. We have for all time pondered over our plight and reflected upon our destiny.

> We are the music-makers
>   And we are the dreamers of dreams
> Wandering by lone sea-breakers
>   And sitting by desolate streams;

World losers and world-forsakers,
  On whom the pale moon gleams:
Yet we are the movers and shakers
  Of the world for ever, it seems. [3:p. 456]

So Sir Arthur Stanley Eddington described us, a picture reminiscent of that painted by Newton.

We have moved farther up the sandy shore than any other of our animal kin. Our emphasis on the digital format has given us many advantages, chief among them our symbolic operation, which allows coded information to be shared with others across large distances of time and space. Our coded information spans many generations. Our information pool, stored in linguistic symbols like our gene pool, interrelates us with the scholars of antiquity. And yet, the digital world must always be a lonely world. In differentiating our world, we differentiate ourselves into unique and finite creatures who must live and die as individuals. Although at times we may wish to participate in the analogic ocean of a merged continuum, we cannot afford the cost. In that limitless world we would lose our most cherished possessions, our selves. And so we stand on the wet sand, frightened of our finiteness and alone.

At times, we may move farther from the shore to glimpse the exciting mirage of worlds beyond the dunes, but as that passion to find the fabeled citadel of certainty begins to fade in the dry heat of reality, we return to the soft waves of the uncertain and, in the end, each individual merges into the continuous all. Perhaps a few, as Longfellow suggested, "leave their footprints in the sands of time," but most of us seem to wander aimlessly, and the ever-shifting winds of process leave little evidence of our passing. Our growing realization of our tiny place in the universe dwarfs our planet and our selves to a grain of salt at the water's edge.

Questions arise as to whether we can forge a frame of reverence out of these nebulous fields of influence or whether we must flow with the Tao in resigned involvement. Our minds, bodies, selves, and souls seem to have dissolved with our gods into uncertain probabilities of information about information about information, reflected in the beeps and bleeps of electronic data processing equipment, their pointer readings, and their digital readouts.

How meek this world of process appears in contrast to the robust tyranny of Zeus and Thor. How sterile are these concepts when compared to the conniving forces of the unconscious. And yet, when all these pointer readings are summed in their entirety, they indicate an almost mystical, eternal process of relating and informing to fashion the fabric of all being and becoming. Since all processes are interrelated, we are simultaneously infinte and finite, differentiated and integrated, and continuous and interrupted. The here and now of our lifetimes are relative and reflect our distortion of a space-time continuum in our fantasies.

References

1. Capra, F: *The Tao of Physics*. Boulder, Colorado: Shambala, 1975
2. Comfort, A: *I and That: Notes of the Biology of Religion*. New York: Crown, 1979
3. Eddington, A S: Reality, causation, science and mysticism. In Commins, S, and

Linscott, R (Eds): *Man and the Universe: The Philosophers of Science.* New York: Washington Square Press, 1947, pp 411–470

4. Long, M: Visions of a new faith. *Science Digest,* November 1981, pp 36–42

5. Pagels, E: *The Gnostic Gospels.* New York: Random House, 1979

6. Russell, B: *History of Western Philosophy.* New York: Simon and Schuster, 1945

7. Stent, G: Limits to the scientific understanding of man. *Science,* Volume 187, March 21, 1975, pp 1052–1057

8. Thomas, L J: *The Lives of a Cell: Notes of a Biology Watcher.* New York: Viking, 1974

9. Watts, A: *The Book: On the Taboo Against Knowing Who You Are.* New York: Vintage Books, 1972

10. Watts, A: *Tao: The Watercourse Way.* New York: Pantheon Books, 1975.

Index